ADVANCES IN MOLECULAR ECOLOGY

NATO Science Series

A Series presenting the results of activities sponsored by the NATO Science Committee.
The Series is published by IOS Press and Kluwer Academic Publishers in conjunction with the NATO Scientific Affairs Division.

General Sub-Series

A Life Sciences	IOS Press
B Physics	Kluwer Academic Publishers
C Mathematical and Physical Sciences	Kluwer Academic Publishers
D Behavioural and Social Sciences	Kluwer Academic Publishers
E Applied Sciences	Kluwer Academic Publishers
F Computer and Systems Sciences	IOS Press

Partnership Sub-Series

1 Disarmament Technologies	Kluwer Academic Publishers
2 Environmental Security	Kluwer Academic Publishers
3 High Technology	Kluwer Academic Publishers
4 Science and Technology Policy	IOS Press
5 Computer Networking	IOS Press

The Partnership Sub-Series incorporates activities undertaken in collaboration with NATO's Partners in the Euro-Atlantic Partnership Council - countries of the CIS and Central and Eastern Europe - in Priority Areas of concern to those countries.

NATO-PCO-DATA BASE

The NATO Science Series continues the series of books published formerly in the NATO ASI Series. An electronic index to the NATO ASI Series provides full bibliographical references (with keywords and/or abstracts) to more than 50 000 contributions from international scientists published in all sections of the NATO ASI Series.
Access to the NATO-PCO-DATA BASE is possible in two ways:
- via online FILE 128 (NATO-PCO-DATA BASE) hosted by ESRIN,
Via Galileo Galilei, I-00044 Frascati, Italy;
- via CD-ROM "NATO-PCO-DATA BASE" with user-friendly retrieval software in English, French and German (© WTV GmbH and DATAWARE Technologies Inc., 1989).
The CD-ROM of the NATO ASI Series can be ordered from PCO, Overijse, Belgium.

Series A: Life Sciences - Vol. 306

ISSN: 1387-6686

Advances in Molecular Ecology

Edited by

Gary R. Carvalho

Molecular Ecology and Fisheries Genetics Laboratory
Department of Biological Sciences, University of Hull, United Kingdom

UNIVERSITY COLLEGE

SCARBOROUGH

IOS
Press

Ohmsha

Amsterdam • Berlin • Oxford • Tokyo • Washington, DC

Published in cooperation with NATO Scientific Affairs Division

Proceedings of the NATO Advanced Study Institute on
Molecular Ecology
Erice, Sicily, Italy
20-31 March 1998

ISBN 90 5199 440 0 (IOS Press)
ISBN 4 274 90250 1 C3045 (Ohmsha)
Library of Congress Catalog Card Number 98-74143

Publisher
IOS Press
Van Diemenstraat 94
1013 CN Amsterdam
Netherlands
fax: +31 20 620 3419
e-mail: order@iospress.nl

Distributor in the UK and Ireland
IOS Press/Lavis Marketing
73 Lime Walk
Headington
Oxford OX3 7AD
England
fax: +44 1865 75 0079

Distributor in the USA and Canada
IOS Press, Inc.
5795-G Burke Center Parkway
Burke, VA 22015
USA
fax: +1 703 323 3668
e-mail: iosbooks@iospress.com

Distributor in Germany
IOS Press
Spandauer Strasse 2
D-10178 Berlin
Germany
fax: +49 30 242 3113

Distributor in Japan
Ohmsha, Ltd.
3-1 Kanda Nishiki-cho
Chiyoda-ku, Tokyo 101
Japan
fax: +81 3 3233 2426

Dedication

To the memory of Goffredo Cognetti (1942-1998), Professor of Cellular Biotechnology, University of Palermo, and Local Organiser of the NATO Advanced Study Institute on *Advances in Molecular Ecology*

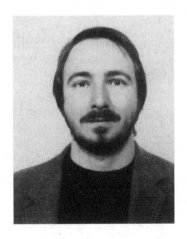

Preface

The past thirty years have witnessed remarkable advances in our ability to describe the structure and dynamics of genetic diversity in wild populations. Beginning with the classical applications of allozyme electrophoresis to populations of *Drosophila* and man, there has been an escalation of molecular methodologies which explore the genetic relationships among individuals, populations and species, a field that has become known as "molecular ecology". The ubiquity across taxa of molecular genetic markers provided by allozymes, restriction fragment length polymorphisms, DNA fingerprinting, microsatellites and DNA sequencing, has enabled wide-scale exploration of problems in ecology and evolution, yielding insights into the origin, maintenance and exploitation of biodiversity.

Much effort has been expended in the development of new molecular technologies, together with concerted attempts to describe the molecular basis and evolutionary dynamics of the various classes of molecular variants utilised. The development of novel methodologies, most notably the discovery of the polymerase chain reaction (PCR) and disclosure of highly repetitive DNA has revolutionised the breadth of tractable problems. Enhanced marker variability, coupled with the relative ease and speed afforded by PCR-based methods, has facilitated opportunities to explore new applications and perspectives. Noteworthy contributions include studies on direct estimates of fitness variation in the wild, the application of ancient DNA to historical population analysis, the mapping of quantitative genetic variation and its ecological significance, and the molecular analysis of microbial population structure and diversity. In view of the wide variety of molecular and analytical methodologies and contemporary applications, it is timely to consider some major contributions and future priorities of the molecular approach, and in particular to enhance our understanding of the markers employed.

It was against this background of escalating activities and outputs in molecular ecology, and a need for consolidation and synthesis, that the NATO Advanced Study Institute (ASI) on Advances in Molecular Ecology was held at the Ettore Majorana, International Centre for Scientific Culture in Erice, Italy, in March 1998. Fifteen lecturers and over seventy students spent ten days engaged in instruction and discussion. The ASI provided the first international opportunity for a comprehensive consideration of how recent advances, most notably, the PCR-based technology had impacted on concepts and applications in ecology and evolution. Researchers across the fields of animals, plants and microbial communities presented a thematic approach, with emphasis on the integration of concepts independently of taxon. A hierarchical structure to the ASI was adopted, starting out with an overview of the molecular methodologies available, including both protein and DNA-based techniques, and proceeding onto deliberations at the individual, population and higher taxonomic levels.

In this book, we present some of the contributions delivered by the NATO lecturers, encompassing aspects of approach and methodology, and illustrated by a diversity of applications. Each author was asked to examine how molecular genetic tools have contributed to their specific area of consideration, identifying novel insights, controversies and future priorities. The coverage is not intended to be comprehensive across all contemporary fields in molecular ecology, but rather illustrative of the diversity of approach and application, and with emphasis on the genetic and evolutionary characteristics of the markers employed. It is only through the use of appropriate sampling design, choice of marker or marker combinations, and apposite statistical analysis of data that meaningful tests and interpretations can be attained. The examples presented here endorse such an approach by considering not only how molecular markers have impacted on concepts and theory, but also by demonstrating through recent developments how they can be employed with effect.

The book begins by placing the approach of molecular ecology into context (Gary Carvalho), pointing out the conceptual contributions of classical ecological genetics, and the impact of advances in DNA technology. Emphasis is placed on the need to consider more widely the genetic and evolutionary characteristics of marker variants as a basis for their effective use. There follows methodological considerations of how frequency data in molecular ecology can be analysed using a phylogenetic approach (David Hillis), and the relative merits of conventional and coalescent approaches to describing population structure and gene flow (Peter Beerli). Arnaud Estoup and Bernard Anders describe the use of variable number of tandem repeats (VNTR) as markers in ecology and evolution in relation to their molecular and evolutionary characteristics. Estoup and Anders conclude that microsatellites offer particularly powerful tools in molecular ecology, including a consideration of contributions at the individual, population and phylogenetic levels. Applications of molecular markers to describe microbial population and community structure are highlighted by Gerard Muyzer. Not only is the wealth of microbial diversity in the wild only now becoming evident, but molecular technology is providing a powerful approach for exploring linkages between bacterial diversity, environmental heterogeneity and bacterial function. Peter Young discusses various recombination mechanisms in bacteria as evidenced by recent applications of the molecular approach, and considers how the nature of bacterial species can offer a new perspective on the general issues surrounding the nature of species. Franco Rollo introduces the concept of ancient DNA, and explains how it can be applied with caution to reveal information on the structure and diversity of ancient bacterial communities, including their association with man. Bob Vrijenhoek reviews the theories to explain the evolution of sex by reference to molecular studies on clonal organisms, and concludes that although clonality is widespread, with few exceptions there is little evidence for the existence of ancient clonal lineages or diversified asexual taxa.

Andrew Schnabel deals with the reconstruction of mating and dispersal processes in natural and experimental plant populations, with emphasis on the methods for assessing parentage of individual progeny and the contribution of molecular markers, especially in relation to estimating relative fertilities of individual parents in populations. Lorenz Hauser and Bob Ward address the contribution that molecular tools have made in the analysis of highly mobile pelagic fishes. They emphasize not only differences in the ability of various markers to detect structuring, but also the influence of ecology and pelagic lifestyle on population structure. Jeffry Mitton reviews how molecular markers can be used to explore the operation of natural selection in the wild, with particular emphasis on some recent allozyme studies, as well as insights provided by mitochondrial and microsatellite markers. Loren Rieseberg describes the contributions of molecular markers to our understanding of hybrid zone structure and dynamics, and how such information has informed our perspectives on introgression, hybrid speciation, species extinction and phylogenetic incongruence. Paul Hebert considers patterns of species diversification in inland waters, and offers molecular evidence for the role that environmental stress may play in modulating mutation and evolutionary rates. Contributions from two other lecturers at Erice, Ciro Rico (animal mating and social systems) and Søren Sorensen (experimental evolution of microbes and GMOs), and are not included in this book.

To increase the practical utility of the book, we conclude with a summary of current software that is available for the analysis of data in molecular ecology, detailing information on names of authors, date of latest update, compatible operating systems, types of data handled and analyses supported. A glossary of terms is provided to facilitate access to unfamiliar topics.

A major advantage of the NATO Advanced Study Institute scheme is the speed of publication of the associated book, allowing a synthesis of contemporary issues, together with an up to date coverage of literature. This is especially valuable in an approach such as molecular ecology, where methodological and analytical methods develop rapidly. The cost, however, has been the demanding schedule imposed on all those who have contributed to the book, either through general organisation of the ASI, those that acted as referees and, of course, those that contributed as authors. The NATO lecturers survived a punishing schedule, and I thank them sincerely for devoting so much time to the ASI, and in providing timely and lively reviews. Additionally, the content and stimulus for respective contributions owe much to the committed and imaginative discussions with the ASI students.

I am especially indebted to the meticulous and speedy peer reviews provided by the following referees: Antoon Akkermans, Mike Arnold, Tim Barraclough, Eliane Beraud-Colomb, Stewart Berlocher, Joseph Bernardo, Louis Bernatchez, Helen Bouter, Terry Brown, Roger Butlin, Tom Cross, John Endler, David Goldstein, Stewart Grant, James Hamrick, Lorenz Hauser, Rus Hoelzel, Roger Hughes, Norman Kaplan, Curt Lively, David Lunt, John Nason, David Parkin, Rémy Petit, Stuart Piertney, Krnelia Smalla, Pam Soltis, George Turner, Larry Weider, and Bruce Weir. I also acknowledge David Threlfall, Head of the Department of Biological Sciences at Hull, for his generous support and cooperation throughout the ASI programme.

Much of the smooth-running of the ASI and its outputs have been due to the dedicated and efficient support of the Hull NATO Secretary, Gillian Dennison, and the general support and editorial assistance of Lorenz Hauser. During final preparation of the book, I relied heavily on the commitment of John Lewis and Miranda Trojanowska, and thank them for taking on the task. I am also grateful to numerous others who have also contributed to the book, either through their involvement at the ASI, or in providing general support, including: Pino Aceto, Giles Davidson, Alberto Gabriele, Maggy Harley, Margherita Randazzo, Elisabetta Rizzo, Paul Shaw, David Taylor, Stefano Velo, Antonia White, Antonio Zichichi, and others who have not been named individually, particularly members of my Research Group at Hull.

Finally, but most importantly, this book is dedicated to the fond memory of the late Professor Goffredo Cognetti, the local organiser of the ASI, who first suggested the idea of an advanced meeting to consider recent advances in molecular ecology. His desire to bring together specialists and students in molecular ecology, and through discussion, explore controversies and future directions, was in keeping with the spirit of the venue and its history, some of which we hope is captured in this book.

Gary Carvalho, Hull, August, 1998

List of Contributors

Bernard Angers
Laboratoire de Génétique des Poissons, INRA, 78352 Jouy-en-Josas, France
e-mail: angers@diamant.jouy.inra.fr

Peter Beerli
Department of Genetics, University of Washington, Seattle, WA 98195-7360, USA
e-mail: beerli@genetics.washington.edu

Gary R. Carvalho
Molecular Ecology and Fisheries Genetics Laboratory, Department of Biological Sciences,
University of Hull, Hull HU6 7RX, UK
e-mail: g.r.carvalho@biosci.hull.ac.uk

Arnaud Estoup
Laboratoire de Modélisation et de Biologie Evolutive, 488 rue Croix Lavit, URBL-INRA,
France
e-mail: estoup@zavez02.ensam.inra.fr

Lorenz Hauser
Molecular Ecology and Fisheries Genetics Laboratory, Department of Biological Sciences,
University of Hull, Hull HU6 7RX, UK
e-mail: l.hauser@biosci.hull.ac.uk

Paul D.N. Hebert
Department of Zoology, University of Guelph, Guelph, Ontario, N1G 2W1, Canada
e-mail: phebert@uogelph.ca

David M. Hillis
Department of Zoology and Institute of Cellular and Molecular Biology, University of
Texas, Austin, TX 78712, USA
e-mail: hillis@phylo.zo.utexas.edu

Jeffry B. Mitton
Department of Environmental, Population and Organismic Biology, University of Colorado
Boulder, CO 80309, USA
e-mail: mitton@colorado.edu

Gerard Muyzer
Netherlands Institute for Sea Research, 1790 AB Den Burg (Texel), The Netherlands
e-mail: gmuyzer@nioz.nl

Loren H. Rieseberg
Biology Department, Indiana University, Bloomington, IN 47405, USA
e-mail: lriesebe@bio.indiana.edu

Franco Rollo
Department of Molecular, Cell and Animal Biology, University of Camerino, I-62032,
Camerino, Italy
e-mail: rollo@cambio.unicam.it

Andrew Schnabel
Department of Biological Sciences, Indiana University South Bend, South Bend, IN 46615,
USA
e-mail: aschnabe@iusb.edu

Robert C. Vrijenhoek
Center for Theoretical & Applied Genetics, Rutgers University, New Brunswick, NJ 08901,
USA
e-mail: vrijen@ahab.rutgers.edu

Robert D. Ward
CSIRO Marine Research, GPO Box 1538, Hobart, Tasmania 7001, Australia
e-mail: bob.ward@marine.csiro.au

J. Peter W. Young
Department of Biology, University of York, PO Box 373, York YO10 5YW, UK
e-mail: jpy1@york.ac.uk

CONTENTS

Advances in Molecular Ecology
G.R. Carvalho (Ed.)
IOS Press, 1998

1

Molecular Ecology: Origins and Approach

Gary R. Carvalho

Molecular Ecology and Fisheries Genetics Laboratory, Department of Biological Sciences,
University of Hull, Hull, HU6 7RX, U.K.
e-mail: g.r.carvalho@biosci.hull.ac.uk

Molecular ecology can be defined broadly as the application of molecular genetic markers to problems in ecology and evolution, encompassing studies on the genetic relationships among individuals, populations and species. As such, its origins can be traced back to the School of Ecological Genetics (1950-1970) pioneered by E.B. Ford, which represented the first concerted attempt to interpret fitness variation in ecologically significant traits within an evolutionary framework. The introduction of allozyme electrophoresis into population genetics in the mid-1960s provided the catalyst to extend direct genetic analysis to wild populations of most species, allowing the subsequent generation of comparative protein variation data sets to address fundamental questions of molecular and adaptive evolution. Subsequent developments in DNA technology, including the use of restriction enzymes, Southern blotting, cloning and sequencing technologies, and the polymerase chain reaction, together with the exploitation of highly repetitive DNA, accelerated the range and sensitivity of molecular genetic assays of genetic variability. Increased levels of molecular polymorphism and heterozygosities facilitated opportunities to link the descriptive (patterns of genetic diversity in space and time) and mechanistic (underlying mechanisms of detected patterns) approaches to molecular ecology, especially through direct estimates of viability and reproductive success in the wild. Greater consideration of the molecular and evolutionary characteristics of different marker systems, their relationships to one another, the molecular analysis of quantitative traits, and an increased focus of applications to detailed case studies are suggested as future priorities.

1. Introduction: the approach of molecular ecology

The application of molecular genetic markers to ecology and evolution, widely know as molecular ecology, has a rich history of successive phases of fashion, each dominated by specific molecular technologies that have been accompanied by the introduction of specialist concepts and terms. The ensuing variety of molecular procedures that are available for tackling fundamental problems such as the dynamics of population structure, or the nature of evolutionary relationships among species, is such that it can lead easily to confusion by prospective users, resulting in wasted effort, inappropriate applications and misinterpretations. Novelty of approach and fashion are driving forces sometimes externally imposed by available expertise or resources, and the preconceptions of funding bodies. Such considerations are not appropriate criteria for the design of studies, especially since the molecular markers available differ fundamentally in their genetic basis and evolutionary dynamics (Avise 1994; Hillis *et al.* 1996a; Li 1997). The probability of choosing inappropriate tools in molecular ecology are particularly high since the approach is based on an amalgam of concepts from diverse fields, including genetics, population biology, molecular biology and systematics, and where theoretical models, statistical inference, experimental studies and field work all may contribute. Moreover, efforts must be made to ensure biological reality in the interpretation of data, by incorporating attributes such as a species' breeding system, mating patterns, dispersal capacity, mode of development, social interactions and population dynamics. This involves not only a consideration of single-species systems, but also interactions among species, where the strength and nature of the interaction may be affected markedly by genetic factors (Endler 1992; Antonovics 1994).

Irrespective of the technical approach adopted, the essence of molecular ecology is to employ heritable, discrete and stable markers to identify genotypes that characterize individuals, populations or species. Such molecular markers typically comprise protein variants or diversity in one of several classes of nucleic acid sequences, so ensuring a ubiquitous application across all taxa, including the analysis of extant individuals or their remains. Through the comparison of inferred genotypes it is possible to gain information on the levels and distribution of genetic variability in relation to mating patterns, life history, population size, migration and environment. It is both the stability of molecular markers, as determined by the fidelity of inheritance, and their diversity, as detected by observable polymorphisms, that provide the basis for their use in tracking the dynamics of genes in time and space. Stability, at least during ecological time-scales, determines the concordance between marker and genotype, whereas diversity supplies the variants for sample comparison. By exploiting methods that estimate genetic similarities and differences among samples, whether conspecific individuals or distinct genera, it is possible to develop hypotheses on their evolutionary relationships.

In order to place the study of molecular ecology into context, and to appreciate its contributions to ecology and evolution, I consider three main questions: 1. What defines the approach of molecular ecology? 2. What are the origins of molecular ecology? 3. What molecular markers are available, and how can we decide which to employ? The objective here is to impart an appreciation of the underlying rationale and complexities in applying molecular tools to studying evolution in the wild, rather than in the available techniques or methods of analysis, for which there already exists several articles (Hoelzel & Dover 1991; Avise 1994; Schierwater *et al.* 1994; Hillis *et al.* 1996a; Ferraris & Palumbi 1996; Smith & Wayne 1996; Givnish & Sytsma 1997; Li 1997).

2. Molecular ecology: what do we mean?

The term "molecular ecology" has come into wide usage since the publication of the journal, *Molecular Ecology*, in May 1992. Prior to, and since that date, the term has been used in different contexts, sometimes encompassing studies on biogeochemical cycling, the biological activity of organic compounds, and ecotoxicology. In the editorial of the first issue of the journal, *Molecular Ecology,* the founding editorial team had the following to say about their new publication:

> "*Molecular Ecology* will publish the results that uses molecular biological approaches to provide innovative insights into any aspect of ecology or population biology. The journal will focus on questions concerning natural and introduced populations and their environments investigated using molecular technologies, and on studies of the ecological release of recombinant organisms".
>
> Burke, Seidler & Smith 1992

Although it is restrictive, and perhaps even misleading for those entering the field to closely associate a particular term with a specific journal, the appearance of the latter was such that it coincided with the explosive use of DNA-based techniques, and it is not surprising that the two have become linked closely. Indeed, within the 1992 editorial was a reference to the "new topic" of molecular ecology. It is here where the approach and journal bearing its name part ways, since although novel molecular technologies were undoubtedly evident at this time, the origins and wide-scale application of the approach stretches back several decades.

In keeping with the usual trend of attempting to delimit the boundaries of a scientific term, it is possible to describe molecular ecology as the application of molecular genetic markers to problems in ecology and evolution, encompassing studies on the genetic relationships among individuals, populations and species (Fig. 1). Although such a broad-based definition may appear all encompassing, certain diagnostic features are identifiable. First, the inclusion only of molecular genetic markers, thus confining studies to the utilization of DNA-based diversity, whether proteins, DNA or RNA sequences. The critical thing is that the markers employed are based on genealogies, thus necessitating a consideration of inheritance and genetic principles. Thus, investigations that examine such topics as the chemical composition or biological activity of organic compounds do not fall within the approach of molecular ecology as defined here.

Second, and this is where the boundaries of molecular ecology are particularly expansive, is the consideration of a plethora of problems in ecology and evolution. These may include such questions as how females choose their mates, how populations adapt to environmental change, the effect of fluctuations in effective population size on adaptive traits, and identifying the likely mechanisms of speciation. Each can be tackled using molecular genetic markers, but the key link that provides the pertinent focus here is the core requirement for information on qualitative and quantitative changes in genetic composition, whether this be over time between generations, or across space among individuals, populations or species. The reference to ecology emphasizes the dependence of traits on environment, whereas its association with evolution underlines the dynamic nature of genotype-environment interactions, necessitating information on the structure and diversity of genes and their transmission.

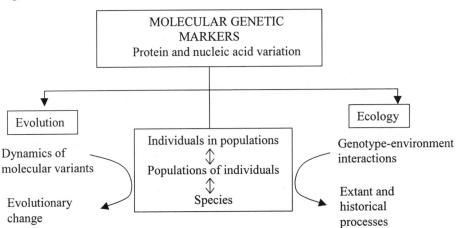

Figure 1: Schematic representation of the approach of molecular ecology. The essence of molecular ecology is to apply DNA-based marker variation to explore the genetic relationships among individuals, populations and species. Use of genetically based variants necessitates the study of changes in genetic structure (evolution) and the associated role of contemporary and historical processes (ecology), including the effects of environmental heterogeneity, demographic change and vicariance events.

The third facet, the genetic relationships among individuals, populations and species, more closely defines the nature and scale of molecular ecological studies. Genetic data on relationships provide the basis for sample comparison, whether this is between parent and putative offspring, or among samples of uncertain species identity. While particular studies may focus on individual- or population-based questions, the availability of markers to tackle all biological levels, including clonal and unitary organisms, has facilitated the integration of the micro- and macroevolutionary domains. It is now possible to explore and interpret processes operating at the level of individuals, such as sexual selection, trophic, or behavioural polymorphisms, as a basis for formulating hypotheses of population differentiation and speciation (Taylor *et al.* 1997; Barraclough *et al.* 1998; Magurran 1998).

Molecular ecology thus describes an approach, rather than a discipline, and necessarily incorporates expertise from diverse fields, but most notably from molecular biology, population and quantitative genetics, ecology, historical biogeography and systematics. From a practical perspective, it is perhaps valuable to consider it as representing a

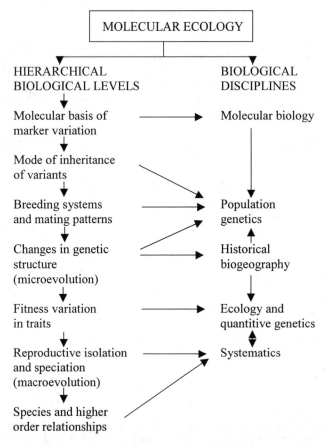

Figure 2: The amalgam of disciplines and levels of biological study employed in molecular ecology. The molecular approach necessitates an integration of information ranging from the origin and molecular basis of the marker variation employed (molecular biology), the transmission genetics of markers, the mechanisms determining the distribution and extent of molecular variation (population genetics), the origins and significance of variance in phenotypic traits (ecology and quantitative genetics), and the mechanisms generating species and study of their evolutionary relationships (biogeography and systematics).

continuum (Fig. 2), that ranges on the one hand from studies examining the molecular basis of observed polymorphisms, linked in turn to the dynamics of genes in space and time, and the effects of evolutionary forces on genes, to the translation of genetic architecture (Bradshaw 1984) into ecologically significant traits such as morphology, behaviour, life history and physiology. Although it is possible to study each of these components in isolation, together they contribute to our understanding of the origins, nature and significance of fitness variation in nature, and as such comprise integral aspects of the molecular ecological approach. Thus, although classical molecular population genetics or molecular biology may appear to be somewhat peripheral to our understanding of the ecological significance of genetic diversity, such considerations are necessary foundations for an understanding of the use and interpretation of the molecular markers employed (e.g. Estoup & Anders, this volume).

3. Molecular ecology: a new term for an established field

Conceptually, molecular ecology embraces an approach for tackling problems in biological diversity that can be traced back before the wide-scale employment of direct DNA-based procedures in the mid-1980s and beyond. The foundations were laid by the Ecological Genetics School of the 1950s-1970s (Cain & Sheppard 1954; Sheppard 1958; Ford 1964), which emphasized studies on the "adjustments and adaptations of wild populations to their environment through combined field and laboratory work" (Ford 1964). Fundamental questions such as the origin of adaptations, the role of genetic polymorphisms, the causes of population differentiation and nature of speciation mechanisms dominated the evolutionary agenda. The ecological genetics approach incorporated several facets that continue to the present day: the dynamic nature of genetic structure in relation to environmental heterogeneity, the focus on populations as evolutionary units, and the value of carefully designed field sampling to describe and monitor diversity. Although studies on visible polymorphisms dominated the original ecological genetic approach, the stage was set for the discovery of a class of markers that not only exhibited clear Mendelian control, but also offered high variability and ubiquity across taxa.

Running parallel to the burgeoning Ecological Genetics School, but largely uninfluenced by it, were studies that examined genetic variation below the level of phenotype, including for example, that which determined diversity of amino acids secreted into urine (Berry *et al*. 1955; Gartler *et al*. 1955) and the identity of blood groups (Harris 1953; Mourant 1954; Stormont 1959; Rasmussen 1962). This work was significant in that it recognized that such molecular, usually referred to as "physiological" variation, could be exploited to reveal allele frequency data, an appropriate currency for population genetic analysis. However, in the same way that visible polymorphisms constrained their application outside the few well-studied cases of molluscs and lepidopterans, the analysis of molecular variation awaited the development of a general methodology that was not taxonomically restrictive.

Such a technology was provided by the procedure of horizontal gel electrophoresis, initially of proteins on starch (Smithies 1955), which when combined with histochemical staining (Hunter & Markert 1957; Markert & Møller 1959), enabled rapid, quantitative and widely applicable surveys of genetic variation in natural populations. Indeed, the same principle of electrophoretic separation underlies most contemporary assays of molecular variation, whether the target samples comprise enzymes, DNA fragments or nucleic acid sequences. Three seminal papers published in 1966 (Hubby & Lewontin 1966; Lewontin & Hubby 1966; Harris 1966) provided the catalyst that led to the widespread application of the molecular approach to wild populations. There are four primary reasons why these much quoted papers on enzyme variation in *Drosophila* (Hubby & Lewontin 1966; Lewontin & Hubby 1966) and in man (Harris 1966) were crucial to the subsequent incorporation of the molecular approach into ecology and evolution. First, was the demonstration that the variants had a clear Mendelian basis. The easily interpretable and stable source of protein variants ensured that meaningful tests based on genetic continuity could be undertaken. Second, the ability to infer genotypes of individuals without any special prior genetic manipulation meant that individuals could be sampled direct from the wild, so securing the necessary consideration of ecology. Third, the use of ubiquitous macromolecules, initially proteins, and latterly nucleic acids, facilitated application across all taxa, so removing the focus on a few model systems where ecological knowledge was sometimes limiting (Dobzhansky 1961). Finally, the detection of much higher levels of genetic variability in nature not only provided, in general, an ample supply of markers, but also necessitated immediate consideration of its maintenance and significance, resulting in a renewed and vigorous appraisal of evolutionary mechanisms (Milkman 1967; Kimura & Ohta 1971; Lewontin & Krakauer 1973). The combined impact was to endorse and generate a plethora of studies incorporating the molecular genetic approach, with emphasis on the dynamics of population genetic structure, the evolution of molecular adaptation, and studies on molecular systematics (Avise 1974; Lewontin 1974; Brown & Wright 1979; Nei 1975; Avise *et al.* 1979).

It was now possible to move beyond explorations of the spots of butterflies, stripes of snails and chromosome polymorphisms of *Drosophila*, and to apply the fundamental approach of ecological genetics, incorporating integrative studies on genotype-environment interactions, population-level questions, and observations from the laboratory and wild, to a range of taxa. In addition to documenting and measuring the magnitude of selection within single populations, it was now possible to consider more readily the impact of changes in population size and structure, the interaction among populations through migration and dispersal, and the interaction between local selection and drift. Thus, the availability of molecular markers, through their objective quantification and genetically stable nature, facilitated a more holistic approach to studying evolutionary change. In particular, there was a stronger emphasis on interactions among selection and other forces, together with greater consideration of the role of environmental heterogeneity, and how such factors shaped phenotypic traits, whether obviously adaptive or not. The rapid accumulation of a comprehensive molecular data base across diverse species and environments also allowed effective application of the comparative approach, and the concomitant search for underlying patterns and processes in the distribution and maintenance of genetic diversity (Powell 1975; Thorpe 1982; Nevo *et al.* 1984; Hamrick & Godt 1989; Ward *et al.* 1992; Skibinski *et al.*1993).

In addition to fuelling the approach that subsequently became known as molecular ecology, the rapid adoption of molecular technology ratified the need during the mid-1960s to reinvigorate the state of population genetics. Limited new theory had appeared since the contributions of Wright, Haldane and Fisher (Dobzhansky 1970; Lewontin 1974), and despite insights from ecological genetic case studies (Ford 1964), it was unclear how much genetic polymorphism occurred in most natural populations, or indeed whether selection was the major determinant of genetic structuring. Indeed, although there was an elaborate theory, there were scarce empirical data to test predictions. The extension of protein electrophoretic techniques to population genetics removed the taxon-specific constraints imposed by studying visible polymorphisms, allowing data generation from virtually any organism; ironically, the accumulation of molecular genetic data has since outpaced the ability of theory to analyse them (Lewontin 1991; Powell 1994).

Other noteworthy landmarks during the early allozyme era, were the extensive electrophoretic studies on the *Drosophila willistoni* group (Ayala 1975), the initial allozymic studies describing population structure and dynamics (Selander & Yang 1969; Selander *et al.* 1971; Selander & Kaufman 1973), and the transfer of electrophoretic technology to plants (Allard *et al.* 1975) and bacteria (Milkman 1973). Such diversity of application allowed general issues to be addressed such as the maintenance of genetic variation in natural populations (neutralist-selectionist controversy; Lewontin 1974; Clarke 1975), the evolutionary significance of sex (Maynard Smith 1976, 1978), the role of gene flow in adaptive evolutionary change (Ehrlich *et al.* 1975; Allard *et al.* 1975; Slatkin 1985), the origins of geographic structuring (Prakash *et al.* 1969; Endler 1977) and the ecological significance of genetic diversity (Soulé & Stewart 1970; Valentine & Ayala 1974; Nei & Graur 1984; Nevo *et al.* 1984). The broad-based integration of theoretical population genetics and empiricism based on allele frequency data collected from wild populations consolidated the ecological genetic approach, though the union of genetic and ecological principles has been slow (Birch 1960; Bradshaw 1984; Berry 1989; Cain & Provine 1992; Berry & Bradshaw 1992). The ingredients were, nevertheless, in place for an expansion of the molecular approach through several technological advances.

Despite the continued value of allozyme polymorphisms as investigative tools in molecular ecology, it became apparent soon after the first flush of publications that limited molecular variability, the relatively slow evolutionary rates of proteins, and the usual destructive sampling of individuals, hindered effective application to many species. Furthermore, the questionable neutrality of allozymes (Lewontin 1974) compromised their use in studies of gene flow estimation and the spatial structuring of populations. Efforts focused increasingly on a search for additional molecular markers, notably those provided by direct analysis of nucleic acids.

4. The DNA era: advances in technology

Four primary developments in DNA recombinant technology revolutionized our ability to analyse the structure and diversity of nucleic acids, unleashing a rich source of marker variation. The first was provided by the discovery of restriction endonucleases (Linn & Arber 1968; Meselson & Yuan 1968) that cleave DNA at a specific sequence of nucleotides, or so-called recognition sites. These "molecular scissors" not only provided the basis for manipulation and fragmentation of the DNA molecule, but also supplied potent tools for assaying nucleotide diversity through the generation of restriction fragment length polymorphisms (RFLPs).

The second was the development of Southern hybridization (or blotting) (Southern 1975) which allowed visualization of specific DNA sequences transferred onto nylon or nitocellulose membranes. Using single-stranded and radioactively labelled DNA probes it was possible to identify, through the procedure of hybridization, target complementary sequences from among the thousands or millions of undetected fragments on a membrane. Without such a procedure, studies of RFLPs would have been restricted to the use of large individuals yielding sufficient DNA for direct visualization on a gel.

Early applications of restriction enzymes, especially for the analysis of animal mitochondrial DNA (mtDNA; Brown & Vinograd 1974; Brown & Wright 1975) revealed high levels of sequence diversity at the species and lower levels, despite strong conservation of gene function and arrangement. Parallel studies on plants were rather slower to emerge, due to the overall greater complexity of structure and transmission of plant mtDNA (Palmer 1985), and the usually slow rate of chloroplast DNA (cpDNA) evolution (Wolfe *et al.* 1987), though considerable intraspecific cpDNA variability has been uncovered (e.g. Soltis *et al.* 1992; Fransisco-Ortego *et al.* 1996; Gauthier *et al.* 1998). Pioneering studies on animal mtDNA (Brown 1980; Lansman *et al.* 1981; Avise *et al.* 1989) characterized the initial applications of DNA markers to natural populations, culminating in the foundation of phylogeographic analysis (Avise *et al.* 1987; Avise 1998) which is concerned with the principles and processes governing geographical distributions of genealogical lineages, especially at the intraspecific level. Phylogeographic studies served to reinforce the integrated approach to analysing molecular marker variation by calling on input from molecular genetics, population genetics, phylogenetics, demography, ethology and historical geography. It additionally served to emphasize the combined effects of extant and historical forces on structuring genetic diversity within species.

The replication of isolated gene sequences by incorporation into a bacterial or viral host through cloning (Maniatis *et al.* 1978) and the development of DNA sequencing (Maxam & Gilbert 1977; Sanger *et al.* 1977) provided a third stimulus for exploring DNA-level diversity. Although somewhat laborious in procedure, cloning enabled the dismantling of genomes into specific genes or sequences, so providing definitive targets for analysis, and the basis for taxonomic comparisons of gene structure and diversity. Clones used as probes could further identify genes of known function or anonymous gene regions taken from single-copy sequences in a genomic library, or from collections of cloned DNA fragments. Although such analyses based on DNA hybridization procedures have been highly informative (Avise 1994), the time and high level of expertise and resources required, hindered wide-scale application at the population level and its adoption by ecologists. DNA sequencing allowed the characterization of specific sequences, ensuring equivocal identification of genes or other nucleotide sequences for direct comparative purposes. Recent automation of DNA sequencing (Hunkapiller *et al.*, 1991) has enhanced significantly its accessibility to molecular ecologists.

The fourth, and perhaps most significant recent technological development was the introduction of the polymerase chain reaction (PCR; Mullis *et al.* 1986; Saiki *et al.* 1988) for *in vitro* amplification of specific DNA sequences. Four characteristics of the PCR were particularly pertinent to the needs of molecular ecology; speed, relative simplicity, non-destructive and minute tissue requirements, and robustness of amplification. Since most intraspecific analysis of genetic diversity is based on allele or genotype frequencies, usually large sample sizes in the order of 30-50 individuals, or greater are required, depending on levels of marker polymorphism. Amplification is essentially an exponential process, such that after twenty PCR cycles taking 2-3 h, over a million copies of a sequence can be produced, generating ample product for detailed genetic analysis. Frequently, however, far fewer copies are required. The ability to proceed from DNA extraction to analysis of nucleotide product in just a few hours renders the PCR approach ideal for rapid screening of large sample sets, as well as often avoiding the need for cloning, thus providing the molecular basis to many current programs in molecular ecology (e.g. Estoup & Angers, this volume; Muyzer, this volume). Moreover, the relatively simple molecular techniques compared to previous hybridization-based procedures, facilitates accessibility to non-molecular biologists.

A further major advantage of the PCR is its non-destructive and minuscule tissue requirements (Whitmore *et al.* 1992), including the analysis of small individuals such as larvae, fin clippings, hair cells and resting propagules. Such non-invasive sampling eases the study of rare or endangered species (Morin & Woodruff 1996), as well as availing opportunities for repetitive sampling of identifiable individuals, imparting a valuable temporal component to the analysis of genetic structure (Purcell *et al.* 1996; Miller & Kapuscinski 1997; Wirgin *et al.* . 1997). Finally, the amplification even of relatively degraded DNA, enables the recovery of nucleic acids from individual remains or their propagules. Studies on recovered or ancient DNA (Hermann & Hummel 1994; Rollo, this volume) provide a new temporal dimension to exploring the dynamics of genetic diversity in relation to environmental change (Nielsen *et al.* 1997; Miller & Kapuscinski 1997; Rivers & Ardren 1998), affording greater opportunities for disentangling natural and anthropogenic effects.

The PCR has additionally facilitated RFLP and sequencing studies through the selective production of specific DNA fragments, so providing in many cases a technically simple and rapid alternative to cloning. The availability of so-called "universal or conserved primers" (Kocher *et al.* 1989) allowing amplification across diverse taxa was of particular benefit by allowing DNA assays without the need for initial sequencing and primer construction.

The late 1980s to early 1990s were characterized by efforts to identify molecular markers that exhibited increasingly higher levels of polymorphism. Although allozymes and the analysis of cytoplasmic and nuclear DNA disclosed sufficient variants to characterize many species (Avise 1994), there remained a need for enhanced discrimination of closely related species and populations, as well as the more effective characterization of individuals, so facilitating the direct study of parentage and genetic relatedness (Strassmann *et al.* 1996). The discovery that many eukaryotic genomes contain highly repetitive DNA sequences (reviewed in Tautz 1993) provided a new source of polymorphic markers that could be exploited for diverse purposes, including applications in forensic science, paternity analysis, estimates of genetic relatedness, population and quantitative genetics (Burke *et al.* 1991; Pena *et al.* 1993). Indeed, the enhanced ability to map quantitative trait loci (Lynch & Walsh 1998; Knott & Haley 1998) provides a major breakthrough in the molecular analysis of traits, and an understanding of their genetic control and evolution.

Foremost among the variety of new methodologies has been the exploitation of nuclear loci with repeat unit lengths of between 1 and 64 bp, or VNTR DNA (variable number of tandem repeats; Tautz & Renz 1984; Nakamura *et al.* 1987). Although the existence of tandemly repetitive DNA sequences had been established (Britten & Kohne 1968), it was the description of so-called minisatellites, and the demonstration of their existence as a general phenomenon (Jeffreys *et al.* 1985a,b), that underpinned the subsequent surge of applications known generically as genetic or DNA fingerprinting. The early multilocus fingerprinting has given way to single-locus VNTR profiling of mini- and microsatellites, which when coupled with PCR (Galvin *et al.* 1995; McGregor *et al.* 1996; O'Connell & Wright 1997), provides a rapid and sensitive assay of nuclear sequence variability, with levels of heterozygosity often in excess of 70%.

Several features of VNTRs render them especially valuable for the molecular analysis of genetic diversity in wild populations. First, they are usually non-coding, and therefore the variation should be largely independent of natural selection, except where they are closely linked to adaptively significant coding sequences. Second, allozyme and many non PCR-based nucleic acid procedures require fresh or frozen tissue, often imposing logistical constraints on sample collection, whereas small amounts of blood or other tissue preserved in alcohol or other DNA-stable solutions, are adequate for analysing repetitive DNA. Third, high levels of heterozygosity (Estoup & Angers, this volume; Hauser & Ward, this volume) usually ensure the provision of abundant variants to characterize individuals and populations, though their effectiveness will depend on the number of loci surveyed and sample size (O'Connell & Wright 1997; Carvalho & Hauser 1998).

Microsatellites, or simple sequence repeats (SSRs: 1-6 bp), are generally more amenable to amplification by PCR than minisatellites because of their smaller size (but see McGregor *et al.* 1996; Galvin *et al.* 1996), and although it is often necessary to develop species-specific primers, there are numerous cases of sufficiently conserved sequence variation in flanking regions to enable amplification of loci across closely related species (Angers & Bernatchez 1996; Rico *et al.* 1996, O'Connell & Wright 1997). Recent advances such as semi-automated multilocus genotyping using colour fluorescent detection with automated DNA sequencers (Olsen *et al*. 1996), and multiplexing of dinucleotide and tetranucleotide loci allowing amplification in the same reaction (O'Reilly *et al*. 1996) have simplified and accelerated the screening of large sample sizes (50-100 individuals). Microsatellites now represent one of the most rapidly expanding source of molecular markers in molecular ecology (Wright & Bentzen 1994; O'Reilly & Wright 1995; Bruford *et al*. 1996; Jarne & Lagoda 1996; O'Connell & Wright 1997; Estoup & Cornuet 1998; Estoup & Angers, this volume). Even where primers for PCR do not exist, it is usually possible to identify and characterize several polymorphic loci within 2-3 months, and if automated facilities are available, an experienced researcher can process up to 150 individuals at four loci in a week.

As a distinct class of markers, microsatellites offer a source of molecular variation amenable to perhaps the widest range of applications in molecular ecology of any hitherto available tool, including analysis at the individual, population and higher taxonomic levels (Estoup & Angers, this volume), though their contribution to phylogenetics may be restricted to rapidly evolving or closely related species (Kornfield & Parker 1997; Sültmann & Mayer 1997).

Despite the undoubted advantages of microsatellites, there are several difficulties in their application, including; the nature of the mutation model which best describes variation at microsatellite loci, the associated choice of statistically appropriate distance measures, the problem of "stuttering" at dinucleotide loci which may often occlude adjacent alleles, the presence of null alleles which may artificially inflate the number of homozygous genotypes, and finally, the choice of appropriate sample size in cases of high allelic diversity (O'Reilly & Wright 1995; Bruford *et al*. 1996; O'Connell & Wright 1997; Carvalho & Hauser 1998; Estoup & Angers, this volume). Nevertheless, the combined advantages of high allelic diversity and heterozygosity, with the potential for rapid automated analysis of large sample sizes, has secured the routine analysis of nucleic acid variation as a core investigative approach in molecular ecology.

5. Descriptive and mechanistic molecular ecology

Two distinct, but interrelated approaches to molecular ecology can be discerned (Fig. 3). Hitherto, the most widely practised has been the descriptive, whereby arrays of gene frequency data have been collected to describe levels and distribution of genetic variability in natural populations. Such data provide the fundamental framework for formulating hypotheses about the underlying causes of patterns observed, but do not necessarily include direct analysis of mechanisms. Often only inferences can be drawn on the contribution of extant and historical forces such as selection or patterns of colonization, especially where laboratory or natural experimentation is constrained. However, the simultaneous comparison of molecular markers differing in their response to microevolutionary forces (Nielsen *et al*. 1997; FitzSimmons *et al*. 1997; Woods & Starman 1997), the employment of a sampling design which incorporates habitat-related (Heithaus & Laushman 1997; Owuor *et al*. 1997) or biologically significant spatial scales (Jones *et al*. 1991; Amos *et al*. 1993; Garza *et al*. 1998; Perry *et al*. 1998; Petrie & Kempenaers 1998), the use of introduced populations (Baker & Moeed 1987; Hauser *et al*. 1995; Carvalho *et al*. 1996), and the temporal analysis of samples (Miller & Kapuscinski 1997) can provide valuable insights into the likely factors shaping the distribution of variants observed.

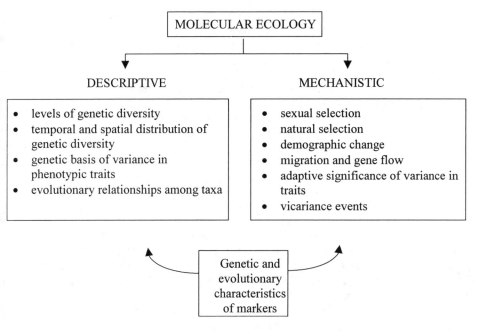

Figure 3: Descriptive and mechanistic approaches in molecular ecology. The descriptive approach employs molecular markers to classify patterns of biodiversity at molecular and phenotypic levels. The mechanistic approach explores directly the relative contributions of extant and historical forces in shaping the patterns of biodiversity observed. Central to both is the requirement to employ appropriate molecular marker sets based on their specific genetic and evolutionary characteristics.

Although the ultimate aim of many early studies employing the molecular approach was to promote an understanding of the origins and significance of fitness variation in natural populations, the current availability of markers exhibiting enhanced polymorphism, especially of VNTR loci, provide greater opportunities for direct analysis in the wild. Sufficient marker variation can usually be revealed to genetically tag individuals and their offspring to compare reproductive success, viability or migration of phenotypes differing in morphology, physiology or behaviour (Meagher & Thompson 1987; Scott & Williams 1994; Fleischer 1996; Taylor *et al.* 1997; Chevillon *et al.* 1998; Schnabel *et al.* 1998; Sunnocks *et al.* 1998; Schnabel, this volume). Such an approach allows direct determination of the consequences of variation in ecologically significant traits, as well as exploration of response to demographic, reproductive or habitat-related processes. There is an identifiable increase in efforts to employ the mechanistic approach in molecular ecology, though descriptive studies will continue to furnish the fundamental database from which patterns can be sought.

6. The molecular genetic toolbox: choices and applications

One of the most difficult decisions in molecular ecology is to decide which molecular marker, or combination of markers, is most appropriate to employ. The difficulty arises not only because of the plethora of options available (Avise 1994; Hillis *et al.* 1996a; Rieseberg this volume), but also because of differences in the ability of different classes of variants to disclose meaningful diversity at the individual, population or higher taxonomic levels (Avise 1994). Furthermore, preconceptions based on novelty and fashion, together with constraints of expertise and resources, often influence the choice made. For example, soon after the initial flush of PCR-based applications in molecular ecology, there was a perception that allozymes would be replaced, and that allozyme electrophoresis was outdated. While it is true that the enhanced variability afforded by direct nucleic acid analysis has revolutionized the effectiveness and range of questions tackled, allozymes continue to be widely employed, and still provide the largest database on genetic diversity within and among species (Thorpe 1982; Nevo et al. 1984; Ward et al. 1992; Skibinski, et al. 1993). Where sufficient allozymic variability exists, it remains a valuable first approach for pilot surveys, as well as in situations where resources or expertise are constrained. Moreover, allozymes are especially suited to particular types of problems such as the analysis of hybridization and hybrid zones (e.g. Schwenk & Spaak 1997; Rieseberg, this volume), determination of mating systems and population structure (e.g. Schnabel, this volume) and the study of molecular adaptation (Powers & Schulte 1996; Mitton, this volume). Much of the popularity of utilising protein variation stems from its ease and simplicity of execution, together with the usually straight forward translation of banding patterns into allele frequencies (Richardson et al. 1986; Murphy et al. 1996).

A further debate is the usage of the randomly amplified polymorphic DNA (RAPD) procedure (Grosberg et al. 1996), where poor reproducibility and marker dominance (Hadrys et al. 1992; Williams et al. 1993) may impede interpretation of data. Although markers such as microsatellites may in many situations be more appropriate, with careful execution and appropriate statistical analysis (Fritsch & Rieseberg 1996; Grosberg et al. 1996), RAPD, or other arbitrary-mediated fingerprinting techniques (Smith & Williams 1994; Vos et al. 1995) can be highly effective, including the molecular analysis of clonal and colonial animals (Okamura et al. 1993; Levitan & Grosberg 1993), plants (Nybom & Schaal 1990; Caetano-Anolles & Gresshoff 1994), in some animal population studies (Fondrk et al. 1993; Bielawski & Pumo 1997) Moreover, it provides a useful tool for isolating genomic sequences (Fani et al. 1993; Ender et al. 1996) . However, because RAPD markers are anonymous and expressed as dominant alleles that may obscure variability, they are generally unsuitable for analysis of breeding systems, the calculation of population genetic parameters such as F statistics, or phylogenetic analysis. It is therefore important to identify criteria to consider when deciding the most appropriate molecular method to employ, recognising the additional constraints often imposed by available resources.

Two related sets of criteria in choosing an appropriate molecular approach can be identified (Figure 4). First, a consideration of the levels of genetic variability revealed by the marker(s) as estimated by polymorphism, allelic diversity or heterozygosity (Avise 1994), and second, the genetic and evolutionary characteristics of different marker sets, including genome ploidy level (Avise et al. 1984), the parental mode of inheritance (biparental or maternal, Moritz 1994), marker inheritance and expression (dominant or co-dominant, Hadrys et al. 1992), response to microevolutionary forces (Avise 1994; Hauser et al. 1995; Kocher & Carleton 1997), mutation rates (Hillis et al. 1996b), and evolutionary rates of divergence (Avise 1994; Hillis et al. 1996a; Kocher & Carleton 1997; Estoup & Anders, this volume). It is worthwhile emphasizing that many studies benefit significantly from the employment of more than a single marker set (Olmstead & Sweere 1994), whether combining the study of coding and non-coding regions of the genome in phylogenetic analysis (Kornfield & Parker 1997; Estoup et al. 1998), or by the joint use of nuclear and mitochondrial markers (Hauser et al. 1995; Brunner et al. 1998). Such analyses may not only reveal the extent of congruence in conclusions reached (Karl & Avise 1992), but also detect different organismal events such as sex-specific dispersal or survival (Bowen et al. 1992; Melnick & Hoelzer 1992). The nature of statistical analysis

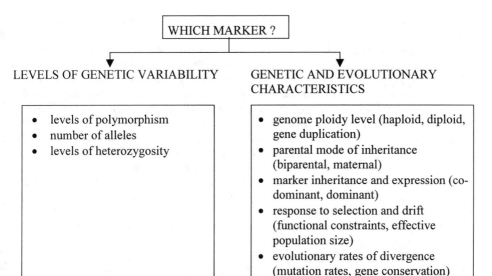

Figure 4: Salient considerations in choosing an appropriate molecular genetic marker in molecular ecology. In matching the molecular tool employed to the question under study, key considerations include identifying the optimal number of markers required, their inheritance, and response to microevolutionary forces and associated evolutionary rates. Optimal choice may be constrained by available resources such as funds, equipment, labour and expertise.

(Chakraborty & Danker-Hopfe 1991; Slatkin 1995; Weir 1996; Hillis *et al.* 1996b) will further determine the ability to address a question effectively.

The level of genetic variability revealed by a procedure depends on its effectiveness in disclosing variants (Avise 1994), the effects of extant and historical microevolutionary forces (Avise *et al.* 1989; Hudson 1990; Slatkin 1993; Avise *et al.* 1992; Moritz 1994; Templeton 1998), and the area of the genome examined (Park & Moran 1994). It is well established that allozyme electrophoresis, for example, reveals only a small proportion of genomic diversity (Singh *et al.* 1976), whereas the more rapidly evolving VNTR loci yield heterozygosities often in excess of 70% (Amos *et al.* 1993). Such high levels of diversity can be especially valuable in situations where multilocus genotypes are required, such as when estimating genetic relatedness (Strassmann *et al.* 1996), parentage analysis (Parker *et al.* 1996), and the mapping of quantitative trait loci (Bachmann & Hombergen 1997). The existence of numerous alleles or haplotypes is also especially useful for the comparison of recently diverged populations or species (Bentzen *et al.* 1996; Kornfield & Parker 1997). The quest to uncover increasingly high levels of marker variation can, however, produce difficulties of interpretation and analysis, and may necessitate the grouping of alleles of similar mobility (O'Reilly & Wright 1995). Moreover, in studies on population structure, the high allelic diversity typical of some microsatellite loci (e.g. Bentzen *et al.* 1996) demands high sample sizes or the use of numerical re-sampling techniques such as bootstrapping, though the latter clearly does not remove the need for adequate sampling.

The one-quarter effective population size of mtDNA due to its haploidy and predominantly maternal inheritance, renders it particularly susceptible to stochastic fluctuations arising from drift, making it an informative approach for detection of population bottlenecks, especially when compared to nuclear-based methods (Hauser *et al.* 1995; Neigel 1996). Despite the higher evolutionary rate of mtDNA compared to many nuclear genes (Wilson *et al.* 1985; Stoneking *et al.* 1991), its single-locus status renders it more likely than multilocus nuclear assays to yield unrepresentative patterns of genomic diversity, necessitating comparisons across genes and nucleotide sequences, or with other marker sets.

Perhaps DNA sequence-based methods provide the most powerful description of genetic variation because they remove the inferential stages necessary in indirect methods such as allozyme electrophoresis or microsatellite analysis, and may overcome to some extent locus-specific biases implicit in most procedures.   Sequences of coding regions offer particular advantages because of the ability to compare silent-site, assumed to be predominantly neutral, and non-silent variation, which is potentially under selection. Sequencing is essential for confirmation of homology in DNA fragments, as well as in assessing phylogenetic relationships, and automated procedures (Hunkapiller *et al.*, 1991) have also increased access for population-level comparisons.   However, despite the high information content of DNA sequencing, care has to exercised in the choice of genes and nucleotide regions analysed. For example, it is known that the distribution of third position transitions and transversions in DNA sequence analysis, and the associated differential impacts of selection, renders existing mutation-based models of sequence evolution inappropriate (Kocher & Carleton 1997).

The plethora of questions in molecular ecology precludes here a detailed consideration of all possible scenarios though it is possible to identify broad approaches in relation to the taxonomic scale of investigation (Mace *et al.* 1996).   For studies at a fine level of resolution, such as the determination of parentage or close family relationships, techniques such as mini- and microsatellites are optimal (Strassmann *et al.* 1996). If limited parental information is available, or if large sample sizes are analysed, microsatellites should be employed, though multilocus fingerprinting of minisatellites remains valuable where analyses can be restricted to within-gel comparisons (Burke 1989; Amos & Pemberton 1992).   Estimates of gene flow and population structuring can be made using a variety of marker systems depending on levels of polymorphism, including the employment of allozymes, mitochondrial DNA RFLPs and microsatellites (Baverstock & Moritz 1996; Niegel 1997; Bossart & Prowell 1998). To detect sex-specific bias due to the maternal inheritance of mtDNA, it is preferable to incorporate direct comparisons with nuclear markers. For the analysis of phylogenetic relationships, DNA sequencing is especially effective, though the choice of sequence is critical (Hillis *et al.* 1996b).   To overcome misinterpretations due to abrupt changes in the evolutionary rates of specific nucleotide sequences, several regions should be sequenced to check for conformity of relationships.

With the ever-growing choice of marker systems available, and the availability of sophisticated methods of statistical analysis that often depend on restrictive assumptions (Neigel 1996; Weir 1996), it is vital to consider fully the molecular and evolutionary characteristics of the chosen method (e.g. for RAPD, Fritsch & Rieseberg 1996; Grosberg *et al.* 1996; for anonymous single-copy nuclear DNA markers, Karl & Avise 1993; Karl 1996; for microsatellites, Estoup & Cornuet 1998; Estoup & Anders this volume; for DNA sequencing, Huelsenbeck *et al.* 1996; Swofford *et al.* 1996; Hillis *et al.* 1996b; Kocher & Carleton 1997). Although practical constraints may exclude the use of an optimal molecular approach, acquisition of such fundamental information remains necessary if only to ensure an objective assessment of reliability on the conclusions reached. It is possible that the conclusions drawn may be more determined by the idiosyncratic nature of the tool employed, than the ecological or evolutionary phenomena under investigation, though the latter is less likely if combined marker data sets are utilized. It is therefore critical at the planning stage of a molecular ecology project to consider carefully, and in detail, the characteristics and diagnostic ability of alternative marker sets in relation to the question tackled.

7. Concluding remarks and future priorities

The Ecological Genetics School (Ford 1964) represented the first concerted attempt to interpret fitness variation in ecologically significant traits within an evolutionary framework, and as such, represents a landmark in the development of molecular ecology. Although classical ecological genetic case studies were restrictive taxonomically, they strengthened the awareness that patterns of biodiversity, especially at the population level, were dynamic in both space and time, and demonstrated the need for interpretations based on an amalgam of ecology and genetics. The availability of ubiquitous genetic markers afforded by protein and nucleic acid variation provides a powerful approach for ensuring the continued integration of these "uneasy bedfellows" (Berry & Bradshaw 1992), as well as providing major opportunities for tackling fundamental problems in adaptive evolution and mechanisms of speciation.

It is not surprising, and in many ways highly appropriate, that vast effort has been expended in the past decade to develop new molecular techniques to assay genetic diversity. There has thus been a concentration of energies on technology, with a corresponding emphasis on understanding the molecular basis of marker variation, and associated development of models and methods of statistical analyses. Advances in technology have not always been met with a commensurate level of applications to natural populations to test predictions, and in particular there has been a continuing dominance of descriptive molecular ecology. As pointed out above, hitherto unprecedented opportunities now exist to examine the influence of changes in gene frequencies on the origin and maintenance of traits affecting viability and reproductive success. It is perhaps in this area that particular additional attention is warranted.

Two notable and related areas in molecular ecology appear poised for major advances; an improved understanding of the evolutionary dynamics of quantitative traits, and the molecular genetic analysis of adaptation. Although it is known that molecular genetic variation evolves at a different rate to the diversity revealed by molecular markers, there has been relatively little attempt to examine the relationship between them (Lynch 1996). With the improved battery of molecular markers available, together with improvements in the mapping of quantitative trait loci (Bachmann & Hombergen 1997; Lynch & Walsh 1998), major opportunities exist to determine the significance of molecular estimates of fitness variation (Spitz 1993; Podolsky & Holtsford 1995; Yang et al. 1996; Waldmann & Andersson 1998). The molecular approach can be extended also to explore the underlying genetic basis of ecologically significant traits and the associated nature and extent of genetic change associated with population divergence and speciation (Bradshaw et al. 1995; Powers & Schulte 1996; Turner et al. 1997). Such studies would address two of the core problems in evolutionary biology; the extent to which genotypic variation influences phenotype, and the nature and extent of genetic change associated with the evolution of adaptation. Both would have significant implications on our predictions of population and species persistence in relation to natural and man-made environmental change.

Although early ecological genetic studies were dominated by study of only a few illustrative examples, much was gained from the availability of comprehensive biological data sets, allowing the effective interpretation of linkages between phenotypic variation, and aspects of environmental heterogeneity, population dynamics, predation, and historical processes. Similarly detailed molecular case studies have emerged (e.g. Magurran et al. 1995; Nielsen 1996; Vrijenhoek 1996; Baldwin 1997; Taylor et al. 1997), though it would be beneficial to increase the focus on particular populations or species that encompass a range of dispersal capacities, mating systems, modes of development, reproductive behaviours, social structures, degrees of physical isolation and demography.

It is only when data from sufficiently detailed disparate examples exist, that meaningful comparative analyses can be undertaken to identify generalities.

In addition to the continued demand for ecological information in relation to patterns of genetic structuring, it is timely to consolidate our understanding of the effectiveness of alternative molecular approaches. An especially informative strategy is to undertake simultaneous comparisons of different marker sets on the same samples, thus not only identifying the optimal combination of molecular tools to address a question, but also for exploring differences in the patterns of genetic diversity revealed under a common set of circumstances. Subsequent integration of such comparative data with knowledge of the evolutionary characteristics of respective markers may then reveal both the constraints and opportunities in their employment.

Amplification of target nucleotides by the PCR, coupled with the availability of automated sequencers, renders direct sequencing an increasingly popular approach for population and phylogenetic analysis, and is likely to expand rapidly in usage. An expansion of such data sets is likely to yield valuable insights into the role of drift and selection on genome structure and organisation, as well as the relative contributions of evolutionary forces in shaping population and species diversity.

Molecular ecology is an established and insightful approach to tackling problems in ecology and evolution. Further advances will, however, depend critically not only on an enhanced understanding of the nature and dynamics of the molecular variation utilized, but also on the effective integration of molecular genetic data with comprehensive information on extant and historical processes. Accessing the latter will demand concentrated effort on additional case studies, though unlike classical ecological genetic approaches, the ubiquity of molecular variation does not restrict such focus to narrow ecological or evolutionary realms.

References

Allard RW, Kahler AL, Clegg MT (1975) Isozymes in plant population genetics. In: *Isozymes. IV. Genetics and Evolution* (ed. Markert CL), pp. 261-272. Academic Press, New York.

Amos W, Pemberton JP (1992) DNA fingerprinting in non-human populations. *Current Opinions in Genetics and Development*, **2**, 857-860.

Amos W, Schlötterer C, Tautz D (1993) Social structure of pilot whales revealed by analytical DNA typing. *Science*, **260**, 670-672.

Angers B, Bernatchez L (1996) Usefulness of heterologous microsatellites obtained from brook charr, *Salvelinus fontinalis* Mitchill, in other *Salvelinus* species. *Molecular Ecology*, **5**, 317-319.

Antonovics J (1994) The interplay of numerical and gene-frequency dynamics in host-pathogen systems. In: *Ecological Genetics* (ed. Real LA), pp. 129-145. Princeton University Press, Princeton, New Jersey.

Ayala FJ (1975) Genetic differentiation during the speciation process. *Evolutionary Biology*, **8**, 1-78.

Avise JC (1974) Systematic value of electrophoretic data. *Systematic Zoology*, **23**, 465-481.

Avise JC (1994) *Molecular Markers, Natural History and Evolution.* Chapman & Hall, London.

Avise JC (1998) The history and purview of phylogeography: a personal reflection. *Molecular Ecology*, 7, 371-379.

Avise JC, Arnold J, Ball RM *et al.* (1987) Intraspecific phylogeography: the mitochondrial DNA bridge between population genetics and systematics. *Annual Review of Ecology and Systematics,* **18**, 489-522.

Avise JC, Lansman RA, Shade RO (1979) The use of restriction endonucleases to measure mitochondrial DNA sequence relatedness in natural populations. I. Population structure and evolution in the genus *Peromyscus. Genetics*, **92**, 279-295.

Avise JC, Neigel JE, Arnold J (1984) Demographic influences of mitochondrial DNA lineage survivorship in animal populations. *Journal of Molecular Evolution*, **20**, 99-105.

Avise JC, Bowen BW, Lamb T (1989) DNA fingerprints from hypervariable mitochondrial DNA genotypes. *Molecular Biology and Evolution*, **6**, 258-269.

Avise JC, Bowen BW, Lamb T, Metlan A, Bermingham E (1992) Mitochondrial DNA evolution at a turtle's pace: evidence for low genetic variability and reduced microevolutionary rate in the Testudines. *Molecular Biology and Evolution*, **9**, 457-473.

Bachmann K, Hombergen E-J (1997) From phenotype via QTL to virtual phenotype in *Microseris* (Asteraceae): predictions from multilocus marker genotypes. *New Phytologist*, **137**, 9-18.

Baker AJ, Moeed A (1987) Rapid genetic differentiation and founder effect in colonizing populations of common mynas (*Acridotheras tristis*). *Evolution*, **41**, 525-528.

Baldwin BG (1997) Adaptive radiation of the Hawaiian silversword alliance: congruence and conflict of phylogenetic evidence from molecular and non-molecular investigations. In: *Molecular Evolution and Adaptive Radiation* (eds. Givnish TJ, Sytsma KJ), pp. 103-128. Cambridge University Press, Cambridge.

Barraclough TG, Vogler AP, Harvey PH (1998) Revealing the factors that promote speciation. *Philosophical Transactions of the Royal Society of London, B*, **353**, 241-249.

Baverstock PR, Moritz C (1996) Project design. In: *Molecular Systematics*, 2nd edn. (eds. Hillis D, Moritz C, Mable BK), pp. 17-28. Sinauer Associates, Massachusetts.

Bentzen P, Taggart CT, Ruzzante DE, Cook D (1996) Microsatellite polymorphism and the population structure of Atlantic cod (*Gadus morhua*) in the northwest Atlantic. *Canadian Journal of Fisheries and Aquatic Sciences*, **53**, 2706-2721.

Berry RJ (1989) Ecology: where genes and geography meet. *Journal of Animal Ecology*, **58**, 733-759.

Berry RJ, Bradshaw, AD (1992) Genes in the real world. In: *Genes in Ecology* (eds. Crawford TJ, Hewitt GM), pp. 431-449. Blackwell Scientific Publications, Oxford.

Berry HK, Dobzhansky T, Gartler SM, Levene H, Osborne RH (1955) Chromatographic studies on urinary excretion patterns in monozygotic and dizygotic twins. I. Methods and analysis. *American Journal of Human Genetics*, **7**, 93-107.

Bielawski JP & Pumo DE (1997) Randomly amplified polymorphic DNA (RAPD) analysis of Atlantic coast striped bass. *Heredity*, **78**, 32-40.

Birch LC (1960) The genetic factor in population ecology. *American Naturalist*, **94**, 9-24.

Bossart JL, Prowell DP (1998) Genetic estimates of population structure and gene flow: limitations, lessons and new directions. *Trends in Ecology and Evolution*, **13**, 202-206.

Bowen BW, Meylan JP, Ross JP, Limpus CJ, Balazs GH, Avise JC (1992) Global population structure and natural history of the green turtle (*Chelonia mydas*) in terms of matriarchal phylogeny. *Evolution*, **46**, 865-881.

Bradshaw AD (1984) The importance of evolutionary ideas in ecology- and vice versa. In: *Evolutionary Ecology* (ed. Shorrocks B), pp. 20-50. Blackwell Scientific Publications, Oxford.

Bradshaw HD, Wilbert SM, Otto KG, Schemske DW (1995) Genetic mapping of floral traits associated with reproductive isolation in monkeyflowers (*Mimulus*). *Nature*, **376**, 762-765.

Britten RJ, Kohne DE (1968) Repeated sequences in DNA. *Science*, **161**, 529-540.

Brown WM (1980) Polymorphism in mitochondrial DNA in humans as revealed by restriction endonuclease analysis. *Proceedings of the National Academy of Sciences USA*, **77**, 3605-3609.

Brown WM, Vinograd J (1974) Restriction endonuclease cleavage maps of animal mitochondrial DNAs. *Proceedings of the National Academy of Sciences USA*, **71**, 4617-4621.

Brown WM, Wright JW (1975) Mitochondrial DNA and the origin of parthenogenesis in whiptail lizards (*Cnemidophorus*). *Herpetological Review*, **6**, 70-71.

Brown WM, Wright JW (1979) Mitochondrial DNA analysis and the origin and relative age of parthenogenetic lizards (Genus *Cnemidophorus*). *Science*, **203**, 1247-1249.

Bruford MW, Cheesman DJ, Coote T *et al.* (1996) Microsatellites and their application to conservation genetics. In: *Molecular Genetic Approaches in Conservation* (eds. Smith TB, Wayne RK), pp. 278-297. Oxford University Press, Oxford.

Brunner PC, Douglas MR, Bernatchez L (1998) Microsatellite and mitochondrial DNA assessment of population structure and stocking effects in Arctic charr *Salvelinus alpinus* (Teleostei: Salmonidae) from central Alpine lakes. *Molecular Ecology*, **7**, 209-224.

Burke T (1989) DNA fingerprinting and other methods for the study of mating success. *Trends in Ecology and Evolution*, **4**, 139-144.

Burke T, Hanotte O, Bruford MW, Cairns E (1991) Multilocus and single locus minisatellite analysis in population biological studies. In: *DNA Fingerprinting: Approaches and Applications* (eds. Burke T, Dolf G, Jeffreys AJ, Wolff R), pp. 154-168. Birkhäuser Verlag, Basel.

Cain AJ, Sheppard PM (1954) Natural selection in *Cepaea. Genetics*, **39**, 89-116.

Cain AJ, Provine WB (1992) Genes and ecology in history. In: *Genes in Ecology* (eds. Crawford TJ, Hewitt GM), pp. 3-28. Blackwell Scientific Publications, Oxford.

Caetano-Anolles G, Gresshoff PM (1994) DNA amplification fingerprinting: a general tool with applications in breeding, identification and phylogenetic analysis of plants. In: *Molecular Ecology: Approaches and Applications* (eds. Schierwater B, Streit B, Wagner GP, DeSalle R), pp. 17-32. Birkhäuser Verlag, Basel.

Carvalho GR, Shaw PW, Hauser L, Seghers BH, Magurran AE (1996) Artificial introductions, evolutionary change and population differentiation in Trinidadian guppies (*Poecilia reticulata*). *Biological Journal of the Linnean Society*, **57**, 219-234.

Carvalho GR, Hauser L (1998) Advances in the molecular analysis of fish population structure. *Italian Journal of Zoology*, **65** (Supplement 1), in press.

Chakraborty R, Danker-Hopfe H (1991) Analysis of population structure: a comparative study of different estimators of Wright's fixation indices. In: *Handbook of Statistics*, Volume 8 (eds. Rao CR, Chakraborty R), pp. 203-254. North-Holland, Amsterdam.

Chevillon C, Rivet Y, Raymond M, Rousset F, Smouse PE, Pasteur N (1998) Migration/selection balance and ecotypic differentiation in the mosquito *Culux pipiens*. *Molecular Ecology*, **7**, 197-208.

Clarke B (1975) The contribution of ecological genetics to evolutionary theory: detecting the direct effects of natural selection on particular polymorphic loci. *Genetics*, **79**, 101-113.

Dobzhansky T (1961) On the dynamics of chromosomal polymorphism in *Drosophila*. *Symposia of the Royal Entomological Society of London*, **1**, 30-42.

Dobzhansky T (1970) *Genetics of the Evolutionary Process*. Columbia University Press, New York.

Ehrlich PR, White RR, Singer MC, McKechnie SW, Gilbert LE (1975) Checkerspot butterflies: A historical perspective. *Science*, **188**, 221-228.

Ender A, Schwenk K, Städler T, Streit B, Schierwater B (1996) RAPD identification of microsatellites in *Daphnia*. *Molecular Ecology*, **5**, 437-441.

Endler JA (1977) *Geographic Variation, Speciation and Clines*. Princeton University Press, Princeton.

Endler JA (1992) Genetic heterogeneity and ecology. In: *Genes in Ecology* (eds. Crawford TJ, Hewitt GM), pp. 315-334. Blackwell Scientific Publications, Oxford.

Estoup A, Cornuet J-M (1998) Microsatellite evolution: inferences from population data. In: *Microsatellites: Evolution and Applications* (eds. Goldstein DB, Schlötterer C). Oxford University Press, Oxford, in press.

Estoup A, Rousset F, Michalakis Y, Cornuet J-M, Adriamanga M, Guyomard R (1998) Comparative analysis of microsatellite and allozyme markers: a case study investigating microgeographic differentiation in brown trout (*Salmo trutta*). *Molecular Ecology*, **7**, 339-353.

Fani R, Damiani G, Di Serio C, Gallori E, Grifoni A, Bazzicalup M (1993) Use of random amplified polymorphic DNA (RAPD) for generating DNA probes for microorganisms. *Molecular Ecology*, **2**, 243-250.

Ferraris JD, Palumbi SR (1996) *Molecular Zoology. Advances, Strategies and Protocols*. Wiley-Liss, New York.

FitzSimmons NN, Moritz C, Limpus CJ, Pope L, Prince R (1997) Geographic structure of mitochondrial and nuclear DNA polymorphisms in Australian green turtle populations and male-biased gene flow. *Genetics*, **147**, 1843-1854.

Fleischer RC (1996) Application of molecular methods to the assessment of genetic mating systems in vertebrates. In: *Molecular Zoology: Advances, Strategies and Protocols* (eds. Ferrais JD, Palumbi SR), pp. 133-162. Wiley-Liss, New York.

Fondrk MK, Page RE, Hunt GJ (1993) Paternity analysis of worker honey bees using random amplified DNA (RAPD). *Naturwissenschaften*, **80**, 226-231.

Ford EB (1964) *Ecological Genetics*. Methuen, London.

Francisco-Ortega J, Janen RK, Mason-Gamer RJ, Wallace RS (1996) Application if chloroplast DNA restriction site studies for conservation genetics. In: *Molecular Genetic Approaches in Conservation* (eds. Smith TB, Wayne RK), pp. 183-201. Oxford University Press, Oxford.

Fritsch P, Rieseberg L (1996) The use of random amplified polymorphic DNA (RAPD) in conservation genetics. In: *Molecular Genetic Approaches in Conservation* (eds. Smith TB, Wayne RK), pp. 54-73. Oxford University Press, Oxford.

Galvin P, McGregor D, Cross T (1995) A single locus PCR amplified minisatellite region as a hypervariable genetic marker in gadoid species. *Aquaculture*, **137**, 31-40.

Galvin P, Taggart J, Ferguson A, O'Farrell M, Cross T (1996) Population genetics of Atlantic salmon (*Salmo salar* L.) in the River Shannon system in Ireland: an appraisal using single locus minisatellite (VNTR) probes. *Canadian Journal of Fisheries and Aquatic Sciences*, **53**, 1933-1942.

Gartler SM, Dobzhansky T, Berry HK (1955) Chromatographic studies on urinary excretion patterns in monozygotic and dizygotic twins. II. Heritability of the excretion rates of certain substances. *American Journal of Human Genetics*, **7**, 108-121.

Garza JC, Dallas J, Duryadi D, Gerasimov S, Croset H, Boursot P (1998) Social structure of the mound-building mouse, *Mus spicilegus*, revealed by genetic analysis with microsatellites. *Molecular Ecology*, **11**, 1009-1018.

Gauthier P, Lumaret R, Bédécarrats (1998) Genetic variation and gene flow in Alpine diploid and tetraploid populations of *Lotus* (*L. alpinus* (D.C.) Scleicher/*L. corniculatus* L.). II. Insights from RFLP of chloroplast DNA. *Heredity*, **80**, 694-701.

Givnish TJ, Sytsma KJ (1997) *Molecular Evolution and Adaptive Evolution*. Cambridge University Press, Cambridge.

Grosberg RK, Levitan DR, Cameron BB (1996) Characterization of genetic structure and genealogies using RAPD-PCR markers: a random primer for the novice and nervous. In: *Molecular Zoology. Advances, Strategies and Protocols* (eds. Ferraris JD, Palumbi SR), pp. 67-100. Wiley-Liss, New York.

Hadrys H, Balick M, Schierwater B (1992) Applications of randomly amplified polymorphic DNA (RAPD) in molecular ecology. *Molecular Ecology*, **1**, 55-63.

Hamrick JL, Godt MJW (1989) Allozyme diversity in plants. In: *Plant Population Genetics, Breeding and Genetic Resources* (eds. Brown AHD, Clegg MT, Kahler AL, Weir BS), pp. 43-63. Sinauer, Massachusetts.

Harris H (1953) *An Introduction to Human Biochemical Genetics.* Eugenics Laboratory Memoirs 37. Cambridge University Press, Cambridge.

Harris H (1966) Enzyme polymorphism in man. *Proceedings of the Royal Society of London B*, **164**, 298-310.

Hauser L, Carvalho GR, Pitcher TJ (1995) Morphological and genetic differentiation of the African clupeid *Limnothrissa miodon* 34 years after its introduction to Lake Kivu. *Journal of Fish Biology*, **47** (Suppl. A),127-144.

Heithaus MR, Laushman RH (1997) Genetic variation and conservation of stream fishes: influence of ecology, life history and water quality. *Canadian Journal of Fisheries and Aquatic Sciences*, **54**, 1822-1836.

Hermann B, Hummel S (1994) *Ancient DNA.* Springer Verlag, New York & London.

Hillis D, Moritz D, Mable BK (1996a) *Molecular Systematics*, 2nd edn. Sinauer Associates, Massachusetts.

Hillis DM, Mable BK, Moritz C (1996b) Applications of molecular systematics: the state of the field and a look to the future. In: *Molecular Systematics*, 2nd edn. (eds. Hillis D, Moritz C, Mable BK), pp. 515-543. Sinauer Associates, Massachusetts.

Hoelzel AR, Dover GA (1991) *Molecular Genetic Ecology.* IRL Press at Oxford University Press, Oxford.

Hubby JL, Lewontin RC (1966) A molecular approach to the study of genic heterozygosity in natural populations. I. The number of alleles at different loci in *Drosophila pseudoobscura. Genetics*, **54**, 577-594.

Hudson RR (1990) Gene genealogies and the coalescent process. *Oxford Surveys in Evolutionary Biology*, **7**, 1-44.

Huelsenbeck JP, Hillis, DM, Jones R (1996) Parametric bootstrapping in molecular phylogenetics: applications and performance. In: *Molecular Zoology. Advances, Strategies and Protocols* (eds. Ferraris JD, Palumbi SR), pp. 19-46. Wiley-Liss, New York.

Hunkapiller T, Kaiser RJ, Koop BF, Hood L (1991) Large-scale and automated DNA sequence determination. *Science*, **254**, 59-68.

Hunter RL, Markert CL (1957) Histochemical demonstration of enzymes separated by zone electrophoresis in starch gels. *Science*, **125**, 1294-1295.

Jarne P, Lagoda PJL (1996) Microsatellites, from molecules to populations and back. *Trends in Ecology and Evolution*, **11**, 424-429.

Jeffreys AJ, Wilson V, Thein SL (1985a) Hypervariable minisatellite regions in human DNA. *Nature*, **314**, 76-79.

Jeffreys AJ, Wilson V, Thein SL (1985b) Individual-specific fingerprints of human DNA. *Nature*, **316**, 76-79.

Jones CS, Lessells CM, Krebs JR (1991) Helpers-at-the-nest in Europen bee-eaters (*Merops apiaster*): a genetic analysis. In: *DNA Fingerprinting: Approaches and Applications* (eds. Burke T, Dolf G, Jeffreys AJ, Wolff R), pp. 169-192. Birkhäuser Verlag, Basel.

Karl SA (1996) Application of anonymous nuclear loci to conservation biology. In: *Molecular Genetic Approaches in Conservation* (eds. Smith TB, Wayne RK), pp. 38-53. Oxford University Press, Oxford.

Karl SA, Avise JC (1992) Balancing selection at allozyme loci in oysters: implications from nuclear RFLPs. *Science*, **256**, 100-102.

Karl SA, Avise JC (1993) PCR-based assays of Mendelian polymorphisms from anonymous single-copy nuclear DNA: techniques and applications for population genetics. *Molecular Biology and Evolution*, **10**, 342-361.

Kimura M, Ohta T (1971) Protein polymorphism as a phase of molecular evolution. *Nature*, **229**, 467-469.

Kocher TD, Thomas WK, Meyer, A (1989) Dynamics of mitochondrial DNA evolution in animals: amplification and sequencing with conserved primers. *Proceedings of the National Academy of Sciences USA*, **86**, 6196-6200.

Kocher TD, Carleton KL (1997) Base substitution in fish mitochondrial DNA: patterns and rates. In: *Molecular Systematics of Fishes* (eds. Kocher TD, Stepien CA), pp. 13-24. Academic Press, London.

Kornfield I, Parker A (1997) Molecular systematics of a rapidly evolving species flock; the *mbuna* of Lake Malawi and the search for phylogenetic signal. In: *Molecular Systematics of Fishes* (eds. Kocher TD, Stepien CA), pp. 25-38. Academic Press, London.

Knott SA, Haley CS (1998) Simple multiple-marker sib pair analysis for mapping quantitative traits. *Heredity*, **81**, 48-54.

Lansman RA, Shade RO, Shapira JF, Avise JC (1981) The use of restriction endonucleases to measure mitochondrial DNA sequence relatedness in natural populations. III. Techniques and potential applications. *Journal of Molecular Evolution*, **17**, 214-226.

Levitan DR, Grosberg RK (1993) The analysis of paternity and maternity in the marine hydrozoan *Hydractinia symbiolongicarpus* using randomly amplified polymorphic DNA (RAPD) markers. *Molecular Ecology*, **2**, 315-326.

Lewontin RC (1974) *The Genetic Basis of Evolutionary Change.* Columbia University Press, New York.

Lewontin RC (1991) Electrophoresis in the development of evolutionary genetics: milestone or millstone? *Genetics*, **128**, 657-662.

Lewontin RC, Hubby JL (1966) A molecular approach to the study of genic heterozygosity in natural populations. II. Amount of variation and degree of heterozygosity in natural populations of *Drosophila pseudoobscura. Genetics*, **54**, 595-609.

Lewontin RC, Krakauer J (1973) Distribution of gene frequency as a test of the theory of selective neutrality of polymorphisms. *Genetics*, **74**, 175-195.

Li W-H (1997) *Molecular Evolution.* Sinauer Associates, Massachusetts.

Linn S, Arber W (1968) Host specificity of DNA produced by *Escherichia coli*. X. *In vitro* restriction of phage fd replicative form. *Proceedings of the National Academy of Sciences USA*, **59**, 1300-1306.

Lynch M (1996) A quantitative-genetic perspective on conservation issues. In: *Conservation Genetics: Case Histories from Nature* (eds. Avise JC, Hamrick JL), pp. 471-501. Chapman & Hall, London.

Lynch M, Walsh B (1998) *Genetics and Analysis of Quantitative Traits.* Sinauer Associates, Massachusetts.

Mace GM, Smith TB, Bruford MW, Wayne RK (1996) An overview of the issues. In: *Molecular Genetic Approaches in Conservation* (eds. Smith TB, Wayne RK), pp. 3-21. Oxford University Press, Oxford.

Magurran AE (1998) Population differentiation without speciation. *Philosophical Transactions of the Royal Society of London, B*, **353**, 275-286.

Magurran AE, Seghers BH, Shaw PW, Carvalho GR (1995) Behavioural and genetic diversity of guppy, *Poecilia reticulata*, populations in Trinidad. *Advances in the Study of Behaviour*, **24**, 155-202.

Maniatis T, Hardison RC, Lacy E *et al.* (1978) The isolation of structural genes from libraries of eucaryotic DNA. *Cell*, **15**, 687-701.

Markert C, Møller F (1959) Multiple forms of enzymes: Tissues, ontogenetic, and species specific patterns. *Proceedings of the National Academy of Sciences USA*, **45**, 753-763.

Maxam AM, Gilbert W (1977) A new method for sequencing DNA. *Proceedings of the National Academy of Sciences USA*, **74**, 560-564.

Maynard Smith J (1976) A short-term advantage for sex and recombination through sib-competition. *Journal of Theoretical Biology*, **63**, 245-258.

Maynard Smith J (1978) *The Evolution of Sex.* Cambridge University Press, Cambridge.

McGregor D, Galvin P, Cross T (1996) PCR amplification of a polymorphic minisatellite VNTR locus in whiting (*Merlangius merlangus* L.). *Animal Genetics*, **27**, 49-51.

Meagher TR, Thompson E (1987) Analysis of parentage for naturally established seedlings of *Chamaelirium luteum* (Liliaceae). *Ecology*, **68**, 803-812.

Melnick DJ, Hoelzer GA (1992) Differences in male and female macaque dispersal lead to contrasting distributions of nuclear and mitochondrial DNA variation. *International Journal of Primatology*, **13**, 379-393.

Meselson M, Yuan R (1968) DNA restriction enzyme from *E. coli. Nature*, **217**, 1110-1114.

Milkman RD (1967) Heterosis as a major cause of heterozygosity in nature. *Genetics*, **55**, 493-495.

Milkman RD (1973) Electrophoretic variation in *E. coli* from natural sources. *Science*, **182**, 1024.

Miller LM, Kapuscinski AR (1997) Historical analysis of genetic variation reveals low effective population size in a northern pike (*Esox lucius*) population. *Genetics*, **147**, 249-258.

Morin PA, Woodruff DS (1996) Noninvasive genotyping for vertebrate conservation. In: *Molecular Genetic Approaches in Conservation* (eds. Smith TB, Wayne RK), pp. 298-313. Oxford University Press, Oxford.

Moritz C (1994) Applications of mitochondrial DNA analysis on conservation: a critical review. *Molecular Ecology*, **3**, 401-411.

Mourant AE (1954) *The Distribution of the Human Blood Groups.* Blackwell, Oxford.

Mullis K, Faloona F, Svharf R, Saiki R, Horn G, Erlich H (1986) Specific enzymatic amplification of DNA *in vitro*: the polymerase chain reaction. *Cold Spring Harbor Symposium on Quantitative Biology*, **51**, 263-273.

Murphy RW, Sites JW Jr, Buth DG, Haufler H (1996) Proteins: Isozyme electrophoresis. *In: Molecular Systematics*, 2nd edn. (eds. Hillis D, Moritz C, Mable BK), pp. 51-120. Sinauer Associates, Massachusetts.

Nakamura Y, Leppert M, O'Connell P *et al.* (1987) Variable number of tandem repeat (VNTR) markers for human gene mapping. *Science*, **235**, 1616-1622.

Nei M (1975) *Molecular Population Genetics and Evolution.* North-Holland, Amsterdam.

Nei M, Graur D (1984) Extent of protein polymorphism and the neutral mutation theory. *Evolutionary Biology*, **17**, 73-118.

Neigel JE (1996) Estimation of effective population size and migration parameters from genetic data. In: *Molecular Genetic Approaches in Conservation* (eds. Smith TB, Wayne RK), pp. 329-346. Oxford University Press, Oxford.

Neigel JE (1997) A comparison of alternative strategies for estimating gene flow from genetic markers. *Annual Review of Ecology and Systematics*, **28**, 105-128.

Nevo E, Beiles A, Ben-Shlomo R (1984) The evolutionary significance of genetic diversity: ecological, demographic and life history correlates. In: *Evolutionary Dynamics of Genetic Diversity* (ed. Mani GS), pp. 13-213. Springer, Berlin.

Nielsen EE, Hansen MM, Loeschke V (1997) Analysis of microsatellite DNA from old scale samples of Atlantic salmon *Salmo salar*: a comparison of genetic composition over 60 years. *Molecular Ecology*, **6**, 487-492.

Nielsen JL (1996) Molecular genetics and the conservation of salmonid biodiversity: *Oncorhynchus* at the edge of their range. In: *Molecular Genetic Approaches in Conservation* (eds. Smith TB, Wayne RK), pp. 383-398. Oxford University Press, Oxford.

Nybom H, Schaal BA (1990) DNA "fingerprints" reveal genotypic distributions in natural populations of blackberries and raspberries (*Rubus*, Rosaceae). *American Journal of Botany*, **77**, 883-888.

O'Connell M, Wright JM (1997) Microsatellite DNA in fishes. *Reviews in Fish Biology and Fisheries*, **7**, 331-364.

Okamura B, Jones CS, Noble LR (1993) Randomly amplified polymorphic DNA analysis of clonal structure and geographic variation in a freshwater bryozoan. *Proceedings of the Royal Society of London B*, **253**, 147-154.

Olmstead RG, Sweere JA (1994) Combining data in phylogenetic systematics: an empirical approach using three molecular data sets in the Solanaceae. *Systematic Biology*, **43**, 467-481.

Olsen GJ, Woese CJ, Overbeek R (1994) The winds of (evolutionary) change- breathing new life into bacteriology. *Journal of Bacteriology*, **176**, 1.

Olsen JB, Wenburg JK, Bentzen P (1996) Semiautomated multilocus genotyping of Pacific salmon (*Oncorhynchus* spp.) using microsatellites. *Molecular Marine Biology and Biotechnology*, **5**, 259-272.

O'Reilly P, Wright JM (1995) The evolving technology of DNA fingerprinting and its application to fisheries and aquaculture. *Journal of Fish Biology*, **47** (Suppl. A), 29-55.

O'Reilly P, Hamilton LC, McConnell K, Wright JM (1996) Rapid analysis of genetic variation in Atlantic salmon (*Salmo salar*) by PCR multiplexing of dinucleotide and tetranucleotide microsatellites. *Canadian Journal of Fisheries and Aquatic Sciences*, **53**, 2292-2298.

Owuor ED, Fahima T, Beiles A, Korol A, Nevo E (1997) Population genetic response to microsite ecological stress in wild barley, *Hordeum spontaneum*. *Molecular Ecology*, **6**, 1177-1187.

Palmer JD (1985) Evolution of chloroplast and mitochondrial DNA in plants and algae. In: *Molecular Evolutionary Genetics* (ed. MacIntyre RJ), pp. 131-240. Plenum Press, New York.

Park LK, Moran P (1994) Developments in molecular genetic techniques in fisheries. *Reviews in Fish Biology and Fisheries*, **4**, 272-299.

Parker P, Waite TA, Peare T (1996) Paternity studies in animal populations. In: *Molecular Genetic Approaches in Conservation* (eds. Smith TB, Wayne RK), pp. 413-423. Oxford University Press, Oxford.

Pena SDJ, Chakraborty R, Epplen JT, Jeffreys AJ (1993) *DNA Fingerprinting: State of the Science*. Birkhäuser Verlag, Basel.

Perry EA, Boness DJ, Fleischer C. (1998) DNA fingerprinting evidence of nonfilial nursing in grey seals. *Molecular Ecology*, **7**, 81-85.

Petrie M, Kempenaers B (1998) Extra-pair paternity in birds: explaining variation between species and populations. *Trends in Ecology and Evolution*, **13**, 52-58.

Podolsky RH, Holtsford TP (1995) Population structure of morphological traits in *Clarkia dudleyana* I. Comparison of *Fst* between allozymes and morphological traits. *Genetics*, **140**, 733-744.

Powell JR (1975) Protein variation in natural populations of animals. *Evolutionary Biology*, **3**, 79-119.

Powell JR (1994) Molecular techniques in population genetics; A brief history. In: *Molecular Ecology: Approaches and Applications* (eds. Schierwater B, Streit B, Wagner GP, DeSalle R), pp. 131-156. Birkhäuser Verlag, Basel.

Powers DA, Schulte PM (1996) A molecular approach to the selectionist/neutralist controversy. In: *Molecular Zoology. Advances, Strategies and Protocols* (eds. Ferraris JD, Palumbi SR), pp. 327-352. Wiley-Liss, New York.

Prakash S, Lewontin RC, Hubby JL (1969) A molecular approach to the study of genic heterozygosity in natural populations. IV. Patterns of genic variation in central, marginal and isolated populations of *Drosophila pseudoobscura*. *Genetics*, **61**, 841-858.

Purcell MK, Kornfield I, Fogarty M, Parker A (1996) Interdecadal heterogeneity in mitochondrial DNA of Atlantic haddock (*Melanogrammus aeglefinus*) from Georges Bank. *Molecular Marine Biology and Biotechnology*, **5**, 185-192.

Rasmussen DI (1962) Blood group polymorphism and inbreeding in natural populations of deer mouse *Peromyscus maniculatus. Evolution*, **18**, 219-229.

Richardson BJ, Baverstock PR, Adams M (1986) *Allozyme Electrophoresis: A Handbook for Animal Systematics and Population Structure.* Academic Press, Sydney.

Rico C, Rico I, Hewitt GM (1996) 470 million years of conservation of microsatellite loci among fish species. *Proceedings of the Royal Society of London,* B, **263**, 549-557.

Rivers PJ, Ardren WR (1998) The value of archives. *Fisheries*, **23 (5)**, 6-9.

Saiki RK, Gelfand DH, Stoffel S *et al.* (1988) Primer-directed amplification of DNA with a thermostable DNA polymerase. *Science*, **239**, 487-491.

Sanger F, Nicklen S, Coulson AR (1977) DNA sequencing with chain-terminating inhibitors. *Proceedings of the National Academy of Sciences USA,* **74**, 5463-5467.

Schnabel A, Nason JD, Hamrick JL (1998) Understanding the population genetic structure of *Gleditsia triacanthos* L: seed dispersal and variation in female reproductive success. *Molecular Ecology*, in press.

Selander RK, Yang SY (1969) Protein polymorphism and genetic heterozygosity in a wild population of house mouse (*Mus musculus*). *Genetics*, **63**, 653-667.

Selander RK, Kaufman DW (1973) Self-fertilization and the genetic population structure in a colonising land snail. *Proceedings of the National Academy of Sciences USA*, **70**, 1186-1190.

Selander RK, Smith MH, Yang SY, Johnson WE, Gentry JB (1971) Biochemical polymorphism and systematics in the genus *Peromyscus.* I. Variation in the old field mouse (*Peromyscus polionotus*). *University Texas Publications*, **7103**, 49-90.

Schierwater B, Streit B, Wagner GP, DeSalle R (1994) *Molecular Ecology and Evolution: Approaches and Applications.* Birkhäuser Verlag, Basel.

Schwenk K, Spaak P (1997) Ecology and genetics of interspecific hybridization in *Daphnia.* In: *Evolutionary Ecology of Freshwater Animals: Concepts and Case Studies* (eds. Streit B, Städler T, Lively CM), pp. 199-230. Birkhäuser Verlag, Basel.

Scott MP, Williams SM (1994) Measuring reproductive success in insects. In: *Molecular Ecology: Approaches and Applications* (eds. Schierwater B, Streit B, Wagner GP, DeSalle R), pp. 61-74. Birkhäuser Verlag, Basel.

Sheppard PM (1958) *Natural Selection and Heredity.* Hutchinson, London.

Singh RS, Lewontin RC, Felton AA (1976) Genetic heterogeneity within electrophoretic "alleles" of xanthine dehydrogenase in *Drosophila pseudoobscura. Genetics ,* **84**, 609-629.

Skibinski DOF, Woodwark M, Ward RD (1993) A quantitative test of the neutral theory using pooled allozyme data. *Genetics*, **135**, 233-248.

Slatkin M (1993) Isolation by distance in equilibrium and non-equilibrium populations. *Evolution*, **47**, 264-279.

Slatkin M (1985) Gene flow in natural populations. *Annual Review of Ecology and Systematics*, **16**, 393-430.

Smith JSC, Williams JGK (1994) Arbitrary primer mediated fingerprinting in plants: case studies in plant breeding, taxonomy and phylogeny. In: *Molecular Ecology: Approaches and Applications* (eds. Schierwater B, Streit B, Wagner GP, DeSalle R), pp. 5-16. Birkhäuser Verlag, Basel.

Smith TB, Wayne RK (1996) *Molecular Genetic Approaches in Conservation.* Oxford University Press, Oxford.

Smithies O (1955) Zone electrophoresis in starch gels: Group variations in the serum proteins of normal adults. *Biochemical Journal*, **61**, 629-641.

Soltis DE, Soltis PS, Milligan BG (1992) Intraspecific chloroplast-DNA variation: systematic and phylogenetic implications. In: *Molecular Systematics of Plants* (eds. Soltis PS, Soltis, DE, Doyle JJ), pp. 117-150. Chapman & Hall, New York.

Soulé M, Stewart, BR (1970) The "niche variation" hypothesis: a test and alternatives. *American Naturalist*, **104**, 85-97.

Southerm EM(1975) Detection of specific sequences among DNA fragments separared by gel electrophoresis. *Journal of Molecular Biology*, **98**, 503-517.

Spitz K (1993) Population structure in *Daphnia obtusa*: quantitative genetic and allozyme variation. *Genetics*, **135**, 367-374.

Stormont C (1959) On the application of blood groups in animal breeding. *Proceedings of the Tenth International Congress in Genetics,* **1**, 206-224.

Stoneking MD, Hedgecock D, Higuchi RG, Vigilant L, Erlich HA (1991) Population variation of human mtDNA control region sequences detected by enzymatic amplification and sequence-specific oligonucleotide probes. *American Journal of Human Genetics*, **48**, 370-382.

Strassmann JE, Solís CR, Peters JM, Queller DC (1996) Strategies for finding and using highly polymorphic DNA microsatellite loci for studies of genetic relatedness and pedigrees. In: *Molecular Zoology: Advances, Strategies and Protocols* (eds. Ferrais JD, Palumbi SR), pp. 163-180. Wiley-Liss, New York.

Sültmann H, Mayer WE (1997) Reconstruction of cichlid phylogeny using nuclear DNA markers. In: *Molecular Systematics of Fishes* (eds. Kocher TD, Stepien CA), pp. 39-52. Academic Press, London.

Sunnucks P, De Barro PJ, Lushai G, Maclean N, Hales D (1998) Genetic structure of an aphid studied using microsatellites: cyclic parthenogenesis, differentiated lineages and host specialization. *Molecular Ecology*, **6**, 1059-1073.

Swofford DL, Olsen GJ, Waddell PJ, Hillis DM (1996) Phylogenetic inference. In: *Molecular Systematics*, 2nd edn. (eds. Hillis D, Moritz C, Mable BK), pp. 407-514. Sinauer Associates, Massachusetts.

Tautz D (1993) Notes on the definition and nomenclature of tandemly repetitive DNA sequences. In: *DNA Fingerprinting: State of the Science* (eds. Pena SDJ, Chakraborty R, Epplen JT, Jeffreys AJ), pp. 21-28. Birkhäuser Verlag, Basel.

Tautz D, Renz M (1984) Simple sequences are ubiquitous repetitive components of eukaryotic genomes. *Nucleic Acids Research*, **12**, 4127-4138.

Taylor EB, McPhail JD, Schluter D (1997) History of ecological selection in sticklebacks: uniting experimental and phylogenetic approaches. In: *Molecular Evolution and Adaptive Radiation* (eds. Givnish TJ, Sytsma KJ), pp. 511-534. Cambridge University Press, Cambridge.

Templeton AR (1998) Nested clade analyses of phylogeographic data: testing hypotheses about gene flow and population history. *Molecular Ecology*, **7**, 318-398.

Thorpe JP (1982) The molecular clock hypothesis: biochemical evolution, genetic differentiation and systematics. *Annual Review in Ecology and Systematics*, **13**, 139-168.

Turner SJ, Lewis GD, Bellamy AR (1997) A genomic polymorphism located downstream of the *gcvP* gene of *Escherichia coli* that correlates with ecological niche. *Molecular Ecology*, **6**, 1019-1032.

Valentine JW, Ayala FJ (1974) Genetic variation in *Frieleia halli*, a deep-sea brachiopod. *Deep Sea Research*, **22**, 37-44.

Vos P, Hogers R, Bleeker M *et al.* (1995) AFLP: a new technique for DNA fingerprinting. *Nucleic Acids Research*, **23**, 4407-4414.

Vrijenhoek RC (1996) Conservation genetics of North American desert fishes. In: *Conservation Genetics: Case Histories from Nature* (eds. Avise JC, Hamrick JL), pp. 367-397. Chapman & Hall, London.

Waldmann P, Andersson S (1998) Comparison of quantitative genetic variation and allozyme diversity within and between populations of *Scabiosa canescens* and *S. columbaria*. *Heredity*, **81**, 79-86.

Ward RD, Skibinski DOF, Woodwark M (1992) Protein heterozygosity, protein structure and taxonomic differentiation. *Evolutionary Biology*, **26**, 73-160.

Weir BS (1996) Intraspecific differentiation. In: *Molecular Systematics*, 2nd edn. (eds. Hillis D, Moritz C, Mable BK), pp. 385-405. Sinauer Associates, Massachusetts.

Whitmore DH, Thai TH, Craft CM (1992) Gene amplification permits minimally invasive analysis of fish mitochondrial DNA. *Transactions of the American Fisheries Society*, **121**, 170-177.

Williams JGK, Hanafey MK, Rafalski JA, Tingey SV (1993) Genetic analysis using random amplified polymorphic DNA markers. *Methods in Enzymology*, **218**, 704-740.

Wilson AC, Cann RL, Carr SM *et al.* (1985) Mitochondrial DNA and two perspectives on evolutionary genetics. *Biological Journal of the Linnean Society*, **26**, 375-400.

Wirgin I, Maceda L, Stabile J, Mesing C (1997) An evaluation of introgression of Atlantic coast striped bass mitochondrial DNA in the Gulf of Mexico population using formaldehyde preserved museum collections. *Molecular Ecology*, **6**, 907-916.

Wolfe KH, Li W-H, Sharp PM (1987) Rates of nucleotide substitution vary greatly among plant mitochondrial, chloroplast and nuclear DNAs. *Proceedings of the National Academy of Sciences USA*, **84**, 9054-9058.

Woods T, Starman SA (1997) Evaluating genetic relationships of Geranium using arbitrary signatures from amplification profiles. *Hortscience*, **32**, 1288-1291.

Wright JM, Bentzen P (1994) Microsatellites: genetic markers for the future. *Reviews in Fish Biology and Fisheries*, **4**, 384-388.

Yang RC, Yeh FC, Yanchuk AD (1996) A comparison of isozyme and quantitative genetic variation in *Pinus contorta* ssp. *Latifolia* by Fst. *Genetics*, **142**, 1045-1046.

Advances in Molecular Ecology
G.R. Carvalho (Ed.)
IOS Press, 1998

Phylogenetic Analysis of Frequency Data in Molecular Ecological Studies

David M. Hillis
Department of Zoology and Institute of Cellular and Molecular Biology,
University of Texas, Austin, Texas 78712 USA, e-mail: hillis@phylo.zo.utexas.edu

The Generalised Parsimony method can be used to analyse virtually any kind of comparative data in a phylogenetic framework. Parsimony methods are highly adaptable, efficient at inferring evolutionary histories, and computationally tractable. However, methods for parsimony analyses of polymorphic population data (of the type often encountered in molecular ecological studies) are rarely utilized and remain poorly known. This chapter describes the rationale of the Generalized Parsimony approach as applied to polymorphic population data, and provides a practical guide to implementing the approach in the program PAUP (Phylogenetic Analysis Using Parsimony; written by David L. Swofford).

1. Introduction

Methods for phylogenetic analysis of molecular data have developed rapidly over the past decade, and several overviews have been published recently (*e.g.* Felsenstein, 1988; Hillis *et al.* 1993; Swofford *et al.* 1996). However, each of these reviews emphasizes methods for dealing with discrete character data, where individual taxa are coded as having discrete states rather than populations coded as having varying frequencies of a given allele. For instance, much of the molecular phylogenetics literature today concerns DNA or protein sequence data, where a single sequence is obtained from each specimen examined, and the operational taxonomic units in the analysis are the individual sequences. The phylogenetic tree then connects these sequences, which may represent genes, individuals, populations, species, or higher taxa. This type of analysis is clearly appropriate for the analysis of individual genes, and if the sequences are all orthologous, it is also appropriate for the analysis of individual organisms (Hillis 1994). At the other end of the hierarchy - relatively distantly related higher taxa - allelic differences within species are likely to be insignificant compared to the differences among species, and once again the analysis of single representative sequences to represent the taxa is appropriate. However, for the analysis of populations or closely related species, some alleles in population A are likely to be more closely related to some alleles in population B than to other alleles in population A. Thus, an analysis of the relationships among the populations can easily be confounded in an allele-by-allele analysis. In many studies in molecular ecology, the relevant data are not discrete differences among populations, but frequency differences in the allelic arrays (*e.g.* mini- or microsatellites or allozymes). Although many methods have been developed for analysing frequency data, many investigators seem unaware that these methods can be incorporated into modern phylogenetics packages to take advantage of recent developments in search algorithms. This chapter presents a description and discussion of an underutilized approach (developed by Swofford & Berlocher 1987; Berlocher & Swofford 1997) that has widespread utility for analysing frequency data from virtually any source.

2. Optimality criteria and search algorithms

There is a common confusion in the phylogenetics literature concerning methods of phylogenetic analysis. There are two distinct components to choosing among the many phylogenetic methods: (1) selecting an optimality criterion; and (2) selecting a search strategy to find optimal or near-optimal trees under the chosen optimality criterion. These distinctions are often blurred in the minds of users of standard software packages, so that one often reads statements such as "results were compared between parsimony and neighbour-joining analyses." This comparison is non-sensical, since parsimony is an optimality criterion, whereas neighbour-joining is a method for finding a point estimate of a tree (without optimising anything). It would be just as meaningful to say that "results were compared between parsimony and stepwise addition" (stepwise addition is another point estimation method that doesn't necessarily produce trees that are optimal under a given optimality criterion).

The first step in a phylogenetic analysis should be to select an optimality criterion. This specifies how we judge the degree to which the data fit a particular phylogenetic hypothesis. There are three commonly used optimality criteria in phylogenetics: parsimony, maximum likelihood, and minimum evolution. These criteria are discussed in detail in Swofford *et al.* (1996). Briefly, the three criteria are: (1) Parsimony: the best phylogenetic hypothesis is the one that minimizes the number of hypothesized evolutionary changes (or a weighted sum of the changes) among the taxa in a tree. (2) Maximum likelihood: the best solution is the tree with the highest log-likelihood score, under an explicit model of evolution. The log-likelihood score for a particular tree is calculated as the log of the probability of observing the data if the tree is true, given an explicit model of evolution. (The log of the probability is used because the probability for any particular set of data under a given hypothesis will be a very small number, so it is more convenient to consider the log of the value). Since the probability will always be less than one, the log likelihood will be a negative number, and the maximum likelihood tree is the tree with a log-likelihood score closest to zero. (3) Minimum evolution: first, observed differences are transformed into a pairwise distance matrix, which may involve a model of evolution to correct for superimposed changes (*e.g.* parallelisms, reversals, and convergences). To evaluate a given tree, the branch lengths on the tree are optimized so that the path-length distances (the distance from one taxon to another along the tree) are as close as possible to the distances in the pairwise distance matrix. After an optimal fit has been found for all the trees to be evaluated, the best tree is the one with the lowest sum of branch lengths. Thus, the minimum evolution criterion is similar to the parsimony criterion in that the optimal tree exhibits the least possible amount of change, but it differs from parsimony in that "change" is evaluated based on a pairwise distance matrix, which may be transformed from the original data according to some model of evolution.

The advantages of parsimony include great versatility (the method is applicable to virtually any comparative data set), high efficiency under a wide range of conditions (good estimates of the correct phylogeny are obtained with a relatively small amount of data), and computational tractability (thorough searches of the solution space are possible, so that optimal or near-optimal trees can be found in a reasonable amount of computation time). Each of the other methods also has advantages under certain conditions (see Hillis 1995, 1997), but the versatility, efficiency, and tractability of parsimony make it the most widely used method in phylogenetics (Sanderson *et al.* 1993). Appropriately, maximum likelihood methods are beginning to be used to a much greater extent with advancements in likelihood models as well as computer software and hardware (*e.g.* see Huelsenbeck & Crandall 1997; Lewis, 1998), but their use is still largely restricted to DNA and protein sequence data. Minimum evolution methods are often applied to population data, because there is a common misconception that parsimony methods are not applicable to populations that differ in the frequencies of the observed states. This chapter discusses the application of parsimony methods in this latter context.

Once an optimality criterion has been chosen, an investigator still needs to select a search strategy for finding the optimal (or a near-optimal) solution. Search strategies are discussed in detail in Swofford *et al.* (1996). For a quick, rough estimate of a near-optimal solution, one can use the stepwise addition or star decomposition algorithms (neighbour joining is a simplification of the latter). These rough estimates can almost always be improved by a process known as branch-swapping, in which trees that are topologically related to the initial tree are evaluated under the chosen optimality criterion. There are also exact algorithms that are guaranteed to find the optimal solution (*e.g.* exhaustive searching and the branch-and-bound algorithm), but these approaches are computationally limited to data sets involving relatively few taxa (generally about 20 or fewer for the branch-and-bound algorithm, and 12 or fewer for exhaustive searches). If a heuristic (non-exact) approach is used, it is important to specify the details of the search so that other investigators can assess the thoroughness of the analysis, replicate the study, and possibly extend the search for better solutions.

3. Selecting an appropriate distance measure

Many different genetic distance measures have been developed for assessing the genetic divergence between two populations that differ in the frequencies of observed alleles (see Wright 1978 for a review). One of the most commonly used genetic distances was proposed by Nei (1972, 1978), but this distance measure has a number of features that make it unsuitable for phylogenetic analysis. If x_i and y_i are the frequencies of the ith allele at a particular locus in taxa X and Y, respectively, then Nei's distance is defined by:

$$D_N = -\ln\left(J_{XY} / \sqrt{J_X J_Y}\right)$$

where J_X, J_Y, and J_{XY} are the arithmetic means across loci of Σx_i^2, Σy_i^2, and $\Sigma x_i y_i$. Among the limitations of Nei's distance is the assumption that the rate of gene substitution is uniform across loci and populations. This assumption probably never holds for real data. A consequence of violation of this assumption is that Nei's distance can vary widely depending on the extent of shared and unshared polymorphisms across taxa; in other words, two pairs of taxa that differ by the same number of loci can have very different Nei's genetic distances (Hillis 1984; Tomiuk & Graur 1988; Frost & Hillis 1990). This particular problem can be overcome by calculating Nei's identity for each locus, and then averaging across loci:

$$D_N^* = -\ln\left[\frac{\sum_L \left(\sum x_i y_i / \sqrt{\sum x_i^2 \sum y_i^2}\right)}{L}\right]$$

where L is the total number of loci (Hillis 1984). However, both the modified and original versions of Nei's distance measure produce distance matrices that violate the triangle inequality (Farris 1981; Hillis 1984), which makes it unsuitable for use with the step-matrix approach described below. Violation of the triangle inequality simply means that the greatest genetic distance between any two of three given populations exceeds the sum of the distances between the other two pairs. If the distance from A to B is 1.5, and the distance from A to C or from C to B is 0.5, then in a parsimony analysis where the total length is being minimized, a transformation directly from A to B will never be reconstructed (because it is shorter to go from A to C to B).

Rogers (1972) proposed using a scaled Euclidean distance between allelic arrays of the populations being compared:

$$D_R = \frac{1}{L} \sum_L \sqrt{\sum (x_i - y_i)^2 / 2}$$

However, a Euclidean distance is not necessarily appropriate for measuring change in frequencies between populations if some of the hypothetical space between the allelic arrays cannot exist in real populations. As an analogy, imagine a resident of a large city, such as Manhattan, who lives at point A in Fig. 1. He wishes to walk to the nearest restaurant; his choices are located at points B and C in Fig. 1. If he evaluates the closest restaurant by measuring the straight-line (Euclidean) distances to B and C from A, he would choose restaurant B, which is five blocks away in Euclidean space. However, the resident cannot walk through Euclidean space, because the blocks between the streets are occupied by tall buildings. Instead, he must stick to the streets, and walk down four blocks and across three, for a total "Manhattan distance" of seven blocks. To reach restaurant C, however, requires a walk of only six blocks. Thus, the relevant measure for the resident is the Manhattan distance, not the Euclidean distance, to the two restaurants from his residence. In a similar manner, the evolutionary distance between two populations can be thought of in terms of the amount of change that is necessary in real allelic space to change the allelic frequencies of one population into another.

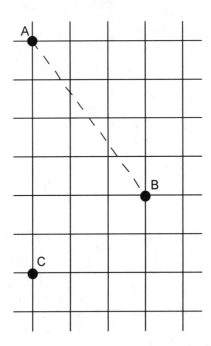

Figure 1: A hypothetical map of Manhattan. The Euclidean distance from residence A to restaurant B is only five city blocks, but the walking (or Manhattan) distance is seven blocks. In contrast, the Euclidean distance from residence A to restaurant C is six blocks (greater than from A to B), but the walking (Manhattan) distance also six blocks (shorter than from A to B).

The Manhattan (or Prevosti) distance is simple to calculate for allelic data. For a single locus, it is calculated by:

$$D_M = \frac{1}{2} \sum |x_i - y_i|$$

(Wright 1978). If a single measure is desired across loci, then the arithmetic average is used. However, for the method considered here, we will treat each locus separately, so the Manhattan distance is calculated between each population at each locus. The Manhattan distance uniformly weights any equivalent change in allelic frequency, so that a change from a frequency of 0.2 to 0.3 receives a weight equal to a change in frequency from 0.6 to 0.7, for instance. Thus the triangle inequality is never violated, and the distance between taxa is dependent only on the degree of divergence, not on the degree of shared or unshared polymorphism. A distance of 1.0 between two populations indicates they share no alleles at that locus, whereas two populations with identical allelic arrays differ by a Manhattan distance of 0.

4. The step matrix

A step matrix describes the relationship among states observed across taxa. For instance, consider the discrete states shown in Fig. 2. Discrete states may be arranged in an ordered transformation series (Fig. 2a), and unordered series (Fig. 2b), a partially ordered series (Fig.2c), or a weighted series (Fig. 2d). In the ordered series shown in Fig. 2a, state "b" isone change way from either state "a" or state "c", but states "a" and "c" are two changes away from each other. We would consider a character to be of this type if it was logically not possible to change from state "a" to state "c" without going through state "b". In

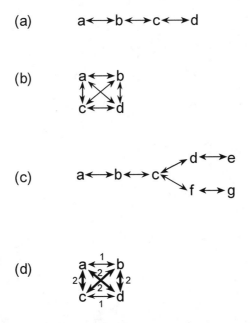

Figure 2: Ordered (a), unordered (b), partially ordered (c), and weighted (d) transformation series of character states.

contrast, in the unordered transformation series shown in Fig. 2b, each state is only one change away from every other state. Transformation series can also be partially ordered; state "c" in Fig. 2c is one change away from states "b", "d", and "f", but two changes away from states "a", "e", and "g". Changes from one state to another can also be weighted so that multiple-step changes do not necessarily go through another observed state, as in Fig. 2d. This latter option is commonly used with DNA sequence data; for instance, transversions between a purine and a pyrimidine are often weighted more heavily than transitions between two purines or two pyrimidines.

The relationships among character states can be expressed in terms of a step matrix (or cost matrix) that summarizes the "cost" of a change from each character state to every other character state (Sankoff 1975; Sankoff & Cedergren 1983; Maddison & Maddison 1992; Swofford *et al.* 1996). For the examples shown in Fig. 2, the step matrices are shown in Fig. 3. This method of generalized parsimony makes parsimony methods applicable to a very wide set of data types and evolutionary conditions.

(a)

	a	b	c	d
a	-	1	2	3
b	1	-	1	2
c	2	1	-	1
d	3	2	1	-

(b)

	a	b	c	d
a	-	1	1	1
b	1	-	1	1
c	1	1	-	1
d	1	1	1	-

(c)

	a	b	c	d	e	f	g
a	-	1	2	3	4	3	4
b	1	-	1	2	3	2	3
c	2	1	-	1	2	1	2
d	3	2	1	-	1	2	3
e	4	3	2	1	-	3	4
f	3	2	1	2	3	-	1
g	4	3	2	3	4	1	-

(d)

	a	b	c	d
a	-	1	2	2
b	1	-	2	2
c	2	2	-	1
d	2	2	1	-

Figure 3: Step (or cost) matrices for the transformation series shown in Fig. 2.

5. Step matrices with frequency data

Swofford and Berlocher (1987) described a parsimony method for use with polymorphic data, in which total change is minimized across a tree. Change was evaluated on a locus-by-locus basis using Manhattan distances (Fig. 4). Swofford and Berlocher described a program, FREQPARS, that implemented the method, but searching algorithms associated with the program were limited. They also described two different optimality criteria for frequency parsimony: the MANAD criterion (*Man*hattan distance, *ad*ditivity requirement), in which the ancestral allelic arrays were constrained only to any possible combination of

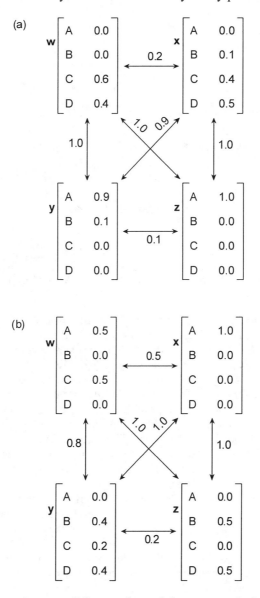

Figure 4: Transformation series among allelic arrays for populations w, x, y, and z for two different loci (a and b). The distance between each array is the Manhattan distance.

(a)

	w	x	y	z
w	-	20	100	100
x	20	-	90	100
y	100	90	-	10
z	100	100	10	-

(b)

	w	x	y	z
w	-	50	80	100
x	50	-	100	100
y	80	100	-	20
z	100	100	20	-

Figure 5: The step matrices for the two loci shown in Fig. 4. The Manhattan distances have been multiplied by a factor of 100 to produce integer values for the matrices (a requirement for step matrices in PAUP). The length of the final trees can be translated back into Manhattan distance by dividing by this same scaling factor.

observed alleles; and the MANOB criterion (*Man*hattan distance, *ob*served allele frequency arrays), in which the ancestral allelic arrays were restricted to the set of arrays observed in the terminal taxa. Although Swofford and Berlocher (1987) recommended the MANAD criterion, they noted that "...the MANOB optimization could be useful as a method for approximating a solution under the MANAD criterion if a more efficient algorithm...could be found." Berlocher and Swofford (1997) showed that generalized parsimony with step matrices (also called Sankoff optimization) could be used to implement the MANOB criterion, and that MANOB trees found in this manner were usually the same trees (or very similar) to those found under the MANAD criterion. The same procedure has been independently implemented by others as well (*e.g.* Wiens 1995), although the connection of the method to Swofford and Berlocher's (1987) MANOB criterion was not clarified until Berlocher and Swofford's (1997) paper.

The basic method involves first calculating a Manhattan distance for each locus between each population, as in Fig. 4. The allelic arrays for each population are treated as character states, and the relationships among the states are described by the Manhattan distances. These relationships can next be coded in a step matrix, as in Fig. 5. In some programs that implement step matrices, such as PAUP (Phylogenetic Analysis Using Parsimony, David L. Swofford, Smithsonian Institution), step matrices must be composed of integers. Manhattan distances can be converted to integers by multiplying by a constant, such as 100, without affecting the results (the final tree and branch lengths can simply be divided by the same constant to return the values back into Manhattan distances).

6. An example using PAUP

Frequency parsimony is easily implemented in PAUP using the generalized parsimony (step matrix) approach. For the four hypothetical populations (**w, x, y** and **z**) and two loci shown in Fig. 4, the input file for PAUP is shown in Fig. 6.

In the input file, note that the character matrix consists of columns of characters in which each different allelic array is assigned a unique state. The relationship among these states is then defined in the assumptions block of the input file, where the matrix for each locus describes the Manhattan distance from each array to every other (in this case multiplied by a constant of 100). The typeset command then assigns the appropriate character types to each of the individual loci; by selecting the character typeset "Manhattan", the character-states are all assigned the appropriate relationships for each locus. The thorough and fast search algorithms of PAUP can then be used in an efficient search for the optimal trees under Swofford and Berlocher's (1987) MANOB criterion. The input file shown in Fig. 6 results in the tree shown in Fig. 7, with branch lengths indicated in Manhattan distance units.

```
#NEXUS

begin data;
     dimensions ntax=4 nchar=2;
     format symbols="1~4";
     matrix

     taxon_w       11
     taxon_x       22
     taxon_y       33
     taxon_z       44

     ;
end;

begin assumptions;
     usertype locus_a = 4
               1     2     3     4
     [1]    .     20   100   100
     [2]    20    .     90   100
     [3]   100    90    .     10
     [4]   100   100    10    .
     ;

     usertype locus_b = 4
               1     2     3     4
     [1]    .     50    80   100
     [2]    50    .    100   100
     [3]    80   100    .     20
     [4]   100   100    20    .
     ;

     typeset Manhattan = locus_a: 1, locus_b: 2;
end;
```

Figure 6: A PAUP input file for conducting a frequency parsimony analysis for the four populations and two loci shown in Fig. 4.

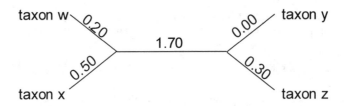

Figure 7: The frequency parsimony tree (with branch lengths shown in Manhattan distances) for the data shown in Fig. 4.

7. Extensions to ecological and behavioural characters

In molecular ecological studies, one often wishes to compare molecular data to ecological or behavioural data. The step matrix approach is highly adaptable to such analyses, and with minor modifications even complex data may be coded using step matrices. For example, Cannatella *et al.* (1998) recently compared data sets from two mitochondrial genes (12S rRNA and cytochrome oxidase I), 26 allozyme loci, morphology, and advertisement calls from a group of frogs in the *Physalaemus pustulosus* species group. They used step matrices to encode both the allozyme data as well as the behavioural (call) data, and conducted parsimony analyses separately and in combination for all of the data sets. One of the questions Cannatella *et al.* (1998) addressed was the degree to which behavioural characters that are involved in mate recognition are reliable indicators of evolutionary relationships. If closely related species undergo strong selection for the divergence of characters involved in mate recognition, then such character complexes may be misleading about evolutionary relationships. However, other investigators have argued that there is no reason to expect behavioural characters to be poor indicators of phylogenetic relationships (see review by Ryan 1996). With frog advertisement calls, there are clear similarities among some lineages of frogs, but most closely related species diverge rapidly (Cocroft and Ryan 1995). Therefore, calls may be least useful for inferring relationships within closely related groups of frogs, even though higher-level groupings may be supported by call data.

The call data analysed by Cannatella *et al.* consist of a series of quantitative measurements of various call parameters, such as the duration of the call and the frequency at the onset of the call. Five of the twelve call variables that they analysed are shown in Table 1. To code these data for comparison to morphological and molecular data, Cannatella *et al.* modified an approach originally developed by Maddison and Slatkin (1990). Each character was scaled to a range of 0 to 25, represented by the letters a through z, respectively. The species mean for each character was then assigned a letter for its character state, according to where the state scaled along the range from a to z. Step matrices were then used to represent the relationships among the character states. For example, imagine a quantitative variable measured in several species (length of a call pulse, for instance), which varied from 22 msec in the species with the shortest call pulse to 178 msec in the species with the longest call pulse. The state "22 msec" would be assigned state a, and "178 msec" would be assigned state z. Likewise, a species whose pulse was 35 msec would be assigned state e, because 35 falls in the fifth bin in a 26-bin scale from 22 to 178. Step matrices are then used to define the relationships among the states. If characters scaled in this manner are included in an analysis with characters scaled differently (nucleotides,

Table 1: Summary of some call statistics for the *Physalaemus pustulosus* group and close relatives, from Cannatella *et al.* (1998). The variables shown are total duration of call (TLDUR, msec), frequency at onset of call (INHZ, Hz), maximum frequency (MXHZ, Hz), time to the maximum frequency (TMMX, msec), and time to mid-frequency (TMHFHZ, msec). The mean is given with the range below. The letter in parentheses following the mean is the character-state code as used in the step matrices. The complete table of call variables is presented in Cannatella *et al.* (1998).

Species	n	TLDUR	INHZ	MXHZ	TMMX	TMHFHZ
sp. A	10	339 (j)	812 (d)	876 (a)	65 (k)	160 (j)
		234-447	800-840	800-920	43-100	150-187
ephippifer	10	266 (g)	900 (h)	944 (e)	62 (j)	140 (i)
		238-308	840-1000	840-1040	43-81	112-162
enesefae	10	747 (z)	944 (j)	976 (g)	162 (z)	386 (z)
		631-903	880-1040	920-1040	81-287	300-456
pustulosus	10	370 (k)	884 (h)	884 (a)	0 (a)	124 (h)
		252-496	840-960	840-960	0-0	87-175
petersi	10	246 (f)	1220 (x)	1220 (w)	0 (a)	28 (b)
		206-350	1040-1400	1040-1400	0-0	18-50
freibergi	10	104 (a)	1253 (z)	1253 (z)	0 (a)	12 (a)
		48.2-140.8	1000-1424	1000-1424	0-0	6-25
coloradorum	9	221 (e)	1031 (o)	1071 (m)	25 (d)	83 (e)
		152-358	960-1080	1000-1160	0-62	50-100
pustulatus	10	206 (d)	964 (k)	964 (f)	0 (a)	88 (f)
		186-230	880-1080	880-1080	0-0	56-118
sp. B	10	395 (l)	740 (a)	888 (a)	112 (r)	115 (g)
		322-608	680-880	840-960	43-150	81-162

for instance), then all the characters can be weighted equally by weighting each character to unity.

For the character states shown in Table 1, the step matrices that represent the scaled relationships among these states are shown in Fig. 8. (Note that only a portion of the original data are shown here; the complete data matrix of DNA sequences, allozymes, morphological data, and call data, including all the step matrices and weights, can be downloaded from http://www.utexas.edu/ftp/depts/systbiol/47_2/physalaemus.nexus).

Are the call data consistent with the overall estimate of phylogeny for the group? The data from DNA sequences, allozymes, and morphology strongly support the phylogeny shown on the left side of Fig. 9, whereas the call data provide weak support for the phylogeny shown on the right side of Fig. 9. There is only one grouping in common between the two analyses (*P. petersi* plus *P. freibergi*). The relatively close apparent relationship among the calls of some relatively distantly related species, as well as the rapid divergence of the calls of some closely related species, provides support for the idea that mate-recognition signals may diverge quickly between sister-species and thus obscure information about evolutionary relationships.

```
USERTYPE Duration STEPMATRIX= 9
            a   d   e   f   g   j   k   l   z
      [a]   .   3   4   5   6   9  10  11  25
      [d]   3   .   1   2   3   6   7   8  22
      [e]   4   1   .   1   2   5   6   7  21
      [f]   5   2   1   .   1   4   5   6  20
      [g]   6   3   2   1   .   3   4   5  19
      [j]   9   6   5   4   3   .   1   2  16
      [k]  10   7   6   5   4   1   .   1  15
      [l]  11   8   7   6   5   2   1   .  14
      [z]  25  22  21  20  19  16  15  14   .
      ;

USERTYPE FreqOnset STEPMATRIX= 8
            a   d   h   j   k   o   x   z
      [a]   .   3   7   9  10  14  23  25
      [d]   3   .   4   6   7  11  20  22
      [h]   7   4   .   2   3   7  16  18
      [j]   9   6   2   .   1   5  14  16
      [k]  10   7   3   1   .   4  13  15
      [o]  14  11   7   5   4   .   9  11
      [x]  23  20  16  14  13   9   .   2
      [z]  25  22  18  16  15  11   2   .
      ;

USERTYPE MaxFreq STEPMATRIX= 7
            a   e   f   g   m   w   z
      [a]   .   4   5   6  12  22  25
      [e]   4   .   1   2   8  18  21
      [f]   5   1   .   1   7  17  20
      [g]   6   2   1   .   6  16  19
      [m]  12   8   7   6   .  10  13
      [w]  22  18  17  16  10   .   3
      [z]  25  21  20  19  13   3   .
      ;

USERTYPE TimetoMax STEPMATRIX= 6
            a   d   j   k   r   z
      [a]   .   3   9  10  17  25
      [d]   3   .   6   7  14  22
      [j]   9   6   .   1   8  16
      [k]  10   7   1   .   7  15
      [r]  17  14   8   7   .   8
      [z]  25  22  16  15   8   .
      ;

USERTYPE TimetoMid STEPMATRIX= 9
            a   b   e   f   g   h   i   j   z
      [a]   .   1   4   5   6   7   8   9  25
      [b]   1   .   3   4   5   6   7   8  24
      [e]   4   3   .   1   2   3   4   5  21
      [f]   5   4   1   .   1   2   3   4  20
      [g]   6   5   2   1   .   1   2   3  19
      [h]   7   6   3   2   1   .   1   2  18
      [i]   8   7   4   3   2   1   .   1  17
      [j]   9   8   5   4   3   2   1   .  16
      [z]  25  24  21  20  19  18  17  16   .
      ;
```

Figure 8: Step matrices for the five characters shown in Table 1, in NEXUS format. The complete data matrix (including character states and step matrices for the DNA, allozymes, morphology, and call data sets) can be seen and downloaded from
http://www.utexas.edu/ftp/depts/systbiol/47_2/physalaemus.nexus.

DNA, allozymes, morphology   **Call data**

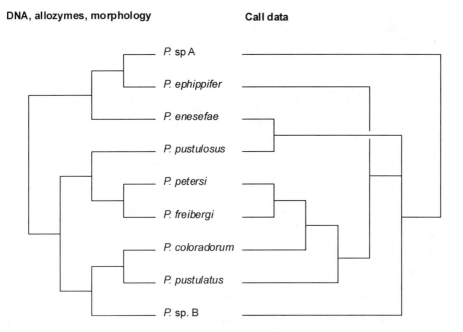

Figure 9: Phylogenetic estimates based on DNA (12S rRNA and cytochrome oxidase I genes), allozymes, and morphology (left) and call data (right). Only one group supported by the morphological and molecular data is also supported by the call data. Based on data in Cannatella *et al.* 1998.

8. Conclusions

Generalized parsimony is an efficient and highly adaptable approach to phylogenetic analysis. The parsimony criterion is easily applied to virtually any comparative data set, and is a computationally tractable and efficient method for estimating phylogenetic history (Hillis *et al.* 1994; Hillis 1996). The use of Manhattan distances to describe relationships among allelic arrays and step matrices to incorporate these relationships into a parsimony analysis provides a straightforward and efficient means of analysing polymorphic population data. The approach is easily adapted to ecological and behavioural character sets, so that phylogenetic comparisons can be drawn among molecular, morphological, ecological, and behavioural data.

References

Berlocher SH, Swofford DL (1997) Searching for phylogenetic trees under the frequency parsimony criterion: An approximation using generalized parsimony. *Systematic Biology*, **46**, 211–215.

Cannatella DC, Hillis DM, Chippindale PT, Weigt L, Rand AS, Ryan MJ (1998) Phylogeny of frogs of the *Physalaemus pustulosus* species group, with an examination of data incongruence. *Systematic Biology*, **47**, 311–335.

Cocroft RB, Ryan MJ (1995) Patterns of advertisement call evolution in toads and chorus frogs. *Animal Behaviour*, **49**, 283–303.

Farris JS (1981) Distance data in phylogenetic analysis. In: *Advances in Cladistics: Proceedings of the First Meeting of the Willi Hennig Society*, (eds. Funk VA, Brooks DR) pp. 3–23. New York Botanical Garden, Bronx.

Felsenstein J (1988) Phylogenies from molecular sequences: inference and reliability. *Annual Review of Genetics*, **22**, 521–565.

Frost DR, Hillis DM (1990) Species in concept and practice: herpetological applications. *Herpetologica*, **46**, 87–104.

Hillis DM (1984) Misuse and modification of Nei's genetic distance. *Systematic Zoology*, **33**, 238–240.

Hillis DM (1994) Homology in molecular biology. In: *Homology: The Hierarchical Basis of Comparative Biology*, (ed. Hall BK) pp. 339–367. Academic Press, New York.

Hillis DM (1995) Approaches for assessing phylogenetic accuracy. *Systematic Biology*, **44**, 3–16.

Hillis DM (1996) Inferring complex phylogenies. *Nature*, **383**, 130-131.

Hillis DM (1997) Primer: phylogenetic analysis. *Current Biology*, 7, 129–131.

Hillis DM, Allard MW, Miyamoto MM (1993) Analysis of DNA sequence data: phylogenetic inference. *Methods in Enzymology*, **242**, 456–487.

Hillis DM, Huelsenbeck JP, Cunningham CW (1994) Application and accuracy of molecular phylogenies. *Science*, **264**, 671-677.

Huelsenbeck JP, Crandall KA (1997) Phylogeny estimation and hypothesis testing using maximum likelihood. *Annual Review of Ecology and Systematics* 28, 437–466.

Lewis PO (1998) A genetic algorithm for maximum-likelihood phylogeny inference using nucleotide sequence data. *Molecular Biology and Evolution*, **15**, 277–283.

Maddison WP, Maddison DR (1992) *MacClade: Analysis of Phylogeny and Character Evolution*, version 3.0. Sinauer Associates, Sunderland, Massachusetts.

Maddison WP, Slatkin M (1990) Parsimony reconstructions of ancestral states do not depend on the relative distances between linearly-ordered character states. *Systematic Zoology*, **39**, 175–178.

Nei M (1972) Genetic distance between populations. *The American Naturalist*, **106**, 283–292.

Nei M (1978) Estimation of average heterozygosity and genetic distance from a small number of individuals. *Genetics*, **89**, 583–590.

Rogers JS (1972) Measures of genetic similarity and genetic distance. *Studies in Genetics, VII, University of Texas Publications*, **7213**, 145-143.

Ryan MJ (1996) Phylogenetics in behavior: some cautions and expectations. In: *Phylogenies and the Comparative Method in Animal Behavior*, (ed. Martins EP), pp. 1–21. Oxford University Press, New York.

Sanderson MJ, Baldwin BG, Bharathan G, *et al.* (1993) The growth of phylogenetic information and the need for a phylogenetic data base. *Systematic Biology*, **42**, 562–568.

Sankoff D (1975) Minimal mutation trees of sequences. *Journal of Applied Mathematics*, **28**, 35–42.

Sankoff D, Cedergren RJ (1983) Simultaneous comparison of three or more sequences related by a tree. In: *Time Warps, String Edits, and Macromolecules: The Theory and Practice of Sequence Comparison*, (eds. Sankoff D, Kruskal JB) pp. 253–263. Addison-Wesley, Reading, Massachusetts.

Swofford DL, Berlocher SH (1987) Inferring evolutionary trees from gene frequency data under the principle of maximum parsimony. *Systematic Zoology*, **36**, 293–325.

Swofford DL, Olsen GJ, Waddell PJ, Hillis DM (1996) Phylogenetic inference. In: *Molecular Systematics 2nd ed.*, (eds. Hillis DM, Mable BK, Moritz C), pp. 407–514. Sinauer Associates, Sunderland, Massachusetts.

Tomiuk J, Graur D (1988) Nei's modified genetic identity and distance measures and their sampling variances. *Systematic Zoology*, **37**, 156–162.

Wiens JJ (1995) Polymorphic characters in phylogenetic systematics. *Systematic Biology*, **44**, 482–500.

Wright S (1978) *Evolution and the Genetics Of Populations*. University of Chicago Press, Chicago.

Advances in Molecular Ecology
G.R. Carvalho (Ed.)
IOS Press, 1998

Estimation of Migration Rates and Population Sizes in Geographically Structured Populations

Peter Beerli

Department of Genetics, University of Washington, Seattle WA 98195-7360, USA,
e-mail: beerli@genetics.washington.edu

The estimation of population parameters from genetic data can help reveal past migration patterns or past population sizes. The transformation of raw genetic data into population parameters requires a model which should reflect the true relationships between subpopulations. Often the models are overly simplified and do not allow, for example, for differences in population sizes and migration rates. I stress here the point that it is important to consider possible asymmetries in migration rates and differences in population sizes. Very recently, several estimators based on the direct use of allele frequencies and based on coalescence theory have been developed. All these outperform migration rate estimators based on F_{ST}.

1. Introduction

The estimation of population parameters such as population size and migration rates between subpopulations of a species is crucial for many ecological studies. Two very different approaches to estimating population parameters are in use: (1) direct methods using direct observations or radio-telemetry data of migrating individuals, and (2) indirect methods using genetic data from samples of individuals in several subpopulations for the inference of migration rates. Direct methods can help to determine the migration pattern of individuals during the study, and can deliver information about very recent history. Under the assumption that the few tracked individuals are picked at random and that their movements are not artefacts of the study, these data can give interesting insights into the migration pattern of a specific population. Limits are also evident, however: small migration rates are undetectable, and the accuracy of the parameter estimates is small when the study is based only on a few individuals. If the study is too short and not repeated we cannot ascertain whether the migration pattern observed was accidental or is general. Current progress in establishing the relationship between individuals using DNA fingerprinting may help to generate accurate information about very recent migration patterns. Using these methods, it is simple to increase the number of individuals studied and to make estimates that are less dependent on the length of the study, because one uses the shared genetic history of parents and offspring. In the future DNA fingerprinting will certainly provide a valuable tool for the detection of very recent migration pattern between small populations Bossart & Prowell 1998).

I will concentrate here on indirect methods that also are based on genetic history. They do not assume that we can find parent-offspring pairs, but instead use probability-based models. The array of possible markers is large and can include allozymes, restriction fragment length polymorphisms, microsatellites, or protein or DNA sequences. These genetic data provide the basis for our inferences on migration patterns. This chapter focuses on models for discrete populations and their assumptions. Interested readers may find more information about the influence of different data types on the parameter estimation in Neigel (1997).

For some methods considered here, we first estimate certain meta-quantities from which we then infer population parameters, such as population sizes and migration rates. These methods all have some advantages compared to the direct approach. One can investigate large sample sizes or many loci and therefore detect small amounts of migration. There is no need to track individuals over time; the estimates are averages over evolutionary time and reveal general, rather than individual, migration patterns. We can use the indirect methods for any organism. There are also disadvantages. We need to assume that the markers are selectively neutral, so that similarity between different subpopulations is a result of migration rather than similar selection pressures. The population parameters are also confounded with the mutation rate. The markers need to show enough variability, so that we can see differences between subpopulations. A marker with a very slow mutation rate will not reveal recent migration events, but may still have some information about migration events far in the past, when compared with geographically more distant populations.

Several groups of approaches using genetic data for the inference of migration rates are recognized: (1) estimators based on allele frequencies and Wright's (1951) F-statistic (reviewed in Michalakis & Excoffier 1996); (2) maximum likelihood estimators based on allele frequencies (Rannala & Hartigan 1996; Tufto *et al.* 1996); and (3) estimators based on genealogies of the sampled individuals (coalescent theory: Kingman 1982b) with migration rates estimated using procedures of Wakeley (1998), Bahlo & Griffiths (1998), or Beerli & Felsenstein (1998). Some estimators are mixtures of these groups. Slatkin & Maddison (1989), for example, developed a method that uses results from coalescent theory and then presents an interpolation table produced by simulating the coalescence with migration, in which the minimal number of migration events found on the best genealogy is related to a migration rate, $4N_em$. Most of these estimators were developed under simplifying assumptions; for example all current "all-purpose" migration rate estimators assume that the population is in migration-mutation equilibrium; in other words they assume that the migration and the mutation rates are constant through time. Additionally, almost all methods assume constant population sizes. There is currently one method, developed by Bahlo & Griffiths (1998), that can allow for subpopulations that are growing. The availability of methods for estimating population parameters under non-equilibrium condition will increase, but development of programs and new methods is often a slow task. Additionally, the more parameters we want to estimate, the more data we need; this makes it perhaps impractical to allow for all possibilities. Methods allowing for non-equilibrium conditions have first to be fully developed and then have to show that they can deliver accurate estimates.

Most migration models are based on the Wright-Fisher population. The Wright-Fisher population model with migration is rather simple (Fig. 1) and has properties that makes its mathematical treatment easy. A subpopulation consists of a constant number of individuals, either haploid or diploid, and here I will describe the diploid case. In each generation each individual produces a large number of gametes. These gametes either stay in a subpopulation or migrate into another subpopulation. New individuals are formed by randomly choosing two gametes in a subpopulation, and these individuals replace their parents.

Subpopulation 1   Subpopulation 2

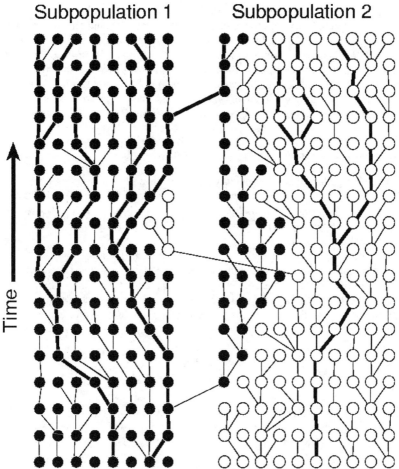

Figure 1: Gene genealogy of a Wright-Fisher population with migration between two subpopulations. Thick lines show the coalescence of lineages from a sample of 4 individuals in each population.

I will focus on some of these estimators and discuss their properties and limitations when subpopulations may exchange migrants at different rates or have different sizes, and in which the mutation rate may vary among loci. Additionally, I will develop an F-statistic framework introduced by Maynard Smith (1970), Maruyama (1970), and Nei & Feldman (1972), so that population sizes and migration rates can be estimated jointly. Finally, I will compare these F_{ST}-based approaches with an approach based on the coalescence theory.

2. How to compare different population parameter estimators

Choosing a method for the estimation of population parameters is a difficult task because many methods are available (see the almost certainly incomplete list of available programs in this book). Each of these different methods has its own set of assumptions; sometimes these are incompatible with the study. Results obtained with real data provide rather unreliable guidance for picking a method, because we normally do not know the underlying true parameter values. With computer generated data sets, however, it is easy to create many replicates with the same population model and the same population parameters. For these arbitrary data generating parameters I will use terms like the "true value" or the "truth". The chosen population parameters should then be recovered from each data set with some error from randomness in the data generation (Hudson 1983) and errors in the analysis. The averages of the parameter estimates from many data sets should converge to the true values when we increase the number of replicates and if the method is unbiased (does not, for example, always yield estimates that are too high). Additionally, a good method should have a small variance and therefore produce small confidence intervals. In short, superior methods have no or little bias and a small variance.

3. Migration rate estimators based on F-statistics

Wright (1951) described a framework that uses his earlier inbreeding coefficient F for a subdivided population with three coefficients: F_{IS}, F_{IT}, and F_{ST}. For the infinite allele model F can be understood as a probability that two randomly chosen alleles are identical by descent, and the F-values are ratios between the F in an individual I, a subpopulation S, and all subpopulations T (Total).

I will focus on F_{ST}, which is the correlation between the probability that two randomly chosen gene copies within a subpopulation share an ancestor in the last generation relative to the probability that two gene copies picked from the total population share an ancestor in the last generation. In other words, this index uses the partitioning of total genetic variability into variability within and between subpopulations. Using insights from Slatkin (1991) and from Michalakis & Excoffier (1996), a highly generalized overview for the relationship of F_{ST} is:

$$F_{ST} = \frac{g(\sigma_W) - g(\sigma_B)}{g(\sigma_B)} \tag{1}$$

where F_{ST} can be replaced by different specific estimators such as θ (Weir 1996), N_{ST} (Lynch & Crease 1990), $<F_{ST}>$ (Hudson et al. 1992), Φ_{ST} (Excoffier & Smouse 1994), ρ_{ST} (Rousset 1996), G_{ST} (Nei 1973), and R_{ST} (Slatkin 1993). The g(x) are correction functions used for the different F_{ST}-estimators scaling the variance within a population (σ_W) or between populations (σ_B). These variances are proportional to the mean coalescence times in a subpopulation and the whole population. This summary statistic, F_{ST}, is interpreted as a measure of the differentiation between subpopulations, where values close to zero indicate that the population is not structured.

F_{ST} is commonly transformed into a more direct measure for migration. Wright (1951) showed that for an n-island population model (Fig. 2) with an infinite number of subpopulations and no mutation, we can use:

$$F_{ST} = \frac{1}{1 + 4N_e m} \tag{2}$$

where N_e is the population size of a Wright-Fisher population (Fig. 1), and m is the migration rate per generation. I use the term effective population size N_e to mark the fact that even when the population is not exactly behaving like a Wright-Fisher population, we still can use N_e to make comparisons with other populations. Relaxing the rather strong assumption of having an infinite number of subpopulations is simple and has been described several times, for example by Li (1976):

$$F_{ST} = \frac{1}{1 + 4N_e m \dfrac{d^2}{(d-1)^2}}$$

(3)

where d is the total number of subpopulations, which is almost certainly different from the number of populations sampled. Charlesworth (1998) pointed out that results for $N_e m$ can be very different depending on which version of F_{ST} is used.

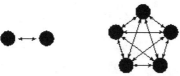

Figure 2: Island population model. Examples with 2 and 5 islands. The relevant population parameters are an overall population size N_e and an immigration rate m that is the same for all subpopulations.

The n-island population model uses only two parameters: the effective population size N_e and the immigration rate per generation m. It is assumed that the subpopulation sizes are the same and that the migration rate is the same between all the subpopulations. These assumptions are often violated in studies of natural populations, for which we know neither the true migration patterns nor the population sizes.

I created simulated data sets using a technique first used by Hudson (1983). One hundred different data sets containing sequence data (500 bp) for 20 individuals in each of 2 subpopulations were created using specific population sizes Θ_1 and Θ_2, and migration rates M_1 and M_2, where Θ is $4N_e \mu \mu$ (Fig. 3). From these data sets $\gamma (\gamma = 4N_e m = \Theta M)$, was estimated using Wright's formula (Equ. 2, 3) with $<F_{ST}>$ (Hudson *et al.* 1992). For this simple two-population situation the estimates for γ are appropriate if subpopulation sizes are the same and migration rates are symmetric; as soon as the assumptions of symmetry of migration rates, or of equal population sizes, is violated, however, the estimates are wrong (Table 1). Relethford (1996) revealed similar problems with approaches that assume that population sizes are equal and develops an alternative approach, that allows for different sizes but not different migration rates, so that $m_{ij} = m_{ji}$. Laurent Excoffier (personal communication 1998) and coworkers have done extensive simulations with different population sizes and have shown that the assumption of equal population sizes is critical to the analysis.

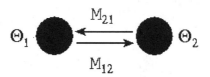

Figure 3: Two population model: Θ_1 is $4N_e^{(1)} \mu$, Θ_2 is $4N_e^{(2)} \mu$, M_{21} is m_{21}/μ, and M_{12} is m_{12}/μ, where N_e is the effective population size, μ is the mutation rate per generation, and m_{ji} is the migration rate per generation from population j to population i.

Table 1: Estimates of migration rates $\gamma = 4N_e m$ based on Wright's formula (Equ. 2, 3) in a two population system (Fig. 3). Averages ± standard deviations of 100 simulated data sets generated with the same population parameters are shown. For each data set 2 populations with 20 sampled individuals with 500bp of sequence data were created according to Hudson (1983). T: the parameter values under which the data sets were created, A: Wright's relation of F_{ST} and migration rate γ without correction for finite and known number of subpopulations (Equ. 2), B: Wright's relation with the correction for two populations (Equ. 3).

	Population 1		Population 2	
	Θ	γ	Θ	γ
T	0.01	1.00	0.01	1.00
A	-	4.56 ± 3.08	-	4.56 ± 3.08
B	-	1.14 ± 0.77	-	1.14 ± 0.77
T	0.01	10.00	0.01	1.00
A	-	31.20 ± 88.78	-	31.20 ± 88.78
B	-	7.80 ± 22.20	-	7.80 ± 22.20
T	0.05	10.00	0.005	1.00
A	-	45.86 ± 74.15	-	45.86 ± 74.15
B	-	11.46 ± 18.54	-	11.46 ± 18.54

The incorporation of asymmetric migration rates in a two-population model seems simple using the framework developed by Maynard Smith (1970), Maruyama (1970), and Nei & Feldman (1972). Interestingly, the equations outlined by Nei & Feldman (1972) could have been used to estimate the effective population size and the migration rate jointly using the F-statistic, but were to my knowledge never used in that context. Their work considered N_e, the mutation rate μ, and the migration rate m, but did not show how to translate these parameters into a more practical estimator, given that the mutation rate is usually unknown. With two populations (Fig. 3) we have three quantities: the probability that two randomly chosen gene copies in subpopulation 1 share the same ancestor in the past generation ($F_W^{(1)}$), a similar probability for subpopulation 2 ($F_W^{(2)}$), and the probability that two copies from different subpopulations have the same ancestor in the past generation (F_B). These statistics can be simply estimated from data using heterozygosity in the subpopulation and an overall heterozygosity; Slatkin & Hudson (1991) outlined a procedure for sequence data. By relating F_B and $F_W^{(i)}$ to population sizes, migration rate and mutation rate, we can use the following recurrence equations, which are adapted from Nei & Feldman (1972), for two populations with different population sizes and migration rates. The exact equations are simplified by removing quadratic terms like μ^2, m^2, μm and divisions by number of individuals in a population (e.g. m/N). For two populations in equilibrium we get the equation system:

$$F_W^{(1)} = \frac{1}{2N_1} + \left(1 - 2\mu - 2m_1 - \frac{1}{2N_1}\right)F_W^{(1)} + 2m_1 F_B,$$

$$F_W^{(2)} = \frac{1}{2N_2} + \left(1 - 2\mu - 2m_2 - \frac{1}{2N_2}\right)F_W^{(2)} + 2m_2 F_B, \qquad (4)$$

$$F_B = F_B\left(1 - 2\mu - m_1 - m_2\right) + m_1 F_W^{(1)} + m_2 F_W^{(2)}$$

where μ is the mutation rate, m_i is the immigration rate into population i, and N_i is the subpopulation size. Because we do not know the mutation rate μ, I follow a common practice in coalescence theory and use a compound parameter Θ which is $4N_e\mu$, and define $M = m/\mu$. Multiplying the equation system by $1/(2\mu)$ we get:

$$F_W^{(1)} = \frac{1}{\Theta_1} - \left(M_1 + \frac{1}{\Theta_1}\right)F_W^{(1)} + M_1 F_B,$$

$$F_W^{(2)} = \frac{1}{\Theta_2} - \left(M_2 + \frac{1}{\Theta_2}\right)F_W^{(2)} + M_2 F_B,$$

$$2F_B = F_B\left(-M_1 - M_2\right) + M_1 F_W^{(1)} + M_2 F_W^{(2)}.$$

(5)

This system can be solved only for three quantities and not for the four quantities we would need to describe the two-population system (Fig. 3). We must either require the population sizes to be the same, but allow different migration rates, or require the migration rates to be the same, but allow different population sizes. For a model with $\Theta = \Theta_1 = \Theta_2$ and two variable migration rates M_1 and M_2 we get:

$$\Theta = \frac{2 - F_W^{(1)} - F_W^{(2)}}{2F_B + F_W^{(1)} + F_W^{(2)}},$$

$$M_1 = \frac{2F_B F_W^{(1)} + F_W^{(1)} - F_W^{(2)} - 2F_B}{\left(F_W^{(1)} - F_B\right)\left(F_W^{(1)} + F_W^{(2)} - 2\right)}, \qquad M_2 = \frac{2F_B F_W^{(2)} + F_W^{(2)} - F_W^{(1)} - 2F_B}{\left(F_W^{(2)} - F_B\right)\left(F_W^{(1)} + F_W^{(2)} - 2\right)},$$

(6)

and for a model with two variable Θ_1 and Θ_2, and $M = M_1 = M_2$ we get:

$$\Theta_1 = \frac{\left(1 - F_W^{(1)}\right)\left(F_W^{(1)} + F_W^{(2)} - 2F_B\right)}{\left(F_W^{(1)}\right)^2 + F_W^{(1)} F_W^{(2)} - \left(2F_B\right)^2}, \qquad \Theta_2 = \frac{\left(1 - F_W^{(2)}\right)\left(F_W^{(1)} + F_W^{(2)} - 2F_B\right)}{\left(F_W^{(2)}\right)^2 + F_W^{(1)} F_W^{(2)} - \left(2F_B\right)^2},$$

$$M = \frac{2F_B}{F_W^{(1)} + F_W^{(2)} - 2F_B}.$$

(7)

These estimators will fail when $F_W^{(i)} \leq F_B$. This can happen more often with more subpopulations and is dependent on the asymmetry of migration rates and on the population sizes (Table 3).

The equation system (5) can be rewritten for more than two populations. One needs, however, to decide whether to base the F_B values on pairwise differences among subpopulations or on an average difference among all pairs of subpopulations. If we want to solve the full model with n population sizes and $n(n-1)$ migration rates we need n^2 quantities. Table 2 shows that we cannot estimate all parameter with one locus. Adding a second locus enables us to solve for all parameters, but complicates the analysis even more. Additionally, we need to assume that the mutation rate is the same for all loci, which is unrealistic for most molecular markers.

Table 2: Variance quantities needed to estimate asymmetric migration rates and population sizes jointly. F_W is the "homozygosity" in a population, F_B is the "homozygosity" between pairs of subpopulations or the averages among all subpopulations.

Populations	Parameters	Quantities			Missing dimension	
		$F_B^{(all)}$	$F_B^{(pairs)}$	F_W	over all	pairwise
2	4	1	1	2	1	1
3	9	1	3	3	5	3
4	16	1	6	4	11	6
.	.	.	.	.	.	.
n	n^2	1	$n(n-1)/2$	n	$n(n-1)-1$	$n(n-1)/2$

Table 3: Estimates of migration rates $\gamma = 4N_e m$ based on equ. 5 in a two population system (Fig. 3). Averages ± standard deviations of 100 simulated data sets with the same population parameters are shown. For each data set 2 populations with 20 sampled individuals with 500bp sequence data were created according to Hudson (1983). T: the parameter values under which the data sets were created, C: Θ is the same for both subpopulations and M can be different for each population (Equ. 7), D: Θ of the two subpopulations can be different, the migration rate M is the same for both subpopulations (Equ.6). N is the number of simulation runs used for calculating the averages and standard deviation. C_1, D_1: cases with negative population parameters were discarded. C_2, D_2: negative results were set to zero.

	Population 1		Population 2		N
	Θ	γ	Θ	γ	
T	0.01	1.00	0.01	1.00	-
C_1	0.0096 ± 0.0056	3.28 ± 6.35	0.0096 ± 0.0056	3.21 ± 8.43	66
C_2	0.0097 ± 0.0059	2.32 ± 5.34	0.0097 ± 0.0059	2.52 ± 7.05	100
D_1	0.0160 ± 0.0214	3.61 ± 6.09	0.0157 ± 0.0271	3.88 ± 12.33	95
D_2	0.0153 ± 0.0211	4.08 ± 7.49	0.0150 ± 0.0266	3.69 ± 12.05	100
T	0.01	10.00	0.01	1.00	-
C_1	0.0063 ± 0.0025	21.66 ± 59.37	0.0063 ± 0.0025	53.43 ± 162.01	34
C_2	0.0064 ± 0.0026	7.79 ± 35.74	0.0064 ± 0.0026	19.75 ± 96.75	100
D_1	0.0349 ± 0.1393	31.48 ± 75.02	0.0186 ± 0.0665	26.64 ± 107.75	46
D_2	0.0166 ± 0.0954	15.89 ± 52.86	0.0106 ± 0.0465	14.83 ± 73.86	100
T	0.05	10.00	0.005	1.00	-
C_1	0.0133 ± 0.0069	22.89 ± 41.42	0.0133 ± 0.0069	9.10 ± 35.20	34
C_2	0.0116 ± 0.0058	7.83 ± 26.27	0.0116 ± 0.0058	3.59 ± 20.73	100
D_1	0.1874 ± 0.7685	58.02 ± 258.86	0.0071 ± 0.0064	2.06 ± 3.29	39
D_2	0.0732 ± 0.4849	22.63 ± 162.88	0.0040 ± 0.0048	2.54 ± 4.35	100

Table 3 gives values for this more complex estimation procedure. The results are not really reassuring. Several of the 100 runs had to be discarded or parameters had to be set to zero because the values for the migration rates were negative for one population. Additionally, the estimates for the migration rates are biased upwards (cf. Beerli & Felsenstein 1998).

4. Maximum likelihood estimators based on allele frequencies

Rannala & Hartigan (1996) and Tufto *et al.* (1996) developed methods based on maximum likelihood to use the allele frequency data of n subpopulations to estimate migration rates directly. Both methods assume a specific probability distribution for the allele frequencies and use this distribution for their likelihood functions. Rannala & Hartigan (1996) used a simpler estimator to calculate the allele frequency estimates and therefore reduced the number of parameters for this approximate likelihood analysis to just one, $4N_e m$. This shortcut makes this method very fast and it is a better estimator of $4N_e m$ than estimators based on F_{ST}. Rannala & Hartigans's implementation (http://mw511.biol.berkeley.edu/homepage.html) has, however, the same limitation as all symmetric estimators and will not deliver correct estimates when the migration rates are asymmetric. Nevertheless, it may be possible to expand it to estimate a full migration matrix to handle asymmetric migration rates. The likelihood method of Tufto *et al.* (1996) is capable of estimating any migration scenario for a finite number of subpopulations. This likelihood method does not make the same assumptions about the allele frequency distribution as the method of Rannala & Hartigan (1996), but needs to estimate the most likely population allele frequencies given the sampled allele frequencies and a migration matrix. It seems that the approach of Tufto *et al.* (1996) would work well for allele frequency data, and Tufto has recently made the method available in form of S-PLUS functions (http://www.math.ntnu.no/jarlet/migration/; S-PLUS is a statistics software package).

5. Estimators using the coalescent

The introduction of coalescence theory (Kingman 1982a, b) changed the field of theoretical population genetics considerably. The coalescence theory is based on an approximation of a sampling process in a Wright-Fisher population (Fig. 1). Looking backwards in time, one can construct a genealogy of the sampled individuals. In a single population this process is only dependent on the effective population size. Kingman showed that the probability of a coalescence of two randomly chosen gene copies from a sample of size k in time interval u which is measured in generations scaled by mutation rate μ, is:

$$\text{Prob}(u \mid N_e, \mu) = \exp\left(-u\frac{k(k-1)}{4N_e}\right)\frac{2}{4N_e}. \tag{8}$$

We can now calculate the probability $\text{Prob}(g \mid N_e, \mu)$ of a whole genealogy g by starting with k sampled alleles or sequences and, going back in time, multiplying the probabilities for each time interval u between nodes on this genealogy. We could now examine all possible genealogies and find the genealogy or a group of genealogies for which the probability, given the population parameters, is highest.

This framework can be expanded and now, for the first time it seems possible to include all possible population parameters into a single consistent framework (Hudson 1990), Kingman's original framework can be easily expanded by incorporating other population parameters (Hudson 1990) such as population growth (Griffiths & Tavaré 1994; Kuhner *et al.* 1998), migration rates (Nath & Griffiths 1996; Bahlo & Griffiths 1998; Beerli & Felsenstein 1998), recombination rates (Griffiths & Marjoram 1996), and selection (Krone & Neuhauser 1997; Neuhauser & Krone 1997). Including migration with a two population system (Fig. 4) changes the equation to:

$$\text{Prob}(u \mid N_e^{(1)}, N_e^{(2)}, m_{21}, m_{12}, \mu) = \exp\left(-u\left[\frac{k_1(k_1-1)}{4N_e^{(1)}} + \frac{k_2(k_2-1)}{4N_e^{(2)}} + k_1m_1 + k_2m_2\right]\right)\beta \tag{9}$$

where β is the actual probability of the event, either a coalescent in population i, with probability $2/4N_e^{(i)}$ or a migration event from population j to i with probability m_{ji}.

Watterson (1975) used the number of segregating sites in a sample of sequences to infer population size. Coalescence theory facilitates finding expectations and variances for population parameters based on the segregating sites method (Wakeley 1998), so that there are two main streams of inference using the coalescent: (1) methods using segregating sites, (2) methods using maximum likelihood analysis based on the coalescence of the total sample. There are additional approximations of the coalescent process (*e.g.* Fu 1994), but they have not been extended to incorporate migration.

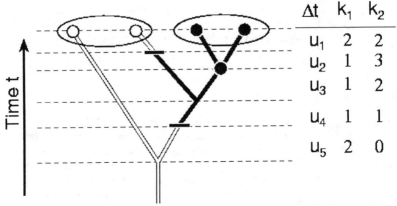

Figure 4: Coalescent genealogy of 4 sampled individuals with migration. Samples from population 1 are shown as blank circles, samples from population 2 in black circles. The migration events are shown as black bars. Δt is the time interval, k_1 and k_2 are the number of lineages in population 1 or 2, respectively, during a time interval u_i. Equ. 8 shows the probability for each given time interval u_i on the genealogy.

5.1. Estimators based on analysis of segregating sites

Wakeley (1998) developed an approximation for the length of a genealogy when there are an infinite number of subpopulations that uses the number of segregating sites of a sample of genes from one to several subpopulations. This approximation to the length of the genealogy is then used to find a new estimator $M_S = 2Nm$ that is dependent on the number of segregating sites within subpopulations and the average number of segregating sites among subpopulations. This estimator is better than those based on F_{ST}, because it has a smaller standard deviation, but shares the same problems: (1) it estimates a symmetric migration rate; and (2) some data sets cannot be analyzed because the estimation of M_S fails when the number of segregating sites in a subpopulation is too large relative to the number of segregating sites over all subpopulations.

5.2. Maximum likelihood estimators using the coalescent

Kingman's probability calculation can be used to construct a maximum likelihood method for the estimation of population parameters. One can weight the probability of a given genealogy g with the likelihood of g which is the probability of the data given the genealogy. This is a quantity well known in phylogenetic studies. Because we do not know the true genealogy of our sample, we use the sum over all possible genealogies and then maximize this function to find the population parameters P:

$$L(P) = \sum_{g \in G} \text{Prob}(g \mid P)\text{Prob}(D \mid g) \tag{10}$$

where D is the sampled data, and P are the population parameters we want to estimate. Taking into account the uncertainty of the genealogy should deliver more accurate parameter values than methods (Slatkin & Maddison 1989) that assume that the topology and the branch length of the genealogy is known.

Griffiths & Tavaré (1994) were the first to use this type of inference of population parameters. There is, however, a problem, that one cannot sample all genealogies, because there are too many. Our group (J. Felsenstein, M. K. Kuhner, J. Yamato, and P. Beerli) uses a Markov chain Monte Carlo Metropolis-Hastings importance sampling scheme to generate an approximation of the likelihood (10) where we integrate over a large sample of genealogies G with different topologies and different branch lengths (Kuhner *et al.* 1995 1998). The approach chosen by Griffiths & Tavaré (1994) and Bahlo & Griffiths (1998) is different from ours (Kuhner *et al.* 1995; Kuhner *et al.* 1998; Beerli & Felsenstein 1998), but estimates the same quantitites. Felsenstein (unpublished data) showed that one can explain the method of Griffiths & Tavaré (1994) in terms used by our group and that it then is very similar to our approach. Both groups have released programs to estimate population parameters. For migration patterns these are GENETREE at the Internet site http://www.maths.monash.edu.au/~mbahlo/mpg/gtree.html, and MIGRATE at http://evolution.genetics.washington.edu/lamarc.html. Both programs use a Markov chain Monte Carlo approach and sample genealogies that are then used to find the maximum likelihood estimate of a full migration matrix with population sizes. MIGRATE estimates the parameters:

$$
P = \begin{pmatrix}
\Theta_1 & M_{21} & \dots & M_{n1} \\
M_{12} & \Theta_2 & \dots & M_{n2} \\
\dots & M_{ji} & \Theta_i & \dots \\
M_{1n} & \dots & \dots & \Theta_n
\end{pmatrix}
\tag{11}
$$

$$
\text{with} \quad \Theta_i = 4 N_e \mu \quad \text{and} \quad M_{ji} = \frac{m_{ji}}{\mu}.
$$

For potential users of these methods, differences in the respective underlying models of evolutionary change are perhaps more important than the similarities between the approaches. Griffiths & Tavaré (1994) and Bahlo & Griffiths (1998) use an infinite sites model that is inappropriate for highly variable sequence data, because it does not allow multiple substitutions at the same site and the researcher needs to discard such sites from the data. This is unfortunate, because discarding variable sites from the data set biases the population parameters; the population size estimates, for example, are too small. Our group uses a more generalized, two parameter mutation model developed by Felsenstein in 1984 (PHYLIP 3.2) (Swofford *et al.* 1996) that is an extension of Kimura's (1980) two-parameter model. Additionally a stepwise mutation model for microsatellites and a model for electrophoretic data are available (Beerli & Felsenstein 1998).

Simulated data sets were analyzed with MIGRATE. As Table 4 shows, MIGRATE delivers less biased estimates and smaller standard deviations than the other methods I have presented (cf. Tables 1, 3) when the population parameters are unequal.

Table 4: Simulation with unequal population parameters of 100 two-locus data sets with 25 individuals in each population and 500 base pairs (bp) per locus. T: Parameter values used to generate the data sets; Migrate: maximum likelihood estimator using the coalescence theory; B: Wright's relation between F_{ST} and γ with the correction for two populations; C_2: Θ is the same for both subpopulations and M can be different for each population (Equ. 7); D_2: Θ of the two subpopulations can be different, the migration rate M is the same for both subpopulations (Equ. 6); negative results in C_2 and D_2 were set to zero.

	Population 1		Population 2	
	Θ	γ	Θ	γ
T	0.05	10.00	0.005	1.00
MIGRATE	0.0476 ± 0.0052	8.35 ± 1.09	0.0048 ± 0.0005	1.21 ± 0.15
B	-	11.46 ± 18.54	-	11.46 ± 18.54
C_2	0.0116 ± 0.0058	7.83 ± 26.27	0.0116 ± 0.0058	3.59 ± 20.73
D_2	0.0732 ± 0.4849	22.63 ± 162.88	0.0040 ± 0.0048	2.54 ± 4.35

6. Variable mutation rate

When we assume that loci are independent and neutral, then each locus delivers an independent estimate of the population parameters N_e and m. It is difficult, however, to exclude the mutation rate from these estimates, so that we normally estimate $\Theta = 4N_e\mu$ and $M = m/\mu$. In principle, this allows us to estimate $\gamma = 4N_e\, m$, which is independent of the mutation rate. For real data, this is only partly true: if there are only a few variable sites, or very few alleles in the data, M will probably be high, but there is much uncertainty because we do not know whether these high values are caused by a high migration rate m or by a very small mutation rate, μ. The estimate of γ therefore has large confidence intervals.

Using more than one locus improves the parameter estimates when the loci are unlinked, because means and variances can be calculated from independent replicates. We still need, however, to assume that the mutation rate is the same for all loci. If one is willing to assume that the mutation rate follows a Gamma-distribution with shape parameter α (Fig. 5), it is then easy to incorporate variable mutation rates into a maximum likelihood framework by integration over all possible mutation rates.

A comparison of MIGRATE with the F_{ST} approach (Table 5) shows that the estimates for Θ are less biased when we take variation of the mutation rate into account. The estimates for the F_{ST}-based migration parameters γ are remarkably good, suggesting that the mutation rates really cancel in γ and that for the parameter values used, F_{ST} is a good estimator for symmetrical migration rates, even when the mutation rate is exponentially distributed.

Table 5: Estimates of population parameters from data with mutation rate variation between loci. The true mutation rate variation follows an exponential distribution ($\alpha = 1$, see Fig. 5). The values are estimates from one single data set for two populations with 30 electrophoretic marker loci. T: the parameter values used to generate the data sets; D: calculation based on equ. 6; Migrate: maximum likelihood estimator based on the coalescence theory. θ is $4N_e\mu$, μ θ can be different for the two subpopulations and the scaled migration rate ($M = m/\mu$) is symmetrical. γ is θM.

	Population 1		Population 2		Shape α
	θ	γ	θ	γ	
T	1.00	1.00	1.00	1.00	1.0
Migrate	1.02	1.03	1.26	1.48	1.7
D	0.70	1.10	0.68	1.07	∞

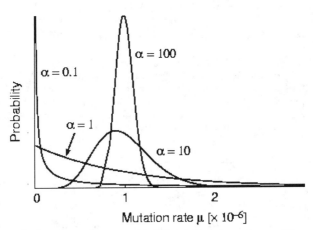

Figure 5: Gamma distributed mutation rates, with different shape parameter α and the same mean μ for all curves. With $\alpha = 1$ the Gamma distribution is an exponential distribution.

7. Testing whether migration rates are symmetric

Given the difficulties of developing a general framework to estimate asymmetric migration rates using F_{ST}, it seems rather cumbersome to develop a test for symmetry of migration rates. A way to solve the problem would be to generate simulated data sets using the estimated migration rates and population sizes (Rousset & Raymond 1997). These simulated data sets could then be used to compare the variances between the different migration rates in an ANOVA.

In the maximum likelihood framework, one would use a log-likelihood ratio test. The standard procedure for testing uses the assumption that with an infinite amount of data log-likelihood curves can be approximated by a normal distribution, so that we can use a χ^2-distribution for the test statistic. This approach may encounter difficulties because the current maximum likelihood estimators (Beerli & Felsenstein 1998; Bahlo & Griffiths 1998) approximate the likelihood using a Markov chain Monte Carlo approach. These methods are known to deliver good point estimates, but these approximate likelihood curves are exact only close to the point estimated. The current speed of computers makes it too time-consuming to generate a data dependent test distribution for these maximum likelihood based estimators.

8. Discussion

The simulation studies for the F_{ST} based estimators (Tables 1, 3) show clearly that, when we violate the assumption that exchange of migrants between subpopulations is symmetrical, the estimates of the migration rates are biased, if not completely wrong. Only those methods allowing the estimation of asymmetric migration rates have a chance of accurately estimating migration pattern in natural populations. This comes at a price, as we need to estimate many more parameters. At least for estimation of growth rate and population sizes, coalescence theory suggests that we need to increase the quantity of data not by sampling more individuals, but by sampling more loci (Kuhner *et al.* 1998). This is probably true even for estimation of migration rates (*cf.* Wakeley 1998; P. Beerli, unpublished data). Adding more individuals will mainly add lineages in the very recent past, so little additional information is gained about historical events at the bottom of the genealogy.

Even when by some external knowledge, for example using direct methods, we know that the subpopulations are approximately equal in size and the migration rates are symmetric, the F_{ST}-based approaches are still superseded by using the pseudo-maximum likelihood approach of Rannala & Hartigan (1996) or using the segregating sites approach of Wakeley (1998). Alternatively, the computationally more demanding but more accurate maximum likelihood methods that sample over all genealogies (Bahlo & Griffiths 1998; Beerli & Felsenstein 1998) can be employed.

9. Conclusion

During the last 60 years many researchers have used and continue to use F-statistics or genetic distances to make inferences about migration patterns. With the advent of newer methods, such as maximum likelihood using allele frequencies and their possible extensions or methods based on coalescence theory, tools now exist that allow us to estimate migration patterns without the unrealistic assumption of symmetry of migration rates or equal population sizes.

References

Bahlo M, Griffiths RC (1998) *GENETREE*. Program and documentation distributed by the authors. Department of Mathematics, Monash University, Sydney, Australia.

Beerli P, Felsenstein J (1998) *MIGRATE   -   Maximum likelihood estimation of migration rates and population numbers.* Program and documentation distributed by the authors. Department of Genetics, University of Washington, Seattle, Washington.

Bosshart JL, Prowell DP (1998) Genetic estimates of population structure and gene flow: limitations, lessons and new directions. *Trends in Ecology and Evolution*, **13**, 202-206.

Charlesworth B (1998) Measures of divergence between populations and the effect of forces that reduce variability. *Molecular Biology and Evolution*, **15** , 538-543.

Excoffier L, Smouse P (1994) Using allele frequencies and geographic subdivision to reconstruct gene trees within species: molecular variance parsimony. *Genetics*, **136**, 343-359.

Fu YX (1994) A phylogenetic estimator of effective population size or mutation rate. *Genetics*, **344**, 685-692.

Griffiths RC, Tavaré S (1994) Sampling theory for neutral alleles in a varying environment. *Philosophical Transactions of the Royal Society London Series B: Biological Sciences*, **344**, 403-410.

Griffiths RC, Marjoram P (1996) Ancestral inference from samples of DNA sequences with recombination. *Journal of Computational Biology*, **3**, 479-502.

Hudson RR (1983) Properties of a natural allele model with intragenic recombination. *Theoretical Population Biology*, **23**, 183-210.

Hudson RR (1990) Gene genealogies and the coalescent process. *Oxford Surveys in Evolutionary Biology*, **7**, 1-44.

Hudson RR, Slatkin M, Maddison WP (1992) Estimation of levels of gene flow from DNA sequence data. *Genetics*, **132**, 583-589.

Kimura M (1980) A simple method for estimating evolutionary rate of base substitutions through comparative studies of nucleotide sequences. *Journal of Molecular Evolution*, **16**, 111-120.

Kingman J (1982a) The coalescent. *Stochastic Processes and their Applications*, **13**, 235-248.

Kingman J (1982b) On the genealogy of large populations. In *Essays in Statistical Science* (eds. Gani J, Hannan E), pp. 27-43. Applied Probability Trust, London.

Krone SM, Neuhauser C (1997) Ancestral processes with selection. *Theoretical Population Biology*, **51**, 210-237.

Kuhner MK, Yamato J, Felsenstein J (1995) Estimating effective population size and mutation rate from sequence data using Metropolis-Hastings sampling. *Genetics*, **140**, 1421-1430.

Kuhner MK, Yamato J, Felsenstein J (1998) Maximum likelihood estimation of population growth rates based on the coalescent. *Genetics*, **149**, 429-434.

Li W-H (1976) Effect of migration on genetic distance. *American Naturalist*, **110**, 841-847.

Lynch M, Crease T (1990) The analysis of population survey data on DNA sequence variation. *Molecular Biology and Evolution*, **7**, 377-394.

Maruyama T (1970) Effective number of alleles in a subdivided population. *Theoretical Population Biology*, **1**, 273-306.

Maynard Smith J (1970) Population size, polymorphism, and the rate of non-Darwinian evolution. *American Naturalist*, **104**, 231-237.

Michalakis Y, Excoffier L (1996) A generic estimation of population subdivision using distances between alleles with special reference for microsatellite loci. *Genetics*, **142**, 1061-1064.

Nath H, Griffiths RC (1996) Estimation in an island model using simulation. *Theoretical Population Biology*, **50**, 227-253.

Nei M (1973) Analysis of gene diversity in subdivided populations. *Proceedings of the National Academy of Sciences USA*, **70**, 3321-3323.

Nei M, Feldman MW (1972) Identity of genes by descent within and between populations under mutation and migration pressures. *Theoretical Population Biology*, **3**, 460-465.

Neigel JE (1997) A comparison of alternative strategies for estimating gene flow from genetic markers. *Annual Review of Ecology and Systematics*, **28**, 105-128.

Neuhauser C, Krone SM (1997) The genealogy of samples in models with selection. *Genetics*, **145**, 519-34.

Rannala B, Hartigan JA (1996) Estimating gene flow in island populations. *Genetical Research, Cambridge*, **67**, 147-158.

Relethford JH (1996) Genetic drift can obscure population history: problem and solution. *Human Biology*, **69**, 29-44.

Rousset F (1996) Equilibrium values of measures of population subdivision for stepwise mutation processes. *Genetics*, **142**, 1357-1362.

Rousset F, Raymond M (1997) Statistical analyses of population genetic data: new tools, old concepts. *Trends in Ecology and Evolution*, **12**, 313-317.

Slatkin M (1991) Inbreeding coefficients and coalescence times. *Genetical Research, Cambridge,* **58**, 167-75.

Slatkin M (1993) A measure of population subdivision based on microsatellite allele frequencies. *Genetics,* **139**, 457-462.

Slatkin M, Hudson R (1991) Pairwise comparisons of mitochondrial DNA sequences in stable and exponentially growing populations. *Genetics,* **129**, 555-562.

Slatkin M, Maddison W (1989) A cladistic measure of gene flow inferred from the phylogenies of alleles. *Genetics,* **123**, 603-613.

Swofford D, Olsen G, Waddell P, Hillis D (1996) Phylogenetic Inference. In: *Molecular Systematics* (eds. Hillis D, Moritz C, Mable B), pp. 407-514. Sinauer Associates, Sunderland, Massachusetts.

Tufto J, Engen S, Hindar K (1996) Inferring patterns of migration from gene frequencies under equilibrium conditions. *Genetics,* **144**, 1911-1921.

Wakeley J (1998) Segregating sites in Wright's island model. *Theoretical Population Biology,* **53**, 166-174.

Watterson GA (1975) On the number of segregating sites in genetical models without recombination. *Theoretical Population Biology,* **7**, 256-276.

Weir SB (1996) *Genetic Data Analysis II.* Sinauer Associates, Sunderland.

Wright S (1951) The genetical structure of populations. *Annals of Eugenics,* **15**, 323-354.

Advances in Molecular Ecology
G.R. Carvalho (Ed.)
IOS Press, 1998

Microsatellites and Minisatellites for Molecular Ecology: Theoretical and Empirical Considerations

Arnaud Estoup[1,2] and Bernard Angers[1]

[1]*Laboratoire de Génétique des Poissons, INRA, 78352, Jouy-en-Josas, France. e-mail: angers@diamant.jouy.inra.fr*

[2] *Present address: Laboratoire de Modélisation et de Biologie Evolutive, 488 rue Croix Lavit, URBL-INRA, France. e-mail: estoup@zavez02.ensam.inra.fr*

Variable number of tandem repeat (VNTR) sequences include both microsatellite and minisatellite loci. We describe qualitative and quantitative features of VNTRs as well as the methods used to isolate these loci and reveal their polymorphism. The relative advantages of VNTRs over other genetic markers and of microsatellites over minisatellites is addressed. A thorough understanding of the mutational events shaping VNTR evolution is necessary to construct sound and accurate theoretical models from which population parameters can be estimated. We examine the mutation models usually considered for VNTR markers along with the statistical tests and experimental data that can be used to evaluate the adequacy of these models. Important additional evolutionary features of VNTRs, namely mutational biases, allele size constraints, size homoplasy and the existence of correlations between structural features and levels of polymorphism, are also examined. Finally, we provide an overview of applications and case studies of VNTR markers in molecular ecology, with particular emphasis on the most promising category of VNTRs in molecular ecology, namely, microsatellites. The high variability of microsatellites presents new perspectives for analyses at the individual level including genetic tagging, classification of individuals to their population of origin, level of relatedness among individuals and parentage assignment. Application of VNTR markers at the population level is also addressed. More specifically, we discuss the methods and statistics available to test and measure population differentiation, to estimate effective population size (N_e), to detect non-equilibrium situations due to N_e fluctuations, and to reconstruct phylogenetic relationships among populations.

1. Introduction

Variable number of tandem repeat (VNTR) sequences include both microsatellite and minisatellite loci depending on the length of the repeated unit. Since their discovery in the early eighties, increasing emphasis has been given to the use of this category of DNA sequences as genetic markers. First applications were made by Jeffreys *et al.* (1985a, b) with multilocus DNA fingerprinting. Since then, technological development has considerably eased the application of VNTR as genetic markers. In particular, PCR-based techniques allowed routine analysis from tiny amounts or even partially degraded DNA, permitting the investigation of numerous issues not previously possible. These technical assets coupled with several attractive evolutionary features explain why VNTR are nowadays increasingly replacing or at least complementing traditional markers such as allozymes for numerous applications in molecular systematics, population genetics and ecology. This is particularly true for microsatellite loci, which present considerable advantages over minisatellites. However, the high potential of VNTR markers may be limited by the time consuming and technically demanding development step, the rudimentary knowledge of their mutation processes, the necessity to develop new methods for data analysis, and limits inherent to the markers themselves in relation to the evolutionary question addressed. The purpose of this chapter is to provide an overview of the recent developments concerning VNTR sequences in molecular ecology.

2. Qualitative, quantitative and technical features

2.1. Qualitative and quantitative features

Satellite DNA was named following the discovery that after CsCl centrifugation a small fraction of total DNA formed a *satellite* band separated from the main genomic band. This DNA fraction was shown to contain simple sequences, less than 500 base pairs (bp) in length, repeated thousands or even millions of times (reviewed by Beridze 1986). Other classes of tandemly repeated DNA with much shorter repeated units were discovered independently from CsCl centrifugation during DNA sequencing of the human insulin gene (Bell *et al.* 1982). They were named minisatellites for the largest ones (repeat unit of 6 to 64 bp, *e.g.* Jeffreys *et al.* 1985a) and microsatellites for the shortest ones (repeat unit of 1 to 5 bp, *e.g.* Hamada & Kakunaga 1992). It is worth noting that the total length of microsatellite arrays is generally quite short (10 to 200 bp) while most minisatellites range from a few hundred to several thousand bp.

Dot-blot hybridization, DNA database searching and cloning procedures revealed that microsatellite sequences were common in most eukaryotic nuclear genomes and in the chloroplastic genome of plants. For instance, the estimated microsatellite frequency in the human genome is one every 6 kb (Beckman & Weber 1992). For reasons that remain unclear, the mean density of microsatellites within species varies widely among taxonomic groups and sometimes among species of a given taxonomic group. For instance, micro- and minisatellites seem generally scarce in several invertebrate groups, *for example,* lepidopterans (Saccheri & Bruford 1993). Microsatellites are also five times less abundant in the genome of plants than in mammals (Lagercrantz *et al.* 1993) and they are six to seven times less frequent in birds than in humans (Primmer *et al.* 1996b). Mono- and di-nucleotide repeats are more common than tri- and tetra-nucleotide repeats in both plants and animals (Lagercrantz *et al.* 1993).

Both *in situ* hybridization and genetic mapping revealed a relatively even distribution of microsatellite over chromosomes, although a slightly lower density is observed in the telomeric and centromeric regions, at least for $(CT)_n$ and $(GT)_n$ repeats (Koch *et al.* 1989; Wintero *et al.* 1992). However, the frequent association of several microsatellites in the same cloned insert indicates a clustering of microsatellites in bees (Estoup *et al.* 1993), a tendency confirmed in several genomic regions by high density maps of the human and mouse genomes (Dib *et al.* 1996; Dietrich *et al.* 1996). In contrast, minisatellite sequences were shown to be preferentially located in sub-telomeric regions (Royle *et al.* 1988; Signer *et al.* 1996).

On the basis of the motif array sequences, microsatellite loci are usually classified as perfect, imperfect or compound sequences (Weber 1990). Perfect microsatellites are composed of uninterrupted stretches of repeat units, while imperfect microsatellites have one to several interrupting bases in an otherwise perfect repeat array. Compound microsatellites consist of neighbouring repeated sequences composed of different repeat types. Sequence analysis of cloned minisatellites has shown that repeat units within a minisatellite are seldom all identical but usually display sequence variation between repeat units (Jeffreys *et al.* 1991; Armour *et al.* 1993).

2.2. Acquisition of individual loci

An extensive number of VNTR loci have already been developed for different purposes in a considerable number of species. In particular, recent genome mapping projects have involved screening for prodigious quantities of microsatellites (reviewed in Pollock *et al.* 1998). However, one of the major drawbacks related to PCR-based VNTR loci is that when no single locus sequence is available in the literature, they must first be isolated from the genome. Several approaches can be used to achieve this objective. Classical methods describing the cloning and characterization of microsatellites and minisatellites are abundant in the literature, for example, Weber (1990) and Estoup *et al.* (1993) for microsatellites, and Wong *et al.* (1986) and Armour *et al.* (1990) for minisatellites. For microsatellite loci, highly detailed protocols provide useful guides for less-experienced geneticists and ecologists: these protocols are available at the Word-Wide-Web addresses http://www.inapg.inra.fr/dsa/microsat/microsat.htm, http://www.nmnh.si.edu/museum/ interdisc.html and http://gator.biol.sc.edu/msats/microsatellites.html. Several additional methods have been published to optimize the task of microsatellite isolation, as enrichment techniques (Ostrander *et al.* 1992; Kijas *et al.* 1994; Nishikawa *et al.* 1995) or methods avoiding genomic library construction (Browne & Litt 1992; Hantula *et al.* 1996; Ender *et al.* 1996). However, these alternative procedures are generally more complex than the usual cloning-screening procedures. Hence, it is preferable to use these methods only for genomes characterized by a low density of microsatellites.

Because microsatellite flanking region are generally conserved among closely related species, an alternative strategy consists in using primers isolated from one species to amplify homologous loci in related species (cross-priming strategy). Cross-priming rates widely vary among taxonomic groups and among loci (Schlötterer *et al.* 1991; Primmer *et al.* 1996b; Rico *et al.* 1996). However, a significant relationship is expected between evolutionary distance and cross-priming performance, both in terms of amplification success and polymorphism (Primmer *et al.* 1996b). The main drawbacks of this strategy is that cross-priming will tend to result in a lower level of polymorphism and a lower PCR pattern quality (presence of non specific PCR products and more intense stutter bands) in the related species. Moreover, cross-priming of related species increases the frequency of null alleles (alleles that give no PCR product). Null alleles result from mutations (base substitution or deletion) which occurred at one or both primer site(s). They can be detected as a departure from Mendelian inheritance in pedigree analyses or as an excess of homozygotes within a population. Once detected, the problem may be resolved by designing new primers (Callen *et al.* 1993; Paetkau & Strobeck 1995).

2.3. Typing

Initially, minisatellite genetic variation was surveyed using multilocus DNA fingerprinting methods that produced complex individual band patterns (Jeffreys *et al.* 1985b). Although this technology found several applications in forensic sciences and ecology such as genetic tagging, the inability to assign bands to a given locus and hence to estimate allele frequencies has limited its application to populations studies considerably. Fingerprinting based on genomic hybridization with locus-specific minisatellite probes was the first method developed to circumvent this major drawback. However, major technical advances became possible with the advent of the polymerase chain reaction (PCR, Mullis *et al.* 1986; Saiki *et al.* 1986). PCR-based techniques offered the possibility to survey greater amounts of genetic variation in the genome with much less effort and expense. However, this method presents a serious drawback for some minisatellite loci because large fragments (> 4-5 Kb) are not readily amplified and detected. Moreover, given the length of some minisatellite arrays compared to the repeat unit size, the percent size difference between many alleles can be too small to detect mobility differences on a gel. This necessitates the grouping or combining of alleles into defined size classes. A common criticism of this practice is that alleles of similar size are often grouped together, thus contributing to an excess of homozygotes and the underestimation of genetic diversity at minisatellite loci. A more sophisticated PCR method termed minisatellite variant repeat (MVR-PCR, Jeffreys *et al.* 1990) was developed based on the fact that repeat units within a minisatellite usually display sequence variation. This method allows detection of both the total number of repeats and the distribution of each repeat unit type comprising the minisatellite allele. This method is particularly adapted for haploid genomes but generates complex banding patterns when analysing diploid heterozygous individuals (O'Reilley & Wright 1995).

The assessment of single-locus variation at any microsatellite loci is based on PCR and high resolution electrophoretic systems. Both the shorter range variation of microsatellite alleles and the use of sequencing-like electrophoretic systems allow an accurate sizing of each microsatellite variant. The reproducibility and accuracy with which microsatellite alleles can be separated have made automated detection and scoring possible (Edwards *et al.* 1991; Zeigle *et al.* 1992; Wenburg *et al.* 1996). Ideally, a set of several loci can be amplified in a single PCR using primers labelled by different fluorescent tags (PCR multiplexing step), and several such sets can be mixed and electrophoresed in a single gel line or capillary (loading multiplexing step), and analysed using a semiautomatic multilocus genotyping system. The benefits over conventional typing methods are numerous: non-radioisotopic visualization of alleles, greater typing yield, reduced labour and laboratory consumable costs, and automated scoring of allele sizes. The drawbacks of semiautomatic genotyping systems are essentially the necessity of having a large choice of loci to optimize the multiplexing PCR and/or loading steps and the high initial financial cost of equipment and fluorescent labelled primers.

A particular feature associated to microsatellite PCR patterns is the occurrence of stutter bands (Hite *et al.* 1996). A positive consequence of such patterns is that they allow the detection of microsatellite alleles without ambiguity. However, they sometimes make it difficult to discriminate between homozygotes and heterozygotes with few repeats between alleles. While tri- and tetranucleotide loci produced less stutter bands than dinucleotide loci, their larger allele size range in bp represents a potential drawback for automatic typing.

2.4. VNTRs as markers for evolutionary studies

Prior to the advent of routine PCR protocols, VNTRs were considered as having limited potential in population genetic studies. With the improvement of PCR technology, former technical limits became assets, and VNTR loci were recognized as one of the most powerful Mendelian markers available. Their main advantages over other markers are: variable but often high levels of polymorphism (heterozygosity usually well above 50% in natural populations), single-locus and codominant inheritance for all microsatellites and some minisatellites, abundance in the genome especially for microsatellites, and no obvious functional role, and hence *a priori* selective neutrality. However, it is worth mentioning that an absence of functionality does not necessarily mean evolutionary neutrality since VNTR markers are potentially genetically linked to selected genes. Moreover, although direct evidence for a general functional role of VNTR loci in eukaryotic genomes is still lacking, several possibilities have been reported (reviewed in Garza *et al.* 1995; Rico *et al.* 1996;

Kashi *et al.* 1997; Kashi & Soller 1998; Meloni *et al.* 1998). Since length variation in VNTRs is usually due to stepwise changes in the repeat unit count (Jeffreys *et al.* 1988; Weber 1990), evolutionary information can also be gained from the number of repeats separating two electromorphs. Finally, the main technical advantages of VNTR over other markers include easy, accurate and potentially automated scoring especially for microsatellites, and small tissue requirements for PCR-based assay techniques.

These numerous advantages explain why VNTRs are nowadays increasingly replacing or at least complementing traditional markers such as allozymes in evolutionary biology and ecology. This is particularly true for microsatellite loci, as they have distinct advantages over minisatellites: a higher density and a more even distribution in the genome, and a higher accuracy of allele sizing. Finally, microsatellites are technically easier to handle than minisatellites and have a higher potential for automated detection and scoring. Hence, although multilocus and single locus minisatellites have been and are still widely used for evolutionary studies (*e.g.* Gilbert *et al.* 1990 and 1991; Galeotti *et al.* 1997; Scribner *et al.* 1997; Wetton & Parkin 1997), the last three years have seen a deluge of publications based on microsatellites (Fig. 1).

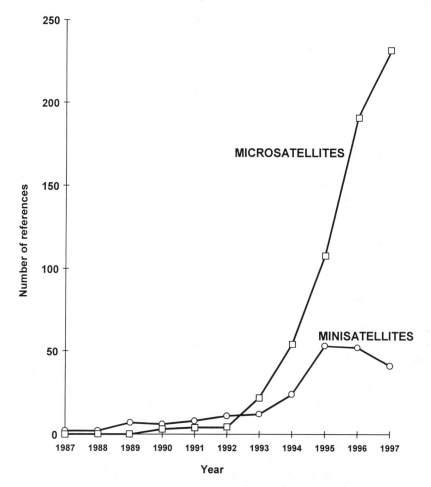

Figure 1: Number of published manuscripts per year since 1987 as referenced in the MEDLINE bibliographic bank when using the key words (microsatellite and (population or ecology or demography)) for square symbols and (minisatellite and (population or ecology or demography)) for circular symbols.

3. Mutation processes

Estimation of numerous population parameters (*e.g.* genetic differentiation, number of migrants per generation, long term effective population size, etc.) is dependent upon the mutation model assumed for the markers. This dependence may be especially strong in the case of VNTRs, since sensitivity to the mutation model increases with the mutation rate (*e.g.* Estoup & Cornuet 1998), which is generally very high for this category of markers. The evolutionary dynamics of VNTR have been examined using various experimental and theoretical methods (see the reviews of Freimer & Slatkin 1996, Jarne & Lagoda 1996; Armour *et al.* 1998; Estoup & Cornuet 1998). Although a number of features suggest that mutation processes at microsatellite and minisatellite loci may differ in important aspects, it is likely that there is a continuum in the mutational processes from the simple sequence repeats of microsatellites to the more complex sequences of minisatellites. In any case, recent studies have shown that the mutation processes of microsatellites and minisatellites may be more complex than previously envisaged.

3.1. Molecular mechanisms involved in repeat number variation

A good knowledge of the molecular mechanisms involved in repeat number variation is essential as they predict different outcomes in terms of the spectrum of size changes expected from mutational events. Two categories of mutation events are considered for VNTR variation: (i) intra-allelic events which can be explained by two simple mechanisms, replication slippage and unequal sister chromatid exchange, (ii) inter-allelic events which involved recombination events such as simple unequal crossover or more complex gene conversion. Indirect evidence suggests that most of the repeat number variations at microsatellites correspond to intra-allelic events involving a replication slippage mechanism (Levinson & Gutman 1987; Schlötterer & Tautz 1992; Primmer *et al.* 1996a). However, the occurrence of rarer inter-allelic events involving crossover or gene conversion cannot be excluded (*e.g.* Estoup *et al.* 1995a). Both intra- and inter-allelic events are common at minisatellite loci (Jeffrey *et al.* 1994; Buard *et al.* 1998). In the majority of cases, inter-allelic recombination events at minisatellites do not seem to be simple unequal crossover but rather appear as non-reciprocal exchange akin to gene conversion events.

3.2. Mutation rates and models

Mutation rates of microsatellites and minisatellites are high compared to rates of point mutation, which are of the order of 10^{-9} to 10^{-10}. Estimates from pedigree analysis in humans suggested a rate of around 10^{-3} events per locus per generation (Weber & Wong 1993) and 6.2×10^{-4} for a set of 5,264 dinucleotide polymorphisms in CEPH families (Dib *et al.* 1996). Similar studies in mice gave estimates of around 10^{-3} to 10^{-4} (Dallas 1992). In *Drosophila*, mutation rates at microsatellites seem to be relatively low at around 6×10^{-6} (Schug *et al.* 1997). Estimates based on allele frequency distributions in populations gave a similar mean values of 7.96×10^{-4} in humans (Goldstein *et al.* 1995b) and 4.75×10^{-4} in honeybees (Estoup *et al.* 1995a). Estimates of microsatellite mutation rates in *in vivo* systems are around 10^{-2} events per locus per replication in *Escherichia coli* (Levinson & Gutman, 1987) and around 10^{-4} to 10^{-5} in yeast (Henderson & Petes, 1992; Strand *et al.* 1993). Most minisatellite loci also show high mutation rates, the most unstable human loci reaching mutation rates of 0.4-7% per gamete (Jeffreys *et al.* 1988; Vergnaud *et al.* 1991; Buard *et al.* 1998), Note that only a very small number of microsatellite loci have been shown to have mutation frequencies in this range (Weber & Wong, 1993; Primmer *et al.* 1996a).

Traditionally, two extreme models of mutation have been considered for VNTR: the infinite allele model (IAM, Kimura & Crow 1964) and the stepwise mutation model (SMM, Kimura & Ohta 1978). The SMM describes the loss or gain of a single tandem repeat, and hence alleles can mutate towards allele states already present in the population. In contrast, under the IAM, a mutation involves any number of tandem repeats and always results in an allele state not previously encountered in the population. More recently, DiRienzo *et al.* (1994) introduced a two phase model (TPM), where the number of repeats gained or lost in each mutation follows a geometric distribution, thus also allowing mutation steps of several repeats. Finally, another classical model, called the K-allele model (KAM), could also be considered (Crow & Kimura 1970). Under this model, there are exactly K possible allelic states and any allele has a constant probability $[\mu/(K-1)]$ of mutating towards any of the other K-1 allelic states.

Direct information about the mutation process of VNTR sequences has been obtained by the analysis of alleles differing by a single mutational event, including single locus or multi-locus pedigree analyses for both categories of markers, and PCR-based analyses of a small pool of spermatozoids for minisatellites. For microsatellites, the distributions of mutation sizes were found to comply with the SMM or the TPM (*e.g.* Weber & Wong 1993; Primmer *et al.* 1996a). For minisatellites, alterations by large numbers of repeats are common (Jeffreys *et al.* 1988, 1994; Buard *et al.* 1998). The theoretical model that would fit length variation at most minisatellite loci should thus be closer to the KAM or the IAM than to the SMM.

Two different approaches have been used to evaluate the adequacy of the above models for microsatellite allelic distributions observed in natural population samples. The first approach is based on the comparison of observed and expected values in the number of alleles and/or the heterozygosity under each mutation model (Shriver *et al.* 1993; Estoup *et al.* 1995a). In the second approach, the population x locus parameter considered is the variance of the number of repeats (Valdes *et al.* 1993; DiRienzo *et al.* 1994). The application of these tests to actual microsatellite population data generated contradictory or inconclusive results. This presumably reflects the involvement of more complex mutation processes than those assumed for the mutation models tested. It also reflects the low power of these tests and the fact that basic assumptions such as mutation-drift equilibrium are not always met due to population size fluctuations. These statistical tests also suggest that mutation processes vary greatly among loci.

3.3. Additional factors relevant to the evolution of VNTRs

The mutation models outlined in the last section do not consider several factors which have recently been identified to be relevant to the evolution of VNTRs. These factors as well as the corresponding references are summarized in Table 1. For a more detailed review of the factors acting on microsatellite evolution see Estoup and Cornuet (1998).

3.3.1. Microsatellites

- *Repeat unit size, composition, count and within-tract interruption.* Although substantial interlocus variation of mutation rates exists, mutation rates are, on average, inversely related to the size of the repeat unit (Chakraborty *et al.* 1997). For a given size of repeat unit, the level of polymorphism of tri- and tetranucleotide microsatellites also seems to depend upon the composition of the repeat unit, in particular to its A/T content (Gastier *et al.* 1995; Sheffield *et al.* 1995). Independently of the repeat type, microsatellite loci with higher repeat counts appear to be associated with higher mutation rates, presumably because the opportunity for a stable misaligned configuration is greater for longer repeat tracts (Weber 1990; Beckmann & Weber 1992; Ostrander *et al.* 1993; Goldstein & Clark

Table 1: Summary of the factors relevant to the evolution of microsatellites and minisatellites

Evolutionary feature	Micro-satellite	Mini-satellite	References
Change of one repeat unit	Frequent	Common	Jeffreys et al. 1988, 1994; Valdes et al.1993; Weber & Wong 1993; Amos et al. 1996; Primmer et al. 1996a, 1998
Change of several repeat units	Relatively rare	Common	Jeffreys et al. 1988, 1994; Weber & Wong 1993; DiRienzo et al. 1994; Estoup et al. 1995a; Amos et al. 1996; Primmer et al. 1996a, 1998
Excess of mutations corresponding to repeat gain	Yes	Yes	Weber & Wong 1993; Jeffreys et al. 1994; Amos et al. 1996; May et al. 1996; Primmer et al. 1996a, 1998; Buard et al. 1998
Influence of repeat size	Yes	No	Chakraborty et al. 1997, Armour 1998
Influence of repeat composition	Yes	No	Gastier et al. 1995; Sheffield et al. 1995; Armour 1998
Influence of the number of repeat units	Yes	Yes	Weber 1990; Jeffreys et al, 1994; Goldstein & Clark, 1995; Buard et al. 1998
Influence of allele purity	Yes	Yes	Chung et al. 1993; Jeffreys et al. 1994; Pépin et al. 1994; Buard et al. 1998
Influence of flanking sequences	?	Yes	Jeffreys & Neumann 1997; Buard et al. 1998
Polarity of the mutation process	?	Yes	Armour et al. 1993; Jeffreys et al. 1994
Constraints on allele size	Yes	Yes	Bowcock et al. 1994; Garza et al. 1995; Armour et al. 1996
Differences in mutability among alleles at the same locus	Yes	Yes	Jeffreys et al. 1994; Monckton et al. 1994; Jin et al. 1996; May et al. 1996; Primmer et al. 1996, 1998
Sex-biased mutation process	Yes	Yes	Weber & Wong 1993; Jeffreys et al. 1994; Armour et al. 1998; Primmer et al. 1998
Mutation rate correlated with allele size difference in heterozygous individuals	Yes (?)	?	Amos et al. 1996; Ellegren et al. 1995, 1997; Crawford et al. 1998; Rubinsztein et al. (1995a and b); Amos, 1998; Primmer et al. 1998

1995). Moreover, interrupting bases appear to stabilize the repeats tract, thus reducing the possibility of misalignment and resulting in lower levels of polymorphism than uninterrupted microsatellites with similar number of repeats (Chung et al. 1993; Pépin et al. 1995). This phenomenon partly explains polymorphism differences among loci as well as within-locus polymorphism differences among species and/or among populations within species. The relationships between variability, repeat count, and within repeat tract interruption also hold for the mutability of alleles at the level of a single microsatellite locus (Jin et al. 1996; Primmer et al. 1996a, 1998; Petes et al. 1997).

- *Mutation biases.* Studies characterising mutations using multilocus or single locus pedigrees in human and the barn swallow (*Hirundo rustica*) suggest that mutations at microsatellite loci involve more gains than losses of repeats, as well as a higher mutation rate in paternal meioses (Weber & Wong 1995; Primmer et al. 1996a, 1998). Male-biased mutation rate can at least be partly attributed to the large difference in the number of cell divisions between spermatogenesis and oogenesis. The gender of the mutating individual may also have a more global influence on the mutation process. At a single hypervariable tetranucleotide locus in the barn swallow, expansions were more common in the male than in the female germline while magnitude of size alteration was larger in females than in males (Primmer et al. 1998). Finally, human family analyses have suggested that mutations are more likely to occur in heterozygous individuals whose alleles differ greatly in repeat counts (Amos *et al.* 1996; Amos 1998). However, this observation has not been confirmed in a study examining germline mutation at a single hypervariable microsatellite locus in barn swallows when alleles of the same repeat count classes were compared (Primmer *et al.* 1998). If the difference in repeat count between alleles in a heterozygote were to increase instability relative to a homozygote, then the mutation rate would correlate with heterozygosity, and loci in larger populations would evolve faster than those in smaller ones. Rubinsztein *et al.* (1995a & b) suggested that microsatellites cloned from humans were on average longer than their chimpanzee homologues and that this could be a result of an ascertainment bias including both an upwardly biased mutation process and a higher mutation rate due to a larger effective population size in humans. However, it has been argued that microsatellite loci will tend to be longer and more polymorphic in the species they were cloned from as a result of the preference for longer repeat arrays during the isolation procedure (Ellegren *et al.* 1995; but see Crawford *et al.* 1998). In any case the ascertainment bias hypothesis still needs to be thoroughly tested (see the review of Amos 1998 for additional details on this question).

- *Size constraints.* A mutation process dependent on the repeat count combined with a propensity for gaining rather than losing repeats would obviously promote an expansion of microsatellite arrays towards a large (virtually infinite) number of repeats. Although a few large repeat arrays have been found in telomeric regions (Wilkie & Higgs 1992), most microsatellite loci have a finite size generally shorter than a few tens of repeat units. This suggests strongly that there must be some size constraints restricting the expansion of repeat arrays. Except for human diseases associated with trinucleotide expansions, there has so far been no direct evidence for selective constraints acting on allele length at microsatellite loci. However, several lines of evidence, mostly based on intra- and interspecific comparison of allele size variance, have been suggested, and several mechanisms, some associated with selection, were proposed as forces counteracting the elongation of microsatellite arrays (Bowcock *et al.* 1994; Garza *et al.* 1995; Samadi *et al.* 1998). Note that if constraints on the repeat count is dependent on the absolute size (in bp) of repeat arrays, they may be stronger for longer repeat units.

3.3.2. Minisatellites

Influences of size and composition of repeat unit on the mutation process of minisatellites have not been shown. However, the influence of repeat count and tract purity on the instability of a single hypervariable minisatellite loci was recently demonstrated (Buard *et al.* 1998). In this case, tract purity corresponded to the level of homogeneity of a repeated region composed of several types of repeat units, and thus to the distribution of repeat unit types within the minisatellite. As for microsatellites, an upward mutation bias and a strong mutational bias in favour of paternal meiosis has also been detected for at least some minisatellite loci (Vergnaud *et al.* 1991; Jeffrey *et al.* 1994; May *et al.* 1996; Armour *et al.* 1998; Buard *et al.* 1998). Interestingly, minisatellites with apparently similar male and female germline mutation rates, appear to undergo different types of mutational process (Jeffreys *et al.* 1994). At several minisatellite loci, population and pedigree analyses provide strong evidence for a large excess of mutation occurring at one extremity of the locus (Armour *et al.* 1993; Jeffreys *et al.* 1994). However, such mutational polarity is not a universal feature since some extremely unstable minisatellite loci undergo mutations along their entire length. The higher homogeneity of the microsatellite repeated regions and the difficulty in application and interpretation of molecular techniques such as the sperm-pool method make the testing for mutation polarity difficult for microsatellite loci. Finally, some size constraints restricting the expansion of minisatellite repeat arrays were postulated, but not demonstrated (Armour et al. 1998).

3.3.3. Incorporation of recent findings into mutation models

At least some of the numerous factors relevant to the evolution of VNTRs are being progressively incorporated into the mutation models that were initially considered (Garza et al. 1995; Kimmel & Chakraborty 1996; Kimmel et al. 1996; Nauta & Weissing (1996); Feldman et al. (1997); Pollock et al. 1998). However, we often do not have the data necessary to estimate accurately the proportion and range of multistep mutations, asymmetry rate in the distributions of mutation, dependence of the mutation rate on the allelic repeat count and purity, and to a lesser extent, constraints on allele size (but see Pollock et al. 1998 for this last factor). Furthermore, the large variance in the mutation parameters among loci, especially microsatellite loci, makes the construction of general theoretical models difficult. Hence, selection of loci with similar and easily assessed mutation parameters appears to be crucial for accurate estimation of population parameters for instance, loci following the SMM for microsatellites and the KAM for minisatellites. Combination of experimental population and molecular studies, and statistical testing of theoretical models, should contribute to this selection of loci as well as to the elaboration of more accurate and realistic models.

3.4. Size homoplasy in VNTR sequences

Variation at microsatellites and some minisatellites is revealed through electrophoresis of PCR products and allelic classes differ by the length (in bp) of the amplified fragments. Two PCR products of the same length may not be identical copies without mutation of the same ancestral sequence, introducing the possibility of size homoplasy (identity by state and not by descent). The occurrence of size homoplasy is associated closely to the way that mutations produce new alleles, and hence to the mutation model. If the mutation model is assumed to be the IAM, there should not be any homoplasy because any new allele created by a mutation is distinct from the existing alleles in the population. All other mutation models (e.g. SMM, TPM and KAM) can generate size homoplasy. Constraints acting on the range of allele size reduce the number of possible allelic states and hence also favour size homoplasy (Nauta & Weissing 1996; Feldman et al. 1997). Finally, the occurrence of homoplasy is expected to increase with mutation rate and time of divergence among populations (Cornuet & Estoup, unpublished data).

As expected, size homoplasy has been detected experimentally by sequencing electromorphs of interrupted or compound microsatellites (Estoup et al. 1995a; Garza & Freimer 1996; Angers & Bernatchez 1997; Primmer & Ellegren 1998; Viard et al. 1998) or flanking regions of perfect microsatellites (Orti et al. 1997; Grimaldi & Crouau-Roy 1997). Because sequence variation among repeat units occurs at many hypervariable minisatellites, size homoplasy was particularly easy to study with this category of VNTR loci (Jeffreys et al. 1991; Armour et al. 1993). Size homoplasy has been frequently detected among populations, in particular among distantly related populations, and to a lesser extent within populations.

Size homoplasy is often considered as a major drawback of microsatellites and minisatellites for population studies. Viard et al. (1998) showed that the detection of size homoplasy through electromorph sequencing may have a substantial effect on the resolution of population structure. When alleles rather than electromorphs were considered, more single-locus pairwise tests of population differentiation were significant and non-stepwise estimators of genetic differentiation (see section 5.2.) were larger. Nevertheless, it is worth stressing that size homoplasy is fully taken into account by several population statistics when a locus follows strictly a SMM (Goldstein et al. 1995b; Slatkin 1995;

Rousset 1996). This is not the case, however, for loci following a TPM or a KAM with unknown parameters (proportion of multistep mutations, variance of the geometric distribution for the TPM, and number of possible alleles for the KAM) and/or when strong allele size constraints exist (but see Feldman *et al.* 1997 and Pollock *et al.* 1998). This reinforces the necessity of selecting SMM loci with a large allelic range for microsatellites, and KAM loci with large k values and hence virtually no size homoplasy for minisatellites.

4. Analyses at the individual level

The variability of VNTR loci is often so high that, even with a small number of loci and a large number of individuals, most individuals have unique multilocus genotypes. For instance, the probability of genotypic identity was estimated to be 1.5×10^{-7} in a genetic tagging study of humpback whales (*Megaptera novaeangliae*) using only six microsatellite loci (Palsboll *et al.* 1997). It is therefore possible to address issues such as discrimination, relationships, structure, relatedness and classification or hierarchy, not only at the population (using allelic frequencies) but also at the individual level (using genotypes). Moreover, individual based analyses potentially allow the analysis of contemporary levels of gene flow (as opposed to gene flow estimates derived from indirect approaches, *e.g.* from F_{st}, see section 5.2, this chapter), providing more tangible estimates of individual movements in an ecologically meaningful time frame. The comparative use of direct and indirect estimates of gene flow is widely discussed in Neigel (1997). It is worth mentioning that the mutation process of VNTR loci is generally of little concern for analyses at the individual level, and levels of polymorphism as determined by the mutation rate and the effective population size are virtually the only factors of importance.

4.1. Genetic tagging

The first application of minisatellites at the individual level involved multilocus DNA fingerprinting in relation to forensic issues (Jeffreys *et al.* 1985a, b). However, since small regions of DNA are more easily PCR-amplified from highly degraded material, microsatellites have replaced minisatellites in most forensic applications (Olaisen *et al.* 1997; de Pancorbo *et al.* 1997).

Since non-lethal sampling is often possible, genetic tagging using microsatellites may also soon replace, or at least complement, classical methods of physical tagging in demography and ecology studies. Genetic tagging using PCR-markers offers at least four advantages over physical tagging. First it ensures temporal stability of individual tags required for long term studies. Second, it allows the tagging of early life-history stages (eggs, larvae), and of species that are difficult to tag physically. Third, it may be used to follow the movement of individuals since DNA can be recovered by non invasive sampling, of shed hair, feathers or faeces (Wasser *et al.* 1997). Finally, when a sufficient number of highly variable markers are typed, the acquisition of information on pattern of relatedness among individuals or on genetic population parameters can facilitate significantly the interpretation of demographic and evolutionary forces operating at the individuals or populations level. On the other hand, microsatellite tagging of individuals remains relatively expensive.

Palsboll *et al.* 's (1997) study on North-Atlantic humpback whales exemplifies the advantages offered by individual genetic tagging using variable PCR-markers. Since the probability that two individuals having identical genotypes was extremely low, the authors were certain that samples with identical genotypes obtained at different locations or time corresponded to the same individual. Therefore, they could track 692 whales spatially (from the West Indies to the Barents sea) and temporally (over seven years), by resampling several times. These data showed that most whales came back each year to the same feeding ground but that a large mixture of individuals from different geographic origin occurred in the reproductive areas (with occasional migrations of up to 8000 km).

4.2. Classification of individuals

While all individuals typed at a sufficient number of VNTR loci have a unique multilocus genotype, individuals within a population are expected to share more alleles than individuals from different populations, and individuals from closely related populations are expected to share more alleles than individuals from distantly related populations. Hence, it should be possible to classify individuals according to the level of similarity of their multilocus genotype. Classification of individual genotypes is relevant to at least three applications: (i) to determine the proportion of individuals which, on the basis of their multilocus genotypes, are correctly assigned to their population of origin, an estimate related to the degree of genetic differentiation among populations, (ii) to assign one individual of unknown origin to its population of origin provided that this population is included in the reference set, and (iii) to detect an admixture of populations in a sample of individuals, and, if such admixture exists, to determine the proportion of the different populations included in the sample. At least three methods are available for classifying individuals according to their multilocus genotype.

The first method is based on the calculation of genetic distances between individuals followed by the application of classical algorithms used in phylogenetic reconstruction (Bowcock et al. 1994; Estoup et al. 1995b; Blouin et al. 1996; Ellegren et al. 1996). The more genetically similar two individuals are, the closer they branch on the tree. An illustration of this method is given in Fig. 2. Bees belonging to the same patriline, that is, progenies of 5 different drones mated to the same queen, cluster together with high bootstrap values (between 80% and 97%), but the 5 patrilines are scattered among other bees from the same population. Note that the high classification resolution of this case may be due to the fact that honey bee drones are haploid and that workers of the same patriline (full-sisters) have 75% of their genes in common (by descent) compared to workers of different patrilines (half-sisters) which share only 25%. Examples given by Chakraborty and Jin (1993) indicate that for an intermediate relationship (parent-offspring, 50% of gene sharing), average heterozygosities higher than 0.7 are required to distinguish parent-offspring from random pairs with 10 loci (see section 4.3, this chapter). Since the population studied has an average heterozygosity of 0.6, it is not surprising, that half sisters, which are more distantly related than parent-offspring, are scattered among the other members of the population. Individual trees potentially also give useful information to assess the origin of new founding populations. For instance, it was argued that wolves (*Canis lupus*) released deliberately from zoos were the source of a new population in Scandinavia. Although the similarity of mtDNA haplotypes argued in favour of this scenario, the hypothesis was rejected when an individual tree constructed using the shared allele distance (D_{AS}, Chakraborty & Jin 1993) of 12 microsatellites revealed that all wild wolves clustered separately from captive animals (Ellegren et al. 1996).

The second classification method consists in assigning an individual to the population in which its multilocus genotype has the highest probability of occurring, assuming Hardy-Weinberg equilibrium and linkage equilibrium in all locus-population combinations (Paetkau et al. 1995). The high efficiency of microsatellites for assigning individuals to their population of origin has been illustrated by a comparative study between microsatellite and allozyme markers on one hatchery and 11 natural populations of resident brown trout (*Salmo trutta*) sampled over a small geographic scale (Estoup et al. 1998a).

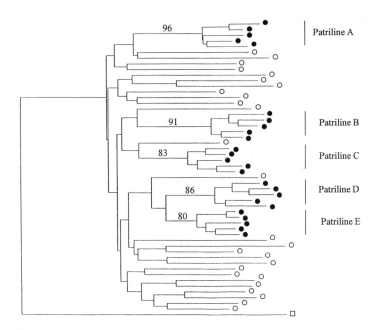

Figure 2: Neighbour-joining tree (12 loci, D_{AS} distance) of individual honey bees (*Apis mellifera*) from Avignon population sample (open circles) and from five different patrilines (A to E, full circles) of a colony also from Avignon (Estoup *et al.* 1995a). A bee from a different population (Forli, open square) has been added as an outgroup. Only bootstrap values equal or superior to 80% are given: they all correspond to patriline clusters.

Eight allozymes and seven microsatellites allowed correct assignment of 52% and 93% of the individual fish to their population of origin respectively. In this case study, a single microsatellite locus (the one with the highest gene diversity) allowed correct assignment of the same proportion of individuals to their population of origin as did eight polymorphic protein loci.

The third classification method, the neural network technique, is a general purpose classification method derived from artificial intelligence. It is based on computer programs which simulate simplified natural neural networks (NN). NN are trained to recognize any groups of objects or individuals, on the basis of their characteristics. Biological application of NN are numerous, for example in the analysis of protein structure, identification of species, automatic counting of fishes or prediction of fish biomass and density (Cornuet *et al.* 1996). Using a data collection of 430 honeybees at various taxonomic levels and 8 microsatellite loci, Cornuet *et al.* (1996) demonstrated the ability of NN to classify individuals on the basis of their genotypes. They also showed that NN performed better than any other general purpose classification methods such as discriminant analysis, in terms of correctly classifying individuals at any taxonomic level.

For all applications, the resolution power of all three methods increases with the level of differentiation of the populations under study as well as with the number and the level of variability of the loci (Bowcock *et al.* 1994; Estoup *et al.* 1995a, 1998a; Paetkau *et al.* 1995; Cornuet *et al.* 1996). Evaluating the power of any method to achieve the objectives of a given application necessitates that individuals of known origin are analysed with a given set of loci. Finally, it is worth mentioning that a major problem for the assignment of individuals of unknown origin to their population of origin, is that the set of reference populations may not include the population from which the unknown individual(s) originates. Therefore, it would be important in such a case to be able to exclude all reference populations (at least the most genetically distant populations), by, for example, setting a minimum threshold for the output statistics (Cornuet *et al.* 1996). To our knowledge, this has yet to be achieved.

4.3. Mating structure, relatedness and parentage assignment

Our understanding of the evolution of social behaviours and mating systems depends on the possibility to differentiate individuals genetically and to estimate with sufficiently high precision the genetic relatedness between groups or pairs of interacting individuals (Queller & Goodnight 1989). Because VNTR loci are particularly suited to analysis at the individual level, they became incorporated rapidly into these research fields (Queller *et al.* 1993; Avise 1994; Estoup *et al.* 1994; Morin *et al.* 1994; Blouin *et al.* 1996; Taylor *et al.* 1997). Interestingly, one of the earliest significant contributions of VNTR loci (especially microsatellites) in this context pertains to establishing mating structures and relatedness relationships within social systems of haplo-diploid insect species (cf. Evans, 1993, 1995; Estoup *et al.* 1994, 1995; Peters *et al.* 1995 for the earliest papers). This is due mainly to the high frequency and variability of sociality in these species, to the poor genetic information at the colony level due to a large deficit of polymorphic protein markers, and to the fact that the haplo-diploid system (males are haploid and females diploid) greatly facilitates genetic analyses (reviewed in Crozier *et al.* 1997).

For any genetic system, the use of highly variable VNTR loci is expected to yield a substantial gain of resolution for any measures and statistics associated with relatedness and parentage assignment. Since the variance of F_{ST} and F_{IT} estimators (see paragraph 5.2) decreases with increasing genetic diversity of markers (Goudet *et al.* 1996), a gain of precision is expected for global statistics such as the average relatedness of individuals within samples compared to the whole [$R = 2F_{ST}/(1+F_{IT})$, Queller & Goodnight 1989]. The ability to assess precisely the genetic relatedness between two individuals of unknown pedigree in a wild population likewise depends on the level of variability of the markers, but also on the number of loci, the category of markers (single-locus or multilocus markers), and the levels of relatedness that one aims at distinguishing (Queller & Goodnight 1989; Blouin *et al.* 1996).

Band sharing indices computed from minisatellite multilocus DNA fingerprints have been used with reasonably high confidence to distinguish between first-order relatives (parent-offspring or full sibs) and unrelated individuals in an outbred population (Piper & Rabenold 1992). It is likely that finer resolution could be achieved with additional probes (Lynch 1991; Piper & Rabenold 1992). Higher resolution should also be possible using data from highly polymorphic single-locus markers, the main restriction being the number of unlinked loci available and the polymorphism level of the loci (Chakraborty & Jin 1993; Brookfield & Parkin 1993; Blouin *et al.* 1996). Typing a realistic set of 20 loci with a mean heterozygosity of 0.75 would still give 2-3% of full-sibs incorrectly classified as unrelated and 15-17% rate of misclassification when comparing full-sibs with half-sibs, or half-sibs with unrelated individuals (Blouin *et al.* 1996). The number of single VNTR loci required would be unrealistically large if one aims at resolving relatedness relationships greater than the first degree with a high degree of confidence (Brookfield & Parkin, 1993). For instance, typing of 40 loci with a mean heterozygosity of 0.75 will still yield a 8% misclassification frequency when comparing unrelated to half sibs (Blouin *et al.* 1996).

Hence, the discrimination ability using realistic sets (say < 20 loci) of single-locus

VNTR markers is only slightly better than what has been accomplished with multilocus DNA fingerprinting using multiple probes and restriction enzymes (Piper & Rabenold 1992; Signer *et al.* 1994). Nevertheless, single-locus VNTRs present at least two advantages over the minisatellite multilocus fingerprint approach : (i) the discriminative ability can be increased by scoring a progressively higher number of loci or more polymorphic loci, whereas both the number of probes and the quantity of DNA available are limited for the multilocus minisatellite approach, and (ii) single-locus markers yield population allele frequencies and hence directly unbiased estimates of relatedness between individuals, while a minisatellite multilocus fingerprint approach gives a measure of bandsharing which must be calibrated for each population using individuals of known relatedness. Among single locus VNTR markers, microsatellites tend to be less polymorphic and hence less informative than minisatellites. However, microsatellites present several advantages which largely compensate for their lower level of polymorphism: they are much easier to obtain in large numbers than minisatellites, their alleles are more accurately sized, and automated detection and scoring are easier. Two multiplexed microsatellite loci with n alleles each will be more informative, for roughly the same amount of laboratory work, than a single minisatellite locus with $2n$ alleles. Indeed, assuming that alleles are equally distributed, two independent loci with n alleles each give $g_1 = n^2(n+1)^2/4$ possible genotypes and a single locus with $2n$ alleles gives $g_2 = n(2n+1)$ possible genotypes, with $g_1 > g_2$ for $n>2$ (Estoup *et al.* 1998b).

Individual polymorphic loci can also be used to identify potential parent-offspring pairs in a population. In a closed population (all potential parents sampled), the simple assignment criterion can be the possibility to generate a given offspring genotype given Mendelian inheritance from a particular pair of parental genotypes (Danzman 1997). More complex probabilistic treatments including typing errors or mutations can also be considered (SanChristobal & Chevalet 1997). Simulations on actual datasets in fish hatchery populations using the method of SanChristobal & Chevalet (1997) illustrate the high power of codominant VNTRs for parentage assignment (Estoup *et al.* 1998b). For example, in a hatchery population of turbot (*Scophtalmus maximus*) directly captured from a natural population, 8 microsatellite loci with a mean heterozygosity of 0.84 allow the correct assignment of any possible offspring genotype to a unique parental pair among 15,000 independent pairs and to a unique father among 520 males in a paternity retrieval scheme (Estoup *et al.* 1998b). In an open population, a first assignment criterion can be that, barring mutation, parent-offspring pairs must share at least one allele at every locus. Using this criterion on a set of 10 (20) simulated loci with a mean heterozygosity of 0.75, 41 % (17 %) of full-sib pairs, 16 % (2 %) of half-sib pairs and 1% (0 %) of unrelated pairs in a population would be misidentified as potential parent-offspring pairs (Blouin *et al.* 1996). Genetic likelihoods for non-excluded parents can then be calculated (using as a baseline the allele frequencies in the local population sample) from the joint genotypic frequencies observed in particular combinations of adults and juveniles. Several packages carry out this last category of treatments. The packages KINSHIP 1.0 (Queller & Goodnight 1989) as well as CERVUS (Marshall *et al.* 1998) perform maximum likelihood tests of pedigree relationships between pairs of individuals in a population. Other algorithms allow to assign not only the best potential father and mother, but the best potential parental couple (Meagher & Thompson 1986, 1987; Thompson & Meager 1987; Prödohl *et al.* 1998). Whatever the assignment criterion, optimal conditions for parentage assignment in an open population system are: small population size, relatively sedentary reproducers, intensive sampling, positional and biological information (age, gender and lactation status) and a large number of highly polymorphic loci (Prödohl *et al.* 1998).

5. Analysis at the population level

5.1. Testing population differentiation, Hardy-Weinberg equilibrium and genotypic linkage disequilibrium

High levels of polymorphism (numerous alleles and high heterozygosity) are particularly useful for studies dealing with microevolutionary events (events that occurred within population or between closely related populations). However, the analysis of large number of alleles has long presented statistical problems, which were largely solved with the recent development of several exact tests and associated computer packages particularly adapted to microsatellite data (*e.g.* Raymond & Rousset 1995; Rousset & Raymond 1997). Interestingly, higher polymorphism levels results in higher asymptotic power for exact tests of population differentiation such as in the recent data analysis package GENEPOP (Raymond & Rousset 1995). Although this issue has rarely been discussed, this conclusion has been supported for an island model population structure (Goudet *et al.* 1996) as well as for other types of analyses *e.g.* Robertson & Hill (1984) or Rousset & Raymond (1995). Thus, microsatellites may allow the detection of genetic differences that less polymorphic markers such as allozymes could not reveal (Estoup *et al.* 1998a). The higher level of polymorphism at microsatellite loci also results in a higher power of GENEPOP exact tests for genotypic linkage disequilibrium (Ott & Rabinowitz 1997; Estoup *et al.* 1998a) and deviations from Hardy-Weinberg equilibrium (Chakraborty & Zhong 1993; Rousset & Raymond 1995).

5.2. Genetic structure among populations

Knowledge of patterns of geographic subdivision and the extent of gene flow among populations is crucial to understand evolutionary processes within species (Ryman 1981; Moritz 1994). Classically, population differentiation can be measured using Wright's F statistics (Wright 1951; Weir & Cockerham 1984, Beerli, this volume) which enable the estimation of number of migrants among populations under a wide variety of conditions if populations are demographically stable (Slatkin & Barton 1989). However, F statistics assume that any new mutation produces a novel allelic state, which implies that they are better suited for IAM markers. However, for stepwise markers such as microsatellites, alleles of similar sizes are not necessarily identical by descent due to size homoplasy. In order to deal with this issue and integrate size differences as a parameter reflecting the extent of population differentiation, new statistics have recently been proposed for microsatellites markers. Slatkin (1995) defined an analogue of G_{ST} (Crow & Aoki 1984) denoted R_{ST}, and Rousset (1996) and Michalakis & Excoffier (1996) an analogue of F_{ST} (Wright 1951) denoted ρ_{ST} and Φ_{ST} respectively. As noted in Rousset (1996), the relationships and differences between R_{ST} and ρ_{ST} are similar to those between G_{ST} and F_{ST}, (both reviewed in Cockerham & Weir 1993). Note that ρ_{ST} weights alleles by their size in bp or repeat count number while any weight including the former is possible for Φ_{ST}; ρ_{ST} may be thus considered as a particular case of Φ_{ST} (Michalakis & Excoffier 1996). For microsatellite loci, Wright's F_{ST} and Φ_{ST} (or ρ_{ST}) can be estimated according to Weir & Cockerham (1984) and Michalakis & Excoffier (1996) respectively. In the multilocus estimators of Φ_{ST} (or ρ_{ST}) the contribution of each locus is weighted proportionally to their allele size variance. Goodman (1997) proposed a multilocus estimator of Φ_{ST} (or ρ_{ST}) for which the weight is independent of the allele size variance.

A major drawback of statistics incorporating allele size differences is their higher variance relative to F_{ST} (Slatkin 1995). The suitability of any genetic measure also largely depends on the degree to which the markers conform to the underlying mutation model assumed for that measure. It is still unclear how departures from the SMM would affect measures of genetic differentiation based on allele size differences such as R_{ST}, Φ_{ST} and ρ_{ST} (but see Kimmel *et al.* 1996 and Angers & Bernatchez 1998 for theoretical and experimental aspects respectively). Hence, it is advisable to compute and compare both categories of statistics (*e.g.* Michalakis & Veuille 1996; Ross *et al.* 1997; Estoup *et al.* 1998a). Slatkin (1995) and Rousset (1996) showed that F_{ST} is similar to R_{ST} and ρ_{ST} when differentiation is roughly independent of the mutation process, that is, with large migration rates and/or recent time of divergence among populations. Contrasted evolutionary case studies revealed that the experimental values of these two categories of statistics were not significantly different, or that F_{ST} values were significantly lower than R_{ST} or ρ_{ST} (Michalakis & Veuille 1996; Barker *et al.* 1997; Estoup *et al.* 1998a). Table 2 reports F_{ST} and ρ_{ST} values for microsatellite loci typed in brown trout (*Salmo trutta*) populations sampled at a microgeographic (Estoup *et al.* 1998a) and macrogeographic scale (Presa, Estoup & Guyomard, unpublished data). Microgeographic sampling is composed of populations which diverged recently (less than 2,500 generations, that is, after the last glaciation), while macrogeographic sampling is composed of sets of populations which diverged more than 125,000 generations ago. Multi-locus F_{ST} and ρ_{ST} values were both high but not significantly different at a microgeographic scale (low migration rate rates but recent time of divergence among populations), while multi-locus ρ_{ST} values were significantly higher than multi-locus F_{ST} values at a macrogeographic scale (low migration rate rates and long time since divergence among populations).

In order to further detail the distribution of the genetic variance among populations and reveal ecological and environmental factors shaping differentiation, it can be helpful to perform hierarchical analysis of population structure (Weir & Cockerham 1984; Excoffier *et al.* 1992). The package ARLEQUIN (Schneider *et al.* 1997) allows to carry out such analyses, optionally taking into account allele size differences among microsatellite alleles.

Finally, it is important to distinguish between testing differentiation (*e.g.* using Fisher exact tests) and measuring differentiation (*e.g.* estimating F_{ST}). The high level of polymorphism at VNTR loci due to their high mutation rate is expected to increase the power for exact tests of population differentiation (see section 5.1.), while it is expected to

Table 2: Single-locus and multi-locus F_{ST} and ρ_{ST} values estimated from microsatellite loci typed in brown trout (*Salmo trutta*) populations sampled at a microgeographic and macrogeographic scale (see text). Multi-locus F_{ST} and ρ_{ST} values are not significantly different (Wilcoxon's signed rank test, P=0.92) and ρ_{ST} values are significantly higher than multi-locus F_{ST} values (Wilcoxon's signed rank test, P=0.018) for the microgeographic and macrogeographic scales respectively.

Microgeographic scale			Macrogeographic scale		
locus	F_{ST}	ρ_{st}	locus	F_{ST}	ρ_{st}
543AE	0.195	0.145	MS-60	0.395	0.640
BS131	0.443	0.445	MS-73	0.484	0.723
T3-13	0.181	0.214	MS-15	0.583	0.734
85	0.361	0.227	MS-791	0.603	0.672
FGT1	0.353	0.365	MS-591	0.567	0.937
43AEL	0.272	0.278	MS-543	0.349	0.683
43AEU	0.082	0.082	MS-85	0.471	0.733
Global	0.279	0.287	**Global**	0.495	0.792

decrease the values of the parameter F_{ST} (Jin & Chakraborty 1995 ; Slatkin 1995 ; Rousset 1996). Hence, comparative studies between low and high mutating markers, *e.g.* allozymes and microsatellites, may eventually show higher proportion of significant tests of differentiation among populations but lower F_{ST} values for microsatellites as compared to enzyme markers. However, since the variance of F_{ST} estimators decreases with increasing genetic diversity of markers (Goudet *et al.* 1996), a gain of precision is expected on this statistics when using highly variable markers such as VNTR. The latest feature would potentially result in a higher number of F_{ST} values significantly higher than zero for microsatellites as compared to allozymes in comparative studies, in particular when analysing slightly differentiated populations. Empirical studies based on a sufficiently large number of both categories of markers and population samples are still needed to experimentally investigate these aspects (Estoup *et al.* 1998a).

5.3. *Effective population size and demographic fluctuations*

Effective population size (N_e) equals the census number of individuals in an ideal population, where all individuals are randomly mated, have the same reproductive potential and discrete generations and where selection, migration and mutations are negligible. However, these conditions rarely hold within real populations. Hence, N_e is defined as the size of an idealized population which would give rise to the variance of change in gene frequency (current N_e) or the rate of inbreeding (long-term N_e) observed in the actual population under consideration (Caballero 1994). N_e is among the most important parameters in evolutionary and conservation biology because it determines the rate of inbreeding and genetic variation decay, and hence the potential for long-term maintenance of genetic variability (Simberloff 1988).

Several methods have been proposed to estimate current N_e from genetic data. The principal methods are based on (i) temporal variation of allelic frequencies (Waples 1989; Jorde & Ryman 1995, 1996), (ii) gametic linkage disequilibrium in cohorts (Hill 1981; Bartley *et al.* 1992), (iii) heterozygote excess (Pudovkin *et al.* 1996) and (iv) maximum likelihood approaches using the Metropolis-Hastings sampling methods (Kuhner *et al.* 1995; Beerli, this volume). Note that some of these methods also take life-history and demographic particularities into account for species with overlapping generations (Jorde & Ryman 1995, 1996). PCR-based markers such as microsatellites allow the use of historical tissue collections. Consequently, precision of temporal-based methods of N_e estimation can be improved by increasing the time interval between samples (Miller & Kapuscinski 1997). The virtually unlimited number of loci that can be analysed is also a significant advantage of microsatellite markers.

In contrast to current N_e, long-term N_e assumes that populations have reached mutation-drift equilibrium and hence, implies hundreds or thousands generations with stable demography. Estimation of long-term N_e is also dependent upon the mutation model and mutation rate assumed for the markers. Regarding microsatellite markers, lower and upper N_e values can be estimated assuming the IAM and the SMM respectively. However, it is worth mentioning that relative estimates of long-term N_e in different populations using the same set of loci is roughly independent of the mutation model (Estoup *et al.* 1995b; Lehmann *et al.* 1998).

Current and long-term N_e of two *Anopheles gambia* populations in Kenya (Assembo and Jego) was estimated by Lehmann *et al.* (1998) from temporal variation at nine microsatellite loci sampled 7 and 9 years apart (current N_e) and from genetic diversity in each sample (long-term N_e). The estimate of current N_e of Assembo and Jego were 6,359 and 4,258 respectively and the lower 95% limits were 2,455 and 1,669 respectively. Thus, despite the typical observation of low density during the dry season, large populations are maintained annually. Current N_e in Assembo was 1.5 fold higher than in Jego, but the difference was not significant. Average long-term N_e in Assembo (22,667 ± 10,251 and 7,572 ± 2,281) was 2.9 and 1.9 fold higher than that in Jego assuming the SMM and the IAM respectively. The difference between populations was significant at both time points regardless of whether long-term N_e values were calculated based on the SMM or the IAM. These results indicate different past demographic histories for the two populations, and illustrate that past demography may not necessarily affect current N_e estimates, and that recent demographic events may not necessarily affect long-term N_e values.

Detection of severe and rapid population size fluctuations such as demographic expansions or demographic reductions (bottleneck), is of importance in population studies since these processes cause rapid changes in genetic structure. If undetected, past population fluctuations can result in misleading interpretation of extant population genetic structure and evolutionary processes. Large fluctuations in effective population size usually translates into changes in the level of genetic variability and distribution of allele frequencies. As microsatellite markers can be amplified from even partly degraded DNA, the genetic structure of past populations can potentially be documented using museum specimens (skins or feathers, Ellegren 1991; Roy et al. 1994; Taylor et al. 1994) or air dried fish scale samples (Nielsen et al. 1997). Temporal change of genetic structure due to population size fluctuation or any other evolutionary phenomenon, such as hybridization (see Rieseberg, this volume), can thus be directly accessed with PCR markers such as microsatellites.

Detection of severe and rapid population size fluctuation is also possible through the analysis of allele frequency distribution within a single population sample. When a population experiences a reduction of its effective size, it generally develops a heterozygosity excess at selectively neutral loci assuming mutation-drift equilibrium and a given mutation model (Cornuet & Luikart 1996). Note that this heterozygosity excess should not be confused with an excess of heterozygotes. The former compares observed and expected heterozygosities, in the sense of Nei's (1978, p. 177) gene diversities, whereas the latter compares the number of heterozygotes with Hardy-Weinberg equilibrium expectation. A population experiencing a population expansion will generally develop a heterozygosity deficiency. The heterozygosity excess (or deficiency) persists only a few generations until a new equilibrium is established. Hence, Cornuet and Luikart's method will only detect recent historical bottlenecks but can be achieved in the absence of historical data. In contrast, Rogers & Harpening (1992) have developed a method for detecting ancient historical bottlenecks using DNA sequences data and a genealogical analysis approach. VNTR markers are very suitable for the detection of population size fluctuations, in particular recent and severe bottlenecks for at least three reasons: (i) they are presumably selectively neutral, (ii) due to their high mutation rates they should be near mutation drift equilibrium in populations whose sizes have not recently been perturbed, and (iii) their high variability, which increases the abundance of polymorphic loci in a post-bottleneck sample. This is particularly true for populations that have suffered a severe size reduction, as postulated in several conservation biology case studies reviewed in Luikart & Cornuet (1998).

Two methods for detecting population expansion were recently developed for microsatellite loci by Reich & Goldstein (1998). The first method is based on the fact that the distribution of allele length at a microsatellite locus of a growing population is expected to be more smoothly peaked (higher kurtosis) than that of a population of constant size. The second method focuses the variability of variances across microsatellite loci, which is expected to be lower for growing populations than for those of constant size. Interestingly, the statistics computed for the second method allow an estimate of the possible dates and ranges of the detected population expansion. The application of both methods to a large human population database of 30 dinucleotide and 30 tetranucleotide microsatellites, showed highly significant evidence for a major expansion in African populations, but no evidence of expansion outside of Africa (Reich & Goldstein 1998). The African expansion is estimated to have occured between 49,000 and 640,000 years ago, certainly before the Neolithic expansions, and probably before the splitting of African and non-African populations. The missing expansion signal outside Africa may be attributed to a population bottleneck associated with the emergence of human groups from Africa, as postulated in the "out of Africa" model of modern human origins.

This last result suggests that it is worth investigating further evolutionary situations corresponding to a founder event and hence a N_e reduction followed by a population flush using both Cornuet & Luikart (1996) and of Reich & Goldstein (1998) approaches. This scenario would indeed correspond to the realistic demographic history experimented by most colonising species.

5.4. Phylogenetic relationships among populations

Assessing phylogenetic relationships among populations can provide useful insights into population evolutionary processes, historical biogeography and conservation issues (Avise 1994; Moritz 1995). In contrast to previous measures of differentiation among populations, phylogenetic reconstruction is based on genetic distances assuming that no gene flow has occurred among populations since they have diverged, and thus differences between populations only result from genetic drift and mutation. In evaluating the performance of a distance measure for phylogenetic reconstruction, linearity with time and coefficient of variation must be considered simultaneously.

The contribution made by microsatellite markers to infer phylogenetic relationships among populations has so far been limited. This is rather surprising since the large number of microsatellite loci available, and their rapid evolutionary rate, should make them particularly useful for inferrring relationships among closely related populations or species (Goldstein *et al.* 1995a,b). Although classical distances such as Cavalli-Sforza & Edwards' (1967) or Nei *et al.*'s (1983) are not based on the SMM or any other mutation model, they were first used for phylogenetic reconstruction using microsatellites. Recently, several genetic distances, which take allele size differences into account, have been specifically developed for phylogenetic inferences based on microsatellites (reviewed by Goldstein & Pollock 1997; Pollock *et al.* 1998).

Divergence among taxa is a continuum, but an arbitrary subdivision between closely related and distantly related populations could be proposed on the criteria of the mean mutation rate of markers. By opposition of closely related taxa, distantly related taxa would correspond to the time frame when mutation has a significant effect on divergence. Because the mean mutation rate of microsatellites (μ) is approximately 5×10^{-4} mutation / locus / generation (see section 4.2.), each microsatellite allele present within taxa separated $1/\mu =$ 2,000 generations ago have mutated once on average. Hence, a divergence time of 2,000 generations could be considered as an upper limit above which mutation at microsatellite loci surely have a substantial effect on divergence among taxa.

5.4.1. Phylogenetic reconstruction among closely related populations

For closely related populations, genetic divergence is essentially due to random drift. For this category of populations, classical distances of Cavalli-Sforza & Edwards (1967) and of Nei *et al.* (1983) have been shown to reconstruct microsatellite phylogenies better than distances that incorporate allele size differences (Takezaki & Nei 1996). This is essentially due to the lower coefficient of variation and to the acceptable linearity with time of these classical distances when short periods of divergence are considered. At this evolutionary scale, the most important aspect seems to be the selection of loci with sufficiently high mutation rates to potentially differentiate even closely related populations. A rough estimate of the variability level (number of alleles and heterozygosity) can be obtained through the typing of a few individuals from a single population (approx. 10 individuals) and should be sufficient for the selection of suitable loci. The reconstruction of a complete topology, including all minor branching patterns among closely related populations surely requires a large number of loci (> 25 loci) (Takezaki & Nei 1996; Estoup *et al.* 1998a). However, relatively robust inferences of major clusters may be obtained with a smaller number of loci.

5.4.2. Phylogenetic reconstruction among distantly related populations / taxa

For distantly related populations, genetic divergence is due to both random drift and mutation. Classical distances are not linear with time and hence do not reflect divergence time over large time scales. This is particularly true when there is no overlap of allele frequency distributions between two populations. Hence, in spite of their high coefficient of variation, distances taking into account allele size differences become more appropriate when analysing distantly related populations.

Three major sources of difficulties in using microsatellites for phylogenetic reconstruction of distantly related populations are considered:

- *Constraints on allele size resulting in a restricted number of allelic states.* The accuracy and linearity with time of all genetic distances are strongly affected by allele size constraints. This is particularly true for loci characterized by reduced allele ranges and high mutation rates (Feldman *et al.* 1997; Goldstein *et al.* 1995a, b; Pollock *et al.* 1998). Several distances taking into account allele size differences were recently proposed to account statistically for these size constraints effects (Feldman *et al.* 1997; Pollock *et al.* 1998). These distances assume similar range constraints and mutation rates across loci (Feldman *et al.* 1997) or can incorporate variable range constraints and mutation rates across loci (Pollock *et al.* 1998). Methods of estimating single locus range constraints and mutation rates or $M=4N_e\mu$, when no information is available on the effective population size, have recently been developed under the assumptions of a SMM (Pollock *et al.* 1998; but see Estoup *et al.* 1994 for an alternative method for the estimation of M)

- *Loci with atypical mutation processes.* Although distances taking into account allele size differences were derived assuming a strict SMM, their linearity with time was shown to be independent of the assumptions of both single-repeat mutation steps and symmetry in the mutation rate (Kimmel *et al.* 1996). However, loci with frequent large mutational changes will have a larger coefficient of variation (Zhivotovsky & Feldman 1995), and thus tend to be less suited for distance calculation and should be avoided.

- *Temporal changes of the evolutionary rate and pattern related to molecular structure.* Over long time periods, substantial structural changes can potentially occur in the repeated region of a given microsatellite locus (Garza *et al.* 1995; Primmer & Ellegren 1998). For loci showing substantial variation in their evolutionary rate across taxa it may be essential to sequence at least a few alleles in different taxa to verify that the repeated motifs have not been interrupted by imperfections (Goldstein & Pollock 1997). Sequencing of alleles is also advisable for loci showing changing patterns of allele size variation. This would serve to verify that the molecular structure of these loci is not heterogeneous across taxa arising for example from the presence of regions with cryptic size variation and/or birth of derivative repeat motifs (Angers & Bernatchez 1997; Primmer & Ellegren 1998). Whatever the origin, loci showing marked changes in evolutionary rate and pattern across populations should be avoided.

Even if these three critical characteristics are not taken into account, increasing the number of microsatellite loci in a phylogenetic reconstruction should reduce the variance of genetic distances and extend their linearity with time. However, the resolving power will be increased most by selectively adding those loci with the greatest accuracy (Pollock *et al.* 1998), including for example SMM microsatellites with large allelic range, low mutation rates and consistent evolutionary rates. We propose a comprehensive and practical methodology aiming at selecting a set of microsatellite loci that will optimize phylogeny reconstruction between distantly related populations. This methodology is summarized in Fig. 3. Step 1 relates to the evolutionary features associated with the molecular structures of microsatellites (see section 3.3.). This simple pre-selection step should increase the proportion of appropriate loci prior to any typing tests. It is difficult to estimate the number of short perfect markers required at step 1 to allow for a final set of at least 25 selected markers for the phylogenetic reconstruction step. However, it is likely that at least 50 short perfect loci will be necessary. It might appear that the costly and labour-intensive cloning and pre-typing steps (steps 1 to 4) are prohibitive, but recent improvements in cloning procedures and automation of genotyping should facilitate these additional steps. This is particularly true when the organism under study is associated with a genome mapping project from which extremely large quantities of microsatellite loci are available (reviewed in Pollock *et al.* 1998). Pilot-studies on such organisms could be achieved in order to (i) estimate experimentally the benefit in term of resolution associated with the suggested choice of loci and (ii) detect molecular features allowing *a priori* selection of microsatellites. For instance, microsatellites with particular repeat size and/or composition may tend to be characterized by suitable range constraints and/or mutation rates (Pollock *et al.* 1998). In any case, the generalization of these results to other organisms may be questionable. Moreover, different categories of loci may tend to follow particular mutation processes, but the variance within each category will be so high that characterization of pre-selected loci will still be necessary. Nevertheless, such pilot studies may be useful to pre-enrich the initial set of markers with a larger proportion of useful loci (before step 1 of Fig. 3).

5.4.3. *Phylogenetic reconstruction among populations with various levels of divergence*

When no information is available on the level of divergence among populations under study, phylogenetic reconstruction often includes populations related by various levels of divergence. In this case, it may be appropriate to use distances taking into account allele size differences after having implemented the locus selection procedure (Fig. 3), but selected loci should have intermediate instead of low mutation rates. In this case, it may be appropriate to first use classical distances (*e.g.* Cavalli-Sforza & Edwards 1967; Nei *et al.* 1983) to construct a tree topology. Branch length estimation calculated with a distance measure taking allele size differences into account can then be imposed on this topology (Takezaki & Nei 1996). This method is illustrated in a phylogenetic study of 26 natural populations of brook charr (*Salvelinus fontinalis*) including closely related populations clustering into divergent genetic groups (Angers & Bernatchez 1998). The tree obtained using this method provides (i) a more reliable topology than a tree based on distances that incorporate allele size differences and (ii) a more accurate estimation of branch lengths than a tree based on the distance of Cavalli-Sforza & Edwards (1967). In particular, the important difference between genetic variances within and among groups as estimated from hierarchical F_{st} and ρ_{ST} is better depicted by branch lengths calculated by distances taking allele size differences into account.

Step 1: Pre-selection on cloned sequences:
→ *Remove compound loci with stretch of different repeat length (heterogeneity in the allelic size changes)*
→ *Avoid interrupted loci (higher risk of evolutionary rate changes across taxa than with perfect loci)*
→ *Select perfect loci with number of repeats < 20 (higher probability of low mutation rate)*

Step 2: Statistical test for conformance to the SMM:
- *Data*: allele size distribution in a single population sample ($N \geq 30$)
- *Methods*: test on several population x locus parameters
      - Heterozygosity or number of alleles (Estoup *et al.* 1994)
      - Variance of allele size (DiRienzo *et al.* 1994; J-M Cornuet, pers. com.)
→ *Remove loci showing strong deviation from the SMM*

Step 3: Estimation of the mutation rate from the parameter M $=4N_e\mu$:
- *Data*: allele size distribution in a single population sample ($N \geq 30$); (data set used for step 2)
- *Methods*:
- Estimate M from the number of alleles in a sample of a given size (Estoup *et al.* 1994; Cornuet & Luikart 1996)
- Estimate M from the variance of the repeat count (Moran 1975; Pollock *et al.* 1998)
→ *Select loci with small values of M and hence small mutation rates*

Step 4: Estimation of the allelic range (R):
- *Data*: Small number of divergent taxa (3-6) with 5 to 10 individuals typed per taxon (Pollock *et al.* 1998)
- *Method*: Estimate R from the difference between the observed maximum and minimum repeat counts among all taxa (Pollock *et al.* 1998)
→ *Select loci with large R*

Step 5: Typing of population samples for phylogenetic inference:
→ *number of diploid individuals per population and number of loci both ≥ 25* (Takezaki & Nei 1996)

Step 6: Detection of changes in evolutionary rate and pattern across taxa (*eg.* occurrence of stabilising interruption(s) or change of repeat unit type):
- *Data*: identification of loci with substantial differences in the amount and/or distribution of allelic variation (*e.g.* occurrence of different allele size change) across taxa, and sequencing of at least one allele in different taxa for these loci
→ *Remove loci with substantial evolutionary/structural changes* across *taxa*

Step 7: Detection of non-equilibrium populations *i.e.* populations which suffered from a recent and strong effective population size fluctuation:
- *Data* produced at step 5
- *Method*: detection of global deficit or excess of heterozygosity assuming a SMM (cf. removal of non-SMM loci at step 1) (Cornuet & Luikart 1996)
→ *Remove non-equilibrium populations*

Step 8: Construction of phylogenetic tree (Neighbor-Joining procedure, but see Hillis, this volume for other procedures) **and/or estimation of time of divergence across taxa** computing the following genetic distances from the set of ≥ 25 loci (and populations) selected after step 6 (and step 7) :
- D_L (Feldman *et al.* 1997) when range constraints and M values are both similar or when M values are similar and R values vary substantially
- D_{GLS} (Pollock *et al.* 1998) when range constraints and M values both vary substantially or when range constraints are similar and M values vary substantially

Figure 3: Suggested methodology for the selection of microsatellite loci for phylogenetic studies among distantly related populations and subspecies, and from different species.

6. Conclusions and future prospects

This chapter provides an overview of the recent developments concerning VNTR sequences in molecular ecology. More specifically, it aims to illustrate why VNTRs are such valuable markers in molecular systematics, population genetics and ecology. Microsatellite loci present significant advantages over minisatellites, and it is likely that the bias in favour of studies based on microsatellite markers will still increase in the future.

Technical challenges associated with VNTR makers are still considerable, in particular the routine analysis of non-invasively sampled and museum material. A higher level of automation and an optimization of cloning procedures would also be useful as they would facilitate the study of larger number of loci and hence give more precise answers to numerous evolutionary questions.

Theoretical mutation models which more accurately represent the evolutionary processes of microsatellites are needed to obtain better estimates of population differentiation measures and demographic parameters inferred from within population variation. This is also vital to more precisely infer past-population history, in particular population expansion or reduction and hybridization between differentiated taxa. It is worth mentioning that the latest category of information, that is, the absence of substantial deviation from mutation-drift equilibrium, is in turn essential for phylogenetic inferences. A combination of large-scale studies on different evolutionary levels ranging from the family to the interspecific level, as well as direct statistical testing of models using population data should contribute to a better knowledge of the mutation processes. In particular, such analyses facilitate the formulation of predictive rules for some important evolutionary features (*e.g.* mutation rate, size constraints, proportion of large step mutations) in relation to certain molecular features of microsatellites (*e.g.* total length, size of repeats, presence of interruptions)

We proposed a comprehensive and practical methodology aimed at selecting a set of microsatellite loci that will optimize phylogeny reconstruction between distantly related populations (Fig. 3). Due to its costly and labour-intensive nature, this stringent methodology should be at present considered as an optimal approach. It should be first tested on organisms from which extremely large quantities of microsatellite loci are or will be available, for example, organisms associated with a genome mapping project. However, improvements in cloning procedures, automation of genotyping and a better knowledge of the mutational processes of microsatellites allowing *a priori* selection of loci should overcome some of these constraints.

In the short term, the most obvious applications of microsatellites in molecular ecology include studies at the individual level (genetic tagging, classification of individuals, reproduction structure, relatedness analysis and parentage assignment). The level of polymorphism of the markers is indeed the only factor of importance for most of these applications. Novel applications interfacing the individual and population levels and based on the mutational process of microsatellites were recently proposed. In particular, allele size variation at microsatellite loci was explored as a tool for measuring how inbred or outbred individuals are in the wild (Coulson *et al.* 1998; Coltman *et al.* 1998). Although this approach still needs to be theoretically formalized and empirically tested, it potentially opens new perspectives for investigating the fitness consequences of inbreeding and outbreeding in natural populations. Finally, because of their abundance and random spacing in the genome, microsatellites will also provide a powerful tool to study the selective forces acting on the genome in greater detail at both the individual and population level.

Acknowledgements

We thank David Goldstein, David Pollock, Paulo Prodöhl, and François Rousset for helpful discussions, Jérôme Buard and David Pollock for sharing unpublished MS, and Jacqui Shykoff and Julie Turgeon for their invaluable help in correcting our English. This chapter also benefited from the constructive comments of Gary Carvalho, Louis Bernatchez and two anonymous reviewers. This work was partly supported by the program "Recherches méthodologiques pour l'amélioration des processus de gestion et de conservation des ressources génétiques animales, végétales et microbiennes" of the Bureau des Ressources Génétiques for A.E., and by a French post-doctoral grant from INRA for B.A.

References

Amos W, Sawcer SJ, Feakes RW, Rubinzstein DC (1996) Microsatellites show directional bias and heterozygote instability. *Nature Genetics*, **13**, 390-391.

Amos W (1998) A comparative approach to the study of microsatellite evolution. In: *Microsatellites: Evolution and Applications*. (eds. Goldstein DB, Schlötterer C), Oxford University Press, Oxford, in press.

Angers B, Bernatchez L (1997) Complex evolution of a salmonid microsatellite locus and its consequences in inferring allelic divergence from size information. *Molecular Biology and Evolution*, **14**, 230-238.

Angers B, Bernatchez L (1998) Combined use of SMM and non-SMM methods to infer fine structure and evolutionary history of closely related brook charr (*Salvelinus fontinalis*, Salmonidae) populations from microsatellites. *Molecular Biology and Evolution*, **15**, 143-159.

Armour JAL, Povey S, Jeremiah S, Jeffreys AJ (1990) Systematic cloning of human minisatellites from ordered array Charomid libraries. *Genomics*, **8**, 501-512.

Armour JAL, Harris PC, Jeffreys AJ (1993) Allelic diversity at minisatellites MS205 (D16S309): evidence for polarized variability. *Human Molecular Genetics*, **2**, 1137-1145.

Armour JAL (1996) Tandemly repeated minisatellites: generating human diversity via recombinational mechanisms. In: *Human Genome Evolution* (eds. M Jackson, T Strachan, G Dover). BIOS Scientific Publishers, Oxford.

Armour JAL, Alonso Alegre S, Miles S, Williams LJ, Badge RM (1998) Minisatellites and mutation processes in tandemly repetitive DNA. In: *Microsatellites: Evolution and Applications*, (eds. Goldstein DB, Schlötterer C), Oxford University Press, Oxford, in press.

Avise JC (1994) *Molecular Markers, Natural History and Evolution.* Chapman & Hall, London UK.

Barker JFS, Moore SS, Hetzel DJS, Evans D, Tan SG, Byrne K (1997) Genetic diversity of Asian water buffalo (*Bubalus bubalis*): microsatellite variation and a comparison with protein-coding loci. *Animal Genetics*, **28**, 103-115.

Bartley D, Bagley M, Gall G, Bentley B (1992) Use of linkage disequilibrium data to estimate effective size of hatchery and natural fish populations. *Conservation Biology*, **6**, 365-375.

Beckman JS, Weber JL (1992) Survey of human and rat microsatellites. *Genomics*, **12**, 627-631.

Bell GI, Selby MJ, Rutter WJ (1982) The highly polymorphic region near the human insulin gene is composed of simple tandemly repeating sequences. *Nature*, **7**, 31-35.

Beridze T (1986) *Satellite DNA*. Springer-Verlag, Berlin.

Blouin MS, Parsons M, Lacaille V, Lotz S (1996) Use of microsatellite loci to classify individuals by relatedness. *Molecular Ecology*, **5**, 393-401.

Bowcock AM, Ruiz-Linares A, Tomfohrde J, Minch E, Kidd JR, Cavalli-Sforza LL (1994) High resolution of human evolutionary trees with polymorphic microsatellites. *Nature*, **368**, 455-457.

Brookfield JFY, Parkin DT (1993) Use of single-locus probes in the establishment of relatedness in wild populations. *Heredity*, **70**, 660-663.

Browne DL, Litt M (1992) Characterization of (CA)n microsatellites with degenerate sequencing primers. *Nucleic Acids Research*, **20**, 141.

Buard J, Bourdet A, Yardley J, Dubrova Y, Jeffreys AJ (1998) Influences of array size and homogeneity on minisatellite mutation. *EMBO Journal*, **17**, 3495-3502.

Caballero A (1994) Developments in the prediction of effective population size. *Heredity*, **73**, 657-679.

Callen DF, Thompson AD, Shen Y, Phillips HA *et al.* (1993) Incidence and origin of "null" alleles in the (AC)n microsatellite markers. *American Journal of Human Genetics*, **52**, 922-927.

Cavalli-Sforza LL, Edwards AWF (1967) Phylogenetic analysis: models and estimation procedures. *American Journal of Human Genetics*, **19**, 233-257.

Chakraborty R, Jin L (1993) A unified approach to study hypervariable polymorphisms: statistical considerations of determining relatedness and population distances. In *DNA fingerprinting: State of the Science*. (eds. Pena SDJ, Chakraborty R, Epplen JT Jeffreys AJ). Birkhauser Verlag Basel/Switzerland.

Chakraborty R, Zhong Y (1993) Statistical power of an exact test of Hardy-Weinberg proportions of genotypic data at a multiallelic locus. *Human Heredity.* **44**, 1-9.

Chakraborty R, Kimmel M, Stivers DN, Davison J, Deka R (1997) Relative mutation rates at di-, tri-, and tetranucleotide microsatellite loci. *Proceedings of the National Academy of Sciences USA,* **94**, 1041-1046.

Chung MY, Ranum MPW, Duvick LA, Servadio A, Zoghbi HY, Orr HT (1993) Evidence for a mechanism predisposing to intergenerational CAG repeat instability in spinocerebellar ataxia type I. *Nature Genetics,* **5**, 254-258.

Cockerham CC, Weir B (1993) Estimation of gene flow from F-statistics. *Evolution,* **47**, 855-863.

Coltman DW, Bowen WD, Wright JM (1998) Birth weight and neonatal survival of harbour seal pups are positively correlated with genetic variation measured by microsatellites. *Proceedings of the Royal Society, London,* B, in press.

Cornuet J-M, Aulagnier S, Lek S, Franck P, Solignac M (1996) Classifying individuals among infra-specific taxa using microsatellite data and neural network. *Comptes Rendus de l'Académie des Sciences,* **319**, 1167-1177.

Cornuet J-M, Luikart G (1996) Description and power analysis of two tests for detecting recent population bottlenecks from allele frequency data. *Genetics,* **144**, 2001-2014.

Coulson T, Pemberton J, Albon S, *et al.* (1998) Microsatellites reveal heterosis in red deer. *Proceedings of the Royal Society, London,* B, in press.

Crawford AM, Kappes SM, Paterson KA *et al.* (1998) Microsatellite evolution: testing the ascertainment bias hypothesis. *Journal of Molecular Evolution,* **46**, 256-260.

Crow JF, Kimura M (1970) *An Introduction to Population Genetics Theory.* Harper and Row, New-York, Evanston and London.

Crow JF, Aoki K (1984) Group selection for a polygenic behavioral trait: estimating the degree of population subdivision. *Proceedings of the National Academy of Sciences of the USA,* **81**, 6073-6077.

Crozier RH, Oldroyd BP, Tay WT(1997) Molecular advances in understanding social insect population structure. *Electrophoresis,* **18**, 1672-1675.

Dallas JF (1992) Estimation of microsatellite mutation rates in recombinant inbred strains of mouse. *Mammalian Genome,* **3**, 452-456.

Danzmann RG (1997) PROBMAX: a computer program for assigning unknown parentage in pedigree analysis from known genotypic pools of parents and progeny. *Journal of Heredity,* **88**, 333.

de Pancorbo MM, Rodriguez-Alarcon J, Castro A *et al.* (1997) Newborn genetic identification: a protocol using microsatellite DNA as an alternative to footprinting. *Clinica Chimica Acta,* **4**, 33-42.

Dib C, Fauré S, Fizames C, Samson D *et al*, (1996) A comprehensive genetic map of the human genome based on 5,264 microsatellites. *Nature,* **380**, 152-154.

Dietrich WF, Miller JC, Steen RG *et al.* (1994) A genetic map of the mousse with 4,006 simple sequence length polymorphism. *Nature Genetics,* **7**, 220-255.

DiRienzo A, Peterson AC, Garza JC, Valdes AM, Slatkin M, Freimer NB (1994) Mutational processes of simple-sequence repeat loci in human populations. *Proceedings of the National Academy of Sciences USA,* **91**, 3166-3170.

Edwards A, Civitello A, Hammond HA, Caskey, CT (1991) DNA typing and genetic mapping with trimeric and tetrameric tandem repeats. *American Journal of Human Genetics,* **49**, 746-756.

Ellegren H (1991) DNA typing of museum birds. *Nature,* **14**, 113.

Ellegren H Primmer CR, Sheldon BC (1995) Microsatellite evolution: directionality or bias. *Nature Genetics,* **11**, 360-362.

Ellegren H, Savolainen P, Rosen B (1996) The genetical history of an isolated population of the endangered grey wolf *Canis lupus*: a study of nuclear and mitochondrial polymorphisms. *Philosophical Transactions of the Royal Society of London B,* **29**, 1661-1669

Ellegren H, Moore S, Robinson N, Byrne K, Ward W, Sheldon BC (1997) Microsatellite evolution: a reciprocal study of repeat lengths at homologous loci in cattle and sheep. *Molecular Biology and Evolution,* **14**, 854-860.

Ender A, Schwenk K, Stadler T, Streit B, Schierwater B (1996) RAPD identification of microsatellites in Daphnia. *Molecular Ecology,* **5**, 437-441.

Estoup A, Solignac M, Harry M, Cornuet, J-M (1993) Characterization of (GT)n and (CT)n microsatellites in two insect species: *Apis mellifera* and *Bombus terrestris. Nucleic Acids Research,* **21**, 1427-1431.

Estoup A, Solignac M, Cornuet J-M (1994) Precise assessment of the number of patrilines and of genetic relatedness in honey bee colonies. *Proceedings of the Royal Society of London,* B, **258**, 1-7.

Estoup A, Tailliez C, Cornuet J-M, Solignac, M (1995a) Size homoplasy and mutational processes of interrupted microsatellites in two bee species, *Apis mellifera* and *Bombus terrestris* (Apidae). *Molecular Biology and Evolution,* **12**, 1074-1084.

Estoup A, Garnery L, Solignac M, Cornuet, J-M (1995b) Microsatellite variation in honey bee (*Apis mellifera* L.) populations: hierarchical genetic structure and test of the infinite allele and stepwise mutation models.

Genetics, **140**, 679-695.

Estoup A, Scholl A, Pouvreau A, Solignac M (1995c) Monoandry and polyandry in bumble bees (Hymenoptera, Bombinae) as evidenced by highly variable microsatellites. *Molecular Ecology*, **4**, 89-93.

Estoup A, Cornuet J-M (1998) Microsatellite evolution: inferences from population data. In: *Microsatellites: Evolution and Applications*. (eds. Goldstein DB, Schlötterer C), Oxford University Press, Oxford, in press.

Estoup A, Rousset F, Michalakis Y, Cornuet J-M, Adriamanga M, Guyomard R (1998a) Comparative analysis of microsatellite and allozyme markers: a case study investigating microgeographic differentiation in brown trout (*Salmo Trutta*). *Molecular Ecology*, **7**, 339-353.

Estoup A, Gharbi K, SanCristobal M, Chevalet C, Haffray P, Guyomard R (1998b) Parentage assignment using microsatellites in turbot (*Scophtalmus maximus*) and rainbow trout (*Oncorhynchus mykiss*) hatchery populations. *Canadian Journal of Fisheries and Aquatic Sciences*, **57**, 715-723.

Excoffier L, Smouse PE, Quattro JM (1992) Analysis of molecular variance inferred from metric distances among DNA haplotytpe: application to human mitochondrial DNA restriction data. *Genetics*, **131**, 479-491.

Evans JD (1993) Parentage analyses in ant colonies using simple sequence repeat loci. *Molecular Ecology*, **2**, 293-297.

Evans JD (1995) Relatedness threshold for the production of female sexuals in colonies of a polygynous ant, *Myrmica tahoensis*, as revealed by microsatellite DNA analysis. *Proceedings of the National Academy of Sciences of the USA*, **92**, 6514-6517.

Feldman MW, Bergman A, Pollock DD, Goldstein DB (1997) Microsatellite genetic distances with range constraints: analytic description and problems of estimation. *Genetics*, **145**, 207-216.

Frankham R (1995) Conservation genetics. *Annual Reviews of Genetics*, **29**, 305-327.

Freimer NB, Slatkin M (1996) Microsatellites: evolution and mutational processes. In: *Variation in the human genome*, (eds, D. Chadwick, G. Cardew),. pp. 51-72. Wiley, Chichester.

Galeotti P, Pilastro A, Tavecchia G, Bonetti A, Congiu L (1997) Genetic similarity in long-eared owl communal winter: a DNA fingerprinting study. *Molecular Ecology*, **6**, 429-435.

Garza JC, Slatkin M, Freimer NB (1995) Microsatellite allele frequencies in humans and chimpanzees, with implications for constraints on allele size. *Molecular Biology and Evolution*, **12**, 594-603.

Garza JC, Freimer NB (1996) Homoplasy for size at microsatellite loci in humans and chimpanzees. *Genome Research*, **6**, 211-217.

Gastier JM, Pulido JC, Sunden S *et al.* (1995) Survey of trinucleotide repeats in the human genome: assessment of their utility as genetic markers. *Human Molecular Genetics*, **4**, 1829-1836.

Gilbert DA, Lehman N, O'Brien SJ, Wayne RK (1990) Genetic fingerprinting reflects population differentiation in the California Channel Island fox. *Nature*, **344**, 764-767.

Gilbert DA, Packer C, Pusey AE, Stephens JC, O'Brien SJ (1991) Analytical DNA fingerprinting in lions: parentage , genetic diversity and kindship. *Journal of Heredity*, **82**, 378-386.

Goldstein DB, Clark GK (1995) Microsatellite variation in north american populations of *Drosophila melanogaster*. *Nucleic Acids Research*, **23**, 3882-3886.

Goldstein DB, Linares AR, Feldman MW, Cavalli-Sforza LL (1995a) An evaluation of genetic distances for use with microsatellite loci. *Genetics*, **139**, 463-471.

Goldstein DB, Linares AR, Feldman MW, Cavalli-Sforza LL (1995b) Genetic absolute dating based on microsatellites and the origin of modern humans. *Proceedings of the National Academy of Sciences, USA*, **92**, 6723-6727.

Goldstein DB, Pollock DD (1997) Launching microsatellites: a review of mutation processes and methods of phylogenetic inference. *Journal of Heredity*, **88**, 335-342.

Goodman SJ (1997) *R*st Calc: a collection of computer programs for calculating estimates of genetic differentiation from microsatellite data and determining their significance. *Molecular Ecology*, **6**, 881-885.

Goudet J, Raymond M, de Meeüs T, Rousset F (1996) Testing differentiation in diploid populations. *Genetics*, **144**, 1933-1940.

Grimaldi MC, Crouau-Roy B (1997) Microsatellite allelic homoplasy due to variable flanking sequences. *Journal of Molecular Evolution*, **44**, 336-340.

Hamada H, Kakunaga T (1992) Potential Z-DNA forming sequences are highly dispersed in the human genome. *Nature*, **352**, 427-429.

Hantula J, Dusabenyagasani M, Hamelin RC (1996) Random amplified microsatellites (RAMS): a novel method for characterizing genetic variation within fungi. *European Journal of Forest Pathology*, **26**, 159-166.

Henderson, ST Petes, TD (1992) Instability of simple sequence DNA in *Saccharomyces cerevisiae*. *Molecular Cell Biology*, **12**, 2749-2757.

Hill WG (1981) Estimation of effective population size from data on linkage disequilibrium. *Genetical Research (Cambridge)*, **38**, 209-216.

Hite JM, Eckert KA, Cheng KC (1996) Factors affecting fidelity of DNA synthesis during PCR amplification of d(C-A)n d(G-T)n microsatellite repeats. *Nucleic Acid Research*, **24**, 2429-2434.

Jarne P, Lagoda JL (1996) Microsatellites, from molecules to populations and back. *Trends in Ecology and Evolution*, **11**, 424-429.

Jeffreys AJ, Wilson V, Thein SL (1985a) Hypervariable 'minisatellite' regions in human DNA. *Nature*, **314**, 67-74.

Jeffreys AJ, Wilson V, Thein SL (1985b) Individual-specific 'fingerprints' of human DNA. *Nature*, **316**, 76-79.

Jeffreys AJ, Royle NJ, Wilson V, Wong Z (1988) Spontaneous mutation rates to new length alleles at tandem-repetitive hypervariable loci in human DNA. *Nature*, **332**, 278-281.

Jeffreys AJ, Neumann R, Wilson V (1990) Repeat unit sequence variation in minisatellites: a novel source of DNA polymorphism for studying variation and mutation by single molecule analysis. *Cell*, **60**, 473-485.

Jeffreys AJ, MacLeod A, Tamaki K, Neil DL, Monckton DG (1991) Minisatellite repeat coding as a digital approach to DNA typing. *Nature*, **354**, 204-209.

Jeffreys AJ, Tamaki K, MacLeod A, Monckton DG, Neil DL, Armour JAL (1994) Complex gene conversion events in germline mutation at human minisatellites. *Nature Genetics*, **6**, 136-145.

Jeffrey AJ, Neuman R (1997) Somatic mutation processes at a human minisatellite. *Human Molecular Genetics*, **56**, 65-76.

Jin L, & Chakraborty R (1995) Population structure, stepwise mutation, heterozygote deficiency and their implications in DNA forensics. *Heredity*, **74**, 274-285.

Jin L, Macaubas C, Hallmayer J, Kimura A, Mignot E (1996) Mutation rate varies among alleles at a microsatellite locus: phylogenetic evidence. *Proceedings of the National Academy of Sciences USA*, **93**, 15285-15288.

Jorde PE, Ryman N (1995) Temporal allele frequency change and estimation of effective size in populations with overlapping generations. *Genetics*, **139**, 1077-1090.

Jorde PE, Ryman N (1996) Demographic genetics of brown trout (*Salmo trutta*) and estimation of effective population size from temporal change of allele frequencies. *Genetics*, **143**, 1369-1381.

Kashi Y, King D, Soller M (1997). Simple sequence repeats as a source of quantitative genetic variation. *Trends in Genetics*, **13**, 74-78.

Kashi Y, Soller M (1998) Functional roles of microsatellites and minisatellites. In: *Microsatellites: Evolution and Applications*, (eds. Goldstein DB, Schlötterer C), Oxford University Press, Oxford, in press.

Kijas JMH, Fowler JCS, Garbett CA, Thomas MR (1994) Enrichment of microsatellites from the citrus genome using biotinylated oligonucleotide sequences bound to streptavidin-coated magnetic particles. *BioTechniques*, **16**, 657-662.

Kimmel M, Chakraborty R (1996). Measures of variation at DNA repeat loci under a general stepwise mutation model. *Theoretical Population Biology*, **50**, 345-367.

Kimmel M, Chakraborty R, Stivers, DN, Deka R (1996) Dynamics of repeat polymorphisms under a forward-backward mutation model: within- and between-population variability at microsatellite loci. *Genetics*, **143**, 549-555.

Kimura M, Crow, JF (1964) The number of alleles that can be maintained in a finite population. *Genetics*, **49**, 725-738.

Kimura M, Ohta T (1978) Stepwise mutation model and distribution of allelic frequencies in a finite population. *Proceedings of the National Academy of Sciences USA*, **75**, 2868-2872.

Koch JE, Kolvraa S, Petersen KB, Gregersen N, Bolund L (1989) Oligonucleotide-priming methods for the chromosome-specific labelling of alpha satellite DNA *in situ. Chromosoma*, **98**, 259-265.

Kuhner MK, Yamato J, Felsenstein J (1995) Estimating effective population size and mutation rate from sequence data using Metropolis-Hastings sampling. *Genetics*, **140**, 1421-1430.

Lagercrantz U, Ellegren H, Andersson L (1993) The abundance of various polymorphic microsatellite motifs differs between plants and vertebrates. *Nucleic Acids Research*, **21**, 1111-1115.

Lehmann T, Hawley WA, Grebert H, Collins FH (1998) The effective population size of *Anopheles gambia* in Kenya: implications for population structure. Molecular Biology and Evolution, *15*, 264-276.

Levinson G, Gutman GA (1987) Slipped-strand mispairing: a major mechanism for DNA sequence evolution. *Molecular Biology and Evolution*, **4**, 203-221.

Luikart G, Cornuet J-M (1998) Empirical evaluation of a test for identifying recently bottleneck populations from allele frequency data. *Conservation Biology*, **12**, 228-237.

Lynch M (1991) Analysis of population genetic structure by DNA fingerprinting. In: *DNA Fingerprinting: Approaches and Applications* (eds. Burke T, Dolf G, Jeffreys AJ, Wolff R), pp. 113-126. Birkhäuser Verlag, Boston.

Marshall TC, Slate J, Kruuk LEB, Pemberton JM (1998) Statistical confidence for likelihood-based paternity inference in natural populations. *Molecular Ecology*, **7**, 639-655.

May CA, Jeffreys AJ, Armour JAL (1996) Mutation rate heterogeneity and the generation of allele diversity at the human minisatellite MS205 (D16S309). *Human Molecular Genetics*, **5**, 1823-1833.

Meagher TP, Thompson EA (1986) The relationship between single parent and parent pair genetic likelihoods in genealogy reconstruction. *Theoretical Population Biology*, **29**, 87-106.

Meagher TP. Thompson EA (1987) Analysis of parentage for naturally established seedlings of *Chamaelirium luteum* (Liliaceae). *Ecology*, **68**, 803-813.

Meloni R, Albanese V, Ravassard P, Treilhou F, Mallet J (1998) A tetranucleotide polymorphic microsatellite, located in the first intron of the tyrosine hydroxylase gene, acts as a transcription regulatory element *in vitro*. *Human Molecular Genetics*, **7**, 423-428.

Michalakis Y, Excoffier L (1996) A generic estimation of population subdivision using distances between alleles with special reference for microsatellite loci. *Genetics*, **142**, 1061-1064.

Michalakis Y, Veuille M (1996) Length variation of CAG/CAA trinucleotide repeats in natural populations of *Drosophila melanogaster* and its relation to the recombination rate. *Genetics*, **143**, 1713-1725.

Miller LM, Kapuscinski, AR (1997) Historical analysis of genetic variation reveals low effective population size in a northern pike (*Esox lucius*) population. *Genetics*, **147**, 1249-1258.

Monckton GG, Neumann R, Guram T *et al.* (1994) Minisatellite mutation rate variation associated with a flanking DNA sequence polymorphism. *Nature Genetics*, **8**, 162-170.

Morin PA, Wallis J, Moore JJ, Woodruff DS (1994) Paternity exclusion in a community of wild chimpanzees using hypervariable simple sequence repeats. *Molecular Ecology*, **5**, 469-478.

Moritz C (1994) Application of mitochondrial DNA analysis in conservation: a critical review. *Molecular Ecology*, **3**, 401-411.

Moritz C (1995) Uses of molecular phylogenies for conservation. *Philosophical Transactions of the Royal Society of London B*, **348**, 113-118.

Mullis K, Faloona F, Scharf S, Saiki R, Horn G, Erlich HA (1986) Specific enzymatic amplification of DNA *in vitro*: the polymerase chain reaction. *Cold Spring Harbour Symposium Quantitative Biology*, **51**, 263-273.

Nauta MJ, Weissing, FJ (1996) Constraints on allele size at microsatellite loci: implications for genetic differentiation. *Genetics,* **143**, 1021-1032.

Nei M (1978) *Molecular Evolutionary Genetics*. Columbia University Press, New York.

Nei M, Tajima F (1981) Genetic drift and estimation effective population size. *Genetics*, **98**, 625-640.

Nei M, Tajima F, Tateno Y (1983) Accuracy of estimated phylogenetic trees from molecular data. *Journal of Molecular Evolution*, **19**, 153-170.

Nielsen EE, Hansen MM, Loeschke,V (1997) Analysis of microsatellite DNA from old samples of Atlantic salmon *Salmo salar*: a comparison of genetic composition over 60 years. *Molecular Ecology*, **6**, 487-492.

Nielsen R (1997) A likelihood approach to populations samples of microsatellite alleles. *Genetics*, **146**, 711-716.

Nishikawa N, Oishi M, Kiyama R (1995) Construction of a human genomic library of clones containing poly(dG-dA).poly(dT-dC) tracts by Mg(2+)-dependent triplex affinity capture. DNA polymorphism associated with the tracts. *Journal of Biology and Chemistry*, **21**, 9258-9264.

Olaisen B, Stenersen M, Mevag B (1997) Identification by DNA analysis of the victims of the August 1996 Spitsbergen civil aircraft disaster. *Nature Genetics*, **15**, 402-405.

O'Reilley P, Wright JM (1995), The evolving technology of DNA fingerprinting and its application to fisheries and aquaculture. *Journal of Fish Biology*, **47** (Suppl. A), 29-55.

Orti G, Pears DE, Avise JC (1997) Phylogenetic assessment of length variation at a microsatellite locus. *Proceedings of the National Academy of Sciences USA*, **94**, 10745-10749.

Ostrander EA, Jong PM, Rine J, Duyk G (1992) Construction of small-insert genomic DNA libraries enriched for microsatellite repeat sequences. *Proceedings of the National Academy of Sciences USA*, **89**, 3415-3423.

Ostrander EA, Sprague GF Jr, Rine J (1993) Identification and characterization of dinucleotide repeat (CA)n markers for genetic mapping in dog. *Genomics,* **16**, 207-213.

Ott J, Rabinowitz D (1997) The effect of marker heterozygosity on the power to detect linkage dissequilibrium. *Genetics*, **147**, 927-930.

Paetkau D, Calvert W, Stirling I, Strobeck C (1995) Microsatellite analysis of population structure in Canadian polar bears. *Molecular Ecology*, **4**, 347-354.

Paetkau D, Strobeck C (1995) The molecular basis and evolutionary history of a microsatellite null allele in bears. *Molecular Ecology*, **4**, 519-520.

Palsboll PJ, Allen J, Bérudé M *et al.* (1997) Genetic tagging of humpback whales. *Nature*, **388**, 767-769.

Pépin L, Amigues Y, Lépingle A, Berthier JL, Bensaid A, Vaiman D (1995) Sequence conservation of microsatellites between cattle (*Bos taurus*), goat (*Capra hircus*) and related species. Examples of use in parentage testing and phylogeny analysis. *Heredity*, **74**, 53-61.

Peters JM, Queller DC, Strassmann JE, Solis CR (1995) Maternity assignment and queen replacement in social wasp. *Proceedings of the Royal Society of London B*, **260**, 7-12.

Petes TD, Greenwell, PW, Dominska M (1997) Stabilization of microsatellite sequences by variant repeats in the yeast *Saccharomyces cerevisiae*. *Genetics*, **146**, 491-498.

Piper WH, Rabenold PP (1992) Use of fragment-sharing estimates from DNA fingerprinting to determine relatedness in a tropical wren. *Molecular Ecology*, **1**, 69-78.

Pollock DD, Bergman A, Feldman MW, Goldstein DB (1998) Microsatellite behavior with range constraints: parameter estimation and improved distances for use in phylogenetic reconstruction. *Theoretical Population Biology*, in press.

Primmer CR, Ellegren H, Saino N, Moller AP (1996a) Directional evolution in germline microsatellite mutations. *Nature Genetics*, **13**, 391-393.

Primmer CR, Moller AP, Ellegren H (1996b) A wide-range survey of cross-species microsatellite amplification in birds. *Molecular Ecology*, **5**, 365-378.

Primmer CR, Ellegren H (1998) Patterns of molecular evolution in avian microsatellites. *Molecular Biology and Evolution*, in press.

Primmer CR, Saino N, Moller AP, Ellegren H (1998) Unravelling the processes of microsatellite evolution through analysis of germline mutations in barn swallows, *Hirundo rustica. Molecular Biology and Evolution*, in press.

Prödohl PA, Loughry WJ, McDonough CM, Nelson WS, Thompson EA, Avise JC (1998) Genetic maternity and paternity in a local population of armadillos assessed by microsatellite DNA markers and field data. *American Naturalist*, **151**, 7-19.

Pudovkin AI, Zaykin DV, Hedgecock D (1996) On the potential for estimating the effective number of breeders from heterozygote-excess in progeny. *Genetics*, **144**, 383-387.

Queller CR, Goodnight KF (1989) Estimating relatedness using genetic markers. *Evolution*, **43**, 258-259.

Queller CR, Strassmann JE, Hughes CR (1993) Microsatellites and kindship. *Trends in Evolution and Ecology*, **8**, 285-288.

Raymond M, Rousset F (1995) Population genetics software for exact test and ecumenicism. *Journal of Heredity*, **86**, 248-249.

Reich DE, Goldstein DB (1998) Genetic evidence for a paleolithic human population expansion in Africa. *Proceedings of the National Academy of Sciences USA*, **95**, 8119-8123.

Rico C, Rico I, Hewitt G (1996) 470 million years of conservation of microsatellite loci among fish species. *Proceedings of the Royal Society of London B*, **263**, 549-557.

Robertson A, Hill WG (1984) Deviations from Hardy-Weinberg proportions: sampling variances and use in estimation of inbreeding coefficients. *Genetics*, **107**, 703-718.

Rogers AR, Harpening H (1992) Population growth makes waves in the distribution of pairwise differences. *Molecular Biology and Evolution*, **9**, 552-569.

Ross KG, Krieger MJ, Shoemaker DD, Vargo EL, Keller L (1997) Hierarchical analysis of genetic structure in native fire ant populations: results from three classes of molecular markers. *Genetics*, **147**, 643-655.

Rousset F (1996) Equilibrium values of measures of population subdivision for stepwise mutation processes. *Genetics*, **142**, 1357-1362.

Rousset F, Raymond M (1995) Testing heterozygote excess and deficiency. *Genetics*, **140**, 1413-1419.

Rousset F, Raymond M (1997) Statistical analyses of population genetic data: new tools, old concepts. *Trends in Evolution and Ecology*, **12**, 313-317.

Roy MS, Girman DJ, Taylor AC, Wayne R. K (1994) The use of museum specimens to reconstruct the genetic variability and relationships of extinct populations. *Experientia*, **15**, 551-557.

Royle NJ, Clarkson RE, Wong Z, Jeffreys AJ (1988) Clustering of hypervariable minisatellites in the proterminal regions of human autosomes. *Genomics*, **3**, 352-360.

Rubinsztein DC, Amos W, Leggo *et al.* (1995a) Microsatellite evolution - evidence for directionality and variation in rate between species. *Nature Genetics*, **10**, 337-343.

Rubinsztein DC, Leggo J, Amos W (1995b) Microsatellites evolve more rapidly in humans than in chimpanzees. *Genomics*, **30**, 610-612.

Ryman N (1981) Conservation of genetics resources: experience from the brown trout (*Salmo trutta*). *Ecological Bulletin* (Stockholm), **99**, 147-151.

Saccheri IJ, Bruford MW (1993) DNA fingerprinting in a butterfly *Bicyclus anynana* (Satyridae). *Journal of Heredity*, **84**, 195-200.

Saiki RK, Bugawan TL, Horn GT, Mullis KB, Erlich HA (1986) Analysis of enzymatically amplified beta-globin and HLA-DQ alpha DNA with allele-specific oligonucleotide probes. *Nature*, **13**, 163-166.

Samadi, S, Erard, F, Estoup, A, Jarne P (1998). The influence of mutation, selection and reproductive systems on microsatellite variability: a simulation approach. *Genetical Research Cambridge*, **71**, 213-222.

SanCristobal M, Chevalet C (1997) Error tolerant parent identification from a finite set of individuals. *Genetical Research.* **70**, 53-62.

Schlötterer C, Amos W, Tautz, D (1991) Conservation of polymorphic simple sequences loci in cetacean species. *Nature*, **354**, 63-65.

Schlötterer C, Tautz D (1992) Slippage synthesis of simple sequence DNA. *Nucleic Acids Research*, **20**, 211-

215.

Schneider S, Kueffer J-M, Roessli D, Excoffier L (1997) Arlequin: a software for population genetic data analysis. Version 1.1. Genetics and Biometry Laboratory, Department. of Anthropology, University of Geneva.

Schug, M.D., Mackay, T.F.C. & Aquadro, C.F. (1997) Low mutation rates of microsatellite loci in *Drosophila melanogaster*. *Nature Genetics*, **15**, 99-102.

Scribner KT, Arntzen JW, Burke T. (1997) Effective number of breeding adults in *Bufo bufo* estimated from age-specific variation at minisatellite loci. *Molecular Ecology*, **6**, 701-712.

Sheffield VC, Weber JL, Buetox KH *et al.* (1995) A collection of tri- and tetranucleotide repeat markers used to generate high quality, high resolution human genome-wide linkage maps. *Human Molecular Genetics*, **4**, 1837-1844.

Shriver MD, Jin L, Chakraborty R, Boerwinkle E (1993) VNTR allele frequency distribution under the stepwise mutation model. *Genetics*, **134**, 983-993.

Signer EN, Gu F, Jeffreys, AJ (1996) A panel of VNTR markers in pigs. *Mammalian Genome*, **7**, 433-437.

Simberloff D (1988) The contribution of population and community biology to conservation science. *Annual Reviews of Ecology and Systematics*, **19**, 473-511.

Slade RW, Moritz C, Heideman A (1994) Multiple nuclear-gene phylogenies: application to pinnipeds and comparison with a mitochondrial DNA genephylogeny. *Molecular Biology and Evolution*, **11**, 341-356.

Slatkin M (1995) A measure of population subdivision based on microsatellite allele frequencies. *Genetics*, **139**, 457-462.

Slatkin M, Barton NH (1989) A comparison of three indirect methods for estimating average levels of gene flow. *Evolution*, **43**, 1349-1368

Strand M, Prolla TA, Liskay RM, Petes, TD (1993) Destabilization of tracts of simple repetitive DNA in yeast by mutations affecting DNA mismatch repair. *Nature*, **365**, 274-276.

Takezaki N, Nei M (1996) Genetic distances and reconstruction of phylogenetic trees from microsatellite DNA. *Genetics*, **144**, 389-399.

Taylor AC, Sherwin WB, Wayne RK (1994) Genetic variation of microsatellite loci in a bottlenecked species: the northern hairy-nosed wombat *Lasiorhinus krefftii. Molecular Ecology*, **3**, 277-290.

Taylor AC, Horsup A, Johnson CN, Sunnucks P, Sherwin B (1997) Relatedness structure detected by microsatellite analysis and attempted pedigree reconstruction in an endangered marsupial, the northern hairy-nosed wombat *Lasiorhinus krefftii. Molecular Ecology*, **6**, 9-19.

Valdes AM, Slatkin M, Freiner NB (1993) Allele frequencies at microsatellite loci: the stepwise mutation model revised. *Genetics,* **133**, 737-749.

Vergnaud G, Mariat D, Apiou F, Aurias A, Lathrop M, Lauthier V (1991). The use of synthetic tandem repeats to isolate new VNTR loci: cloning of a human hypermutable sequence. *Genomics,* **11**, 135-144.

Viard F, Franck P, Dubois M-P, Estoup A, Jarne P (1998) Variation of microsatellite size homoplasy across electromorphs, loci and populations in three invertebrate species. *Journal of Molecular Evolution*, **47**, 42-51.

Waples RS (1989) A generalized approach for estimating effective population size from temporal changes in allele frequency. *Genetics*, **121**, 379-391.

Wasser SK, Houston CS, Koehler GM, Cadd GG, Fain SR (1997) Techniques for application of faecal DNA methods to field studies of Ursids. *Molecular Ecology*, **6**, 1091-1097.

Weber JL (1990) Informativeness of human (dC-dA)n.(dG-dT)n polymorphisms. *Genomics,* **7**, 524-530.

Weber JL, Wong C (1993) Mutation of human short tandem repeats. *Human Molecular Genetics*, **2**, 1123-1128.

Weir BS, Cockerham CC (1984) Estimating *F*-statistics for the analysis of population structure. *Evolution*, **38**, 1358-1370.

Wenburg JK, Olsen JB, Bentzen P (1996) Multiplexed systems of microsatellites for genetic analysis in costal cutthroat trout (*Oncorhynchus clarki clarki*) and steelhead (*Oncorhynchus mykiss*). *Molecular Marine Biology and Biotechnology*, **5**, 273-283.

Wetton JH, Parkin DT (1997) A suite of falcon single-locus minisatellite probes: a powerful alternative to DNA fingerprinting. *Molecular Ecology*, **6**, 119-128.

Wilkie AOM, Higgs DR (1992) An unsually large (CA)n repeat in the region of divergence between subtelomeric alleles of human chromosome 16p. *Genomics*, **13**, 81-88.

Wintero AK, Fredholm M, Thomsen PD (1992) Variable (dG-dT)n.(dC-dA)n sequences in the porcine genome. *Genomics*, **12**, 281-288.

Wong Z, Wilson V, Jeffreys AJ, Thein SL (1986) Cloning a selected fragment from a human DNA 'fingerprint': isolation of an extremely polymorphic minisatellite. *Nucleic Acids Research*, **14**, 4605-4616.

Wright S (1951) The genetical structure of populations. *Annual Eugenics*, **15**, 323-354.

Zhivotovshy LA, Feldman MW (1995) Microsatellite variability and genetic distances. *Proceedings of the National Academy of Sciences USA,* **92**, 11549-52.

Ziegle JS, Su Y, Corcoran KP *et al.* (1992) Application of automated DNA sizing technology for genotyping microsatellite loci. *Genomics*, **14**, 1026-1031.

Advances in Molecular Ecology
G.R. Carvalho (Ed.)
IOS Press, 1998

Structure, Function and Dynamics of Microbial Communities: the Molecular Biological Approach

Gerard Muyzer

Max-Planck-Institute for Marine Microbiology, D-28359 Bremen, Germany
Present address: Netherlands Institute for Sea Research, Nl-1790 AB Den Burg (Texel),
The Netherlands. e-mail: gmuyzer@nioz.nl

Molecular biological methods, such as PCR, fluorescent *in situ* hybridization and DNA sequencing, are nowadays routinely used to detect and identify microorganisms in their natural environment and to explore microbial diversity. The use of these methods has become necessary, because it is now recognized that cultivation-based methods do not retrieve the enormous microbial diversity existing in nature. Although successful the molecular methods are not free from limitations and biases. This paper describes the potentials and problems of molecular methods, and gives examples of their application to study the structure, function, and dynamics of microbial communities. Regarding the limitations of both the microbiological as well as the molecular approach, I would argue for an integrated approach combining both approaches with a detailed investigation of environmental parameters, to fully understand the role of microbes in ecosystem functioning.

1. Introduction

For several reasons, microbial communities are ideal systems to study ecological concepts and to test hypotheses. Microorganisms play an important role in the cycling of geochemical elements, such as carbon, sulphur and nitrogen, and in the degradation and removal of pollutants. All metabolic processes, such as autotrophic and heterotrophic growth under both aerobic and anaerobic conditions, and the utilization of organic and inorganic carbon sources, are used within the microbial world. Furthermore, microbial communities can be easily manipulated. Toxic compounds can be added to these systems, in order to study their effects on the bacterial populations, which is difficult to do with macroecosystems for ethical reasons. In addition, the response time of bacterial populations on perturbations is fast, measured in seconds, minutes, or hours rather than in days, months or years, which is the case for macroecosystems, such as plant communities (Gwynfryn Jones 1996).

Although many papers have been published in journals dedicated to microbial ecology, microbial communities have seldom been studied in an ecological context. In 1986, Thomas Brock wrote a critical paper on microbial ecological research, stating that most studies to date did not fit the definition of microbial ecology, which describes the study of interrelationships between microorganisms and their living and nonliving environment (Atlas and Bartha 1987), because most studies used pure cultures, mixed cultures or involved viable counts. Although pure culture studies are necessary to obtain an insight into the physiology, biochemistry, and genetics of isolated microorganisms, the ecological relevance of the isolated strains has rarely been determined. It is now well recognized among microbiologists that only a small fraction of all bacteria in nature can be isolated in pure cultures (Giovannoni et al. 1990; Ward et al. 1990a,b). Comparison between the number of culturable bacteria and total cell counts showed that in most environments, such as seawater, freshwater, sediments, and soil, less than 1% can be cultured (summarized in Amann et al. 1995). Only for a habitat such as activated sludge was a maximum of 15% culturability obtained. This discrepancy is mainly caused by our inability to mimic the environmental conditions for growing most bacteria in the laboratory. Intrinsic interdependency of organisms upon each other, as in the case for endosymbionts, or bacteria living in consortia, most likely contribute to the observed low culturability typical of most studies. An additional problem in microbial ecological studies is the difficulty of species identification. Microorganisms are small, and in general, lack conspicuous morphological features. They have been grouped by their morphology, such as a coccoid, helical, vibroid, rod or curved shape, or by possessing a stalk, a sheath or appendages (Holt et al. 1994). However, classification on morphological traits mostly does not reflect evolutionary relationships between microorganisms. Another reason for the lack of 'real' ecological studies in microbiology is the absence of interaction between microbiologists and ecologists, as emphasized by Pedrós-Alió and Guerrero (1994).

To improve significantly our understanding of the role of microbial diversity in ecosystem functioning the following questions has to be addressed. Who is there? How many of them? Where are they located? What are they doing? How do populations respond to changing environmental conditions? What is the relationship between diversity and community stability? To answer these questions, we need other approaches, which complement the microbiological approach, to classify and identify microorganisms.

The development of techniques to analyse nucleic acids, DNA and RNA, allows us to study microbial diversity at a different level, the genetic level. Microorganisms are detected, identified, and enumerated by the analysis of genes. Although in principle every gene can be used, the 16S ribosomal RNA gene is an excellent molecular marker for this purpose, because (i) it is present in all organisms, (ii) it has conserved as well as variable sequence regions, which makes it possible to design general and specific primers and probes, (iii) it has sufficient sequence information for phylogenetic inference, and (iv) it is an important cellular compound, which facilitates detection. Furthermore, approximately 10,000 sequences are available from public nucleotide sequence databases, such as GenBank (Benson et al. 1997) and the RDP (Maidak et al. 1997), or are included in phylogenetic programs, such as ARB (Strunk et al. 1998). Woese (1987) and others used 16S rRNA sequences to study bacterial evolution, and created a phylogenetic framework for the identification of both culturable and non-culturable microorganisms. This *Tree of Life* consists of 3 domains, *Bacteria* (eubacteria), *Archaea* (archaebacteria), and *Eukarya* (eukaryotes) (Fig. 1). Phylogenetic relationships of microorganisms based on other molecular markers, such as the 23S rRNA, the elongation factor EF-Tu, or the ATPase - subunit, gave similar trees (Ludwig et al. 1998), which justifies the use of 16S rRNA sequences for phylogenetic inference.

Pace and co-workers (Olsen et al. 1986; Pace et al. 1986) were the first to realize that this phylogenetic framework of 16S rRNA sequences could also be used to design primers and probes, and to apply these to study microbes in their natural habitat. Fig. 2 shows a schematic diagram of the different steps in the application of molecular biological techniques to study the structure and function of microbial communities. The different techniques are discussed below, and their potentials and problems are highlighted. Emphasis will be placed on the use of genetic fingerprinting techniques to study population dynamics caused by daily and seasonal fluctuations or by environmental stress. Nearly all molecular microbial ecological studies start with the extraction of nucleic acids, DNA and

Figure 1: *Tree of Life* based on complete 16S rRNA sequences. The main groups in the domains *Eukarya* (eukaryotes), *Archaea* (archaebacteria), and *Bacteria* (eubacteria) are shown. The tree is produced with the ARB program developed by Strunk and coworkers (1998).

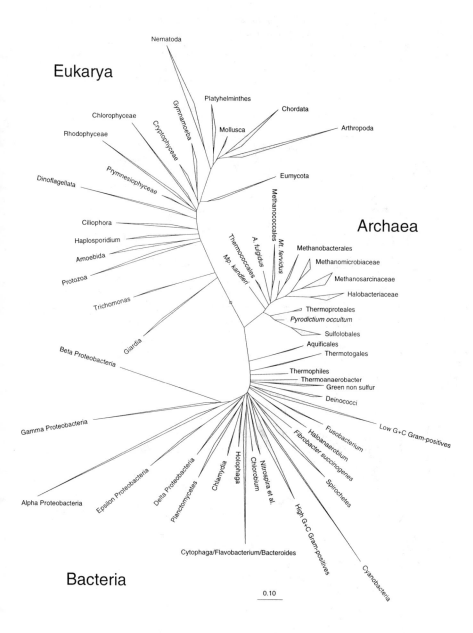

Figure 2: Flow diagram of the different steps in the application of molecular biological techniques to study the structure, function and dynamics of microbial communities. Nucleic acids are extracted from environmental samples, dislodged cells or from enrichment cultures, and subsequently examined using different methods to determine the presence (by analysing their DNA) or activity (by analysing their rRNA or mRNA) of microbial populations. Mixtures of PCR products obtained after enzymatic amplification of genomic DNA or reverse transcribed RNA (cDNA) can be analysed by cloning or genetic fingerprinting. Comparative analysis of cloned sequences or of sequenced DGGE bands will reveal the phylogenetic affiliation of the community members, and can be used to design taxon-specific oligonucleotide probes for fluorescence *in situ* hybridisation (FISH) or quantitative rRNA slot-blot hybridisation (rRNA-SBH). In addition, the fingerprinting techniques, can be used to monitor the isolation of ecologically relevant bacteria in pure cultures, and to screen clone libraries for redundancy. The complexity of the investigated microbial communities can be reduced by cell or genomic DNA fractionation.

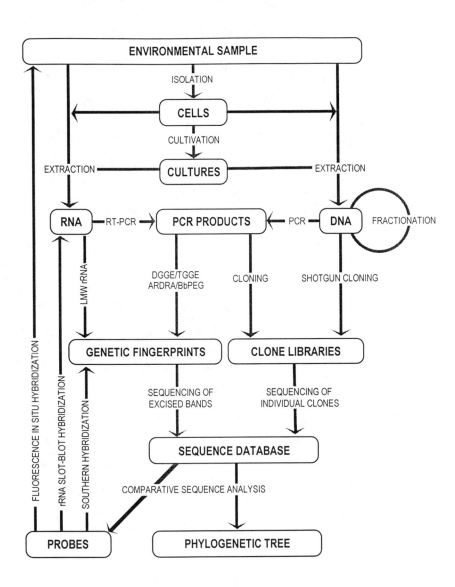

RNA, which are then further used as target molecules in, for instance, 'shotgun' cloning, LMW-RNA fingerprinting, rRNA slot-blot hybridization, or in the polymerase chain reaction (PCR; Saiki et al. 1988). The analysis of DNA can provide insights into the species composition or 'structure' of microbial communities, while the analysis of RNA, that is, rRNA and mRNA, may reveal the metabolic activity or 'function' of particular microbial populations. Apart from these 'cell destructive' approaches, there is the 'whole cell' or in situ hybridization approach using oligonucleotide probes labelled with an enzyme or fluorescent compound to enumerate bacterial cells by epifluorescence or bright-field microscopy, and to determine their spatial distribution in their natural environment.

2. Cloning of 16S rRNA encoding genes

So far, most of the molecular microbial ecological studies have focused on the exploration of microbial diversity by sequencing of cloned 16S rDNA fragments. For this purpose, DNA fragments, produced either by restriction digestion of genomic DNA, by reverse transcription of rRNA, or by PCR amplification of the 16S rRNA encoding genes, are ligated in a suitable vector, and introduced into E. coli host cells. Subsequently, the E. coli cell suspension is plated onto agar plates at a density to form individual colonies. Sequencing of the vector inserts, followed by comparative sequence analysis reveals the phylogenetic affiliation of the bacteria present in the environmental sample.

Schmidt et al. (1997) used the so-called 'shotgun' cloning approach to analyse the phylogenetic diversity of bacterioplankton in the north central Pacific Ocean. For this purpose, bacterial cells were collected from approx. 8,000 litres seawater by tangential flow filtration. Total genomic DNA was isolated from the cells, and subsequently digested in fragments with a restriction endonuclease. The fragments were size fractionated and cloned into the bacteriophage lambda vector. Filter replicates of the recombinant bacteriophage library plates were made, and hybridized with a radioactively-labelled, mixed-kingdom rRNA probe to screen for 16S rDNA inserts. By using this approach the authors obtained 16 unique rDNA clones out of 3.2×10^4 insert containing recombinants. Four sequences were affiliated to cyanobacterial sequences obtained from a similar study on picoplankton from the Atlantic Ocean (Giovannoni et al. 1990), and to two marine Synechococcus isolates. Eleven sequences belonged to different subdivisions of the class Proteobacteria, and one sequence was similar to the 16S rRNA sequence of a dinoflagellate. The disadvantage of this approach is that only a very low percentage (0.32%) of the clones contained 16S rDNA inserts, which makes extensive screening necessary. On the other hand, an important advantage is that in principle the complete genomic information of all bacteria in the environment is retrieved and enabling the study of additional genes (Pace 1997).

Ward and co-workers (Weller & Ward 1989; Ward et al. 1990a,b; Weller et al. 1991) used a variant approach, by cloning and sequencing the 16S rcDNA fragments, to determine the species composition of cyanobacterial communities from hot springs in the Yellowstone National Park. Ribosomal RNA was extracted from community members by the application of harsh mechanical cell lysis methods, such as French press or bead beating (Ward et al. 1995). The isolated small subunit rRNA was subsequently reverse transcribed into ribosomal-copy-DNA (rcDNA) by the enzyme reverse transcriptase and a synthetic oligonucleotide complementary to a universally conserved region at the 3'-end of the 16S rRNA as primer for cDNA synthesis (Weller & Ward 1989). The fragments were cloned into a plasmid vector. Sequence analysis of the cloned 16S rcDNA inserts revealed the presence of many new bacteria that had not been recognized before (Ward et al. 1990a,b; Weller et al. 1991). The main advantage of this approach over the 'shotgun' cloning approach was the selective recovery of 16S rRNA. A problem, however, was the early termination of rcDNA synthesis, because of the strong secondary structure of the 16S rRNA molecule. The use of random hexanucleotides instead of a specific primer improved rcDNA synthesis, resulting in longer rcDNA fragments, thus yielding more phylogenetic information (Weller et al. 1991).

Far more successful than the former two approaches is the cloning of PCR-amplified 16S rRNA genes. In this approach, total genomic DNA is isolated from an environmental sample, and used as template DNA in the PCR with primers specific for the 16S rRNA encoding genes of Bacteria or Archaea. Thereafter, the amplicons are cloned into a plasmid vector, and the inserts are sequenced. Giovannoni and co-workers (Giovannoni et al. 1990; Britschgi & Giovanni 1991) were the first to use this approach for the phylogenetic analysis of bacterioplankton in the Sargasso Sea, a central gyre in the Atlantic Ocean. They found sequences grouping together in clusters, such as the SAR 7 cluster, which is affiliated to the oxygenic phototrophs. Another cluster of sequences, the SAR 11 cluster, formed a subgroup within the alpha subdivision of the class Proteobacteria. Hybridization analysis of DNA with an oligonucleotide probe specific for this latter cluster of sequences indicated that these bacteria were abundant in this habitat. Table 1 shows a summary of the cloning results from different studies on the exploration of microbial diversity in various habitats. From these results certain general patterns can be seen, such as the presence of phylogenetically related bacteria, such as those belonging to the SAR 11 cluster, in different oceans, and the absence of members of the β-subdivision of the Proteobacteria in the marine environment. It also shows that habitats, such as hot springs, which were assumed to be low in prokaryotic diversity, because of extreme environmental conditions, showed an enormous bacterial (Hugenholz et al. 1998) as well as archaeal (Barns et al. 1996) diversity.

In summary, the cloning approach of 16S rDNA fragments has revealed marked microbial diversity in nature, and concomitantly the inability of current microbiological techniques to isolate most of the ecologically relevant bacteria in pure cultures. It circumvents the isolation of microorganisms for their detection and classification, and can be used to describe the species composition ('species richness') of microbial ecosystems. However, although successful in the exploration of microbial diversity, the cloning approach is neither suitable for studying many different microbial communities simultaneously. It is also inappropriate for quantifying the abundance ('species evenness') and spatial distribution of particular bacterial populations, or the behaviour of a microbial community over time, because the technique is time-consuming, cumbersome, and impractical for analysis of multiple samples. For this purpose other molecular biological techniques are needed.

3. Ribosomal RNA slot-blot hybridization

One of the techniques for quantifying the abundance of particular populations in environmental samples is rRNA slot-blot hybridization (rRNA-SBH). In this approach, ribosomal RNA isolated from natural samples is spotted onto nylon membranes, and hybridized with group-specific radioactive 16S rRNA-targeted oligonucleotide probes. The relative abundance of the taxon (species, genus, family, etc.) can be estimated by comparing the hybridization signal obtained with the taxon-specific probe to the signal obtained with an universal probe. Fig. 3 shows an example of a rRNA slot-blot hybridization to compare the abundance of Archaea in two different anaerobic bioreactors. Comparison of the signal intensity of the samples incubated with the universal probe and

Table 1: Prokaryotic diversity in different habitats as revealed by sequence analysis of cloned 16S rDNA

Habitat	Target group	Phylogenetic affiliation of cloned sequences[a]	Citation
open ocean (Pacific)	Bacteria	α, γ, Cb	Mullins et al. 1995[b]
open ocean (Pacific)	Bacteria	Fb/Gs	Gordon and Giovannoni 1996
open ocean (Pacific, Atlantic)	all life forms	α, γ, Arc, Cb, CFB, HG⁺,	Fuhrman et al. 1993
marine snow	Bacteria	α, γ, δ, ε, CFB, LG⁺, Pm, Vm	Rath et al. 1998
marine aggregates	Bacteria	α, γ, Cb, CFB, Pm, Ua	DeLong et al. 1993
Antarctic sea ice	Bacteria	α, γ, CFB, HG⁺	Bowman et al. 1997
marine sediment	Bacteria	α, γ, δ, HG⁺, LG⁺, Pm	Grey and Herwig 1996
mountain lake	Bacteria	α, β, γ, Cb, CFB, HG⁺, Hp, Vm	Hiorns et al. 1997
freshwater puddle	Bacteria	α, β, δ, GnS, G⁺, Fb, Vm	Wise et al. 1997
agricultural soil	all life forms	α, β, γ, δ, Cb, CFB, Euc, Fb, HG⁺, LG⁺, Pm, 4 Ua	Borneman et al. 1996
Amazonian soil	all life forms	α, β, δ, Cb, CFB, Cr, Fb, HG⁺, LG⁺, Cm, Pm, Vm, Ua	Borneman and Triplett 1997
grassland soil	Bacteria	α, β, HG+, Hp, LG+, Vm	Felske et al. 1998
activated sludge	Bacteria	α, β, γ, ε, Pm/Cm, LG+	Snaidr et al. 1997
anaerobic biodigester	Bacteria	α, β, γ, δ, CFB, Pm/Cm, GnS, HG+, LG+, Sp, Syn	Godon et al. 1997
hydrothermal vent	Bacteria	γ, δ, ε, Syn	Moyer et al. 1995
hot spring	Bacteria	Cb, GnS, Gs, Pm, Pr, Sp	Ward et al. 1994[c]
hot spring	Bacteria	α, β, δ, Af, CFB, Dc, Dg, GnS, Gs, HG⁺, Hp, Ns, Pm, Tdb, Tt, Vm, 12 Ua	Hugenholtz et al. 1998
hot spring	all life forms	α, β, Af, G+	Yamamoto et al. 1998
hot aquifer	Bacteria	β, γ, δ, Arc, Af, Cb, Dc, Fu, HG⁺, LG⁺, GnS, Pm, Sp, Tt	Byers et al. 1998
termite gut	Bacteria	β, γ, δ, CFB, G⁺	Ohkuma and Kudo 1996
Antarctic seawater	Archaea	GImC, GIImE	DeLong et al. 1994
salt marsh sediment	Archaea	Hb, Mc, Mcu, Ml, Mg, GIImE	Munson et al. 1997
hot spring	Archaea	Arf, Cr, Ua	Barns et al. 1994
hot spring	Archaea	GImC, Eur, Kor	Barns et al. 1996
holothurian (sea cucumber) gut	Archaea	GImC	McInerney et al. 1995

[a] α, β, γ, δ, ε, alpha, beta, gamma, delta, and epsilon subdivisions of the class Proteobacteria; Af, Aquificales; Arc, Archaea; Arf, Archaeoglobus fulgidus; Cb, Cyanobacteria; CFB, Cytophaga-Flavobacteria-Bacteroides; Cm, Chamydia; Cr, Crenarchaeta; Dc, Deinococcus/Thermus; Dg, Dictoglomus; Euc, Eucarya; Eur, Euryarchaeota; Fb, Fibrobacter; Fu, Fusobacterium; GnS, Green non-sulfur bacteria; Gs, Green sulfur bacteria; GImC, group I marine Crenarchaeta; GIImE, group II marine Euryarchaeota; Hb, Halobacteriaceae; HG⁺, high G+C Gram positive bacteria; Hp, Holophaga/Acidobacterium; Kor, Korarchaeota; Mb, Methanobacterales; Mc, Methanococcoides; Mcu, Methanoculleus; Mg, Methanogenium; Ml, Methanolobus; Ms, Methanosarcinaceae; Ns, Nitrospira; Pm, Planctomyces; Pr, Proteobacteria; Sp, Spirochetes; Syn, Synergistes; Vm, Verrucomicrobium; Tdb, Thermodesulfobacterium; Tt, Termotogales; Ua, unknown affiliation. See also Figure 1, the Tree of Life.
[b] Extension of earlier work published by Giovannoni et al. (1990) and by Britschi and Giovannoni (1991).
[c] Summary of the results published in earlier papers.

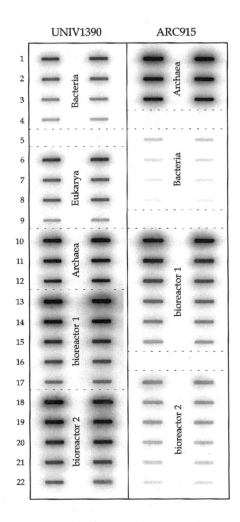

Figure 3: Slot-blot hybridisation of rRNA from 2 different anaerobic bioreactors. Serial dilutions of RNAs of the bioreactor samples and of the standards, *Escherichia coli* (Bacteria), *Methanobacterium thermoautotrophicum* (Archaea), and calf liver (Eukarya), were spotted in duplicate. The left blot was incubated with a radiolabelled oligonucleotide probe targeting the rRNA of all life forms (UNIV1390); the right blot with a probe specific for the rRNA of Archaea (ARC915). Archaea are present in bioreactor 1, but not in bioreactor 2.

with a probe specific for Archaea indicates the presence of substantial amounts of archaeal ribosomal RNA in bioreactor 1, but not in bioreactor 2.

The rRNA-SBH approach has been used to study the microbial ecology of the bovine rumen (Stahl *et al.* 1988), and to resolve the abundance and diversity of *Fibrobacter* species in gut contents (Lin & Stahl 1995). In another study, Lin *et al.* (1997) used 16S rRNA-targeted oligonucleotide probes to compare the microbial community structure in the gastrointestinal (GI) tracts of domestic animals, such as cow, goat, pig, sheep and cattle. Bacterial, eukaryotic (*e.g.* fungi and protozoa), and archaeal (*i.e.* methanogen) rRNA accounted for 60-90%, 3-30% and 0.5-3%, respectively, of the total rRNA in the GI tracts of most of the animals. By using probes specific for different orders of the *Archaea,* the authors showed that members of the *Methanobacteriacea* were most abundant in the GI tracts of ruminal animals, followed by populations belonging to the *Methanomicrobiales*. No (reliable) signals were obtained with probes for members of the *Methanococceae* and the *Methanosarcinales*. The abundance of another important group of anaerobic microorganisms, the mesophilic Gram-negative sulphate-reducing bacteria (SRB), was also determined. *Desulfovibrio* species were found to be most abundant, while members belonging to the *Desulfobacter* group were only found at low levels. Ribosomal RNA of *Desulfobulbus* was not detected, and the presence of Gram-positive SRB, such as *Desulfotomaculum ruminis*, could not be tested, because no probe was available. A recent study found similar results for methanogenic populations in the rumen, with the highest relative abundance for representatives of the *Methanobacteriales*, followed by members of the *Methanomicrobiales* (Sharp *et al.* 1998). In addition, the authors found that the abundance of the first group was correlated to the number of the protozoa; a reduction in abundance was observed after the loss of protozoa from the rumen.

Raskin and co-workers used rRNA slot-blot hybridization to quantify different methanogens in anaerobic bioreactors (Raskin *et al.* 1994a,b), to characterize filamentous foaming in activated sludge systems (De los Reyes *et al.* 1997), and to study the competition and coexistence of sulphate reducing bacteria and methanogens in anaerobic biofilms (Raskin *et al.* 1995, 1996). The latter study convincingly demonstrated the power of this approach in studying population dynamics after environmental perturbations. Hybridization analysis with group-specific probes detected a dramatic shift in the relative numbers of methanogens and SRB in a sulphate-free bioreactor to which sulphate was added. The relative abundance of the methanogens changed from 25% prior to sulphate addition to 8% after addition, while the number of SRB increased from 15% to approximately 35%, confirming the hypothesis of competitive advantage of SRB over methanogens in environments with high sulphate concentrations. Risatti *et al.* (1994) used rRNA-SBH to determine the distribution and abundance of different sulphate reducing bacterial populations in a microbial mat community. They showed that mats are stratified by detecting different phylogenetic groups of SRB at different depths in the mat, indicating depth-specific metabolic functions. In the upper layer (1-2 mm depth) populations belonging to the *Desulfococcus* group were the most abundant, followed by *Desulfovibrio* species (members of both groups can oxidize different substrates, such as lactate, ethanol, and fatty acids), while the acetate-oxidising *Desulfobacter* and *Desulfobacterium* species were restricted to greater depths. The presence of SRB in the photooxic zone, complements the finding of high sulphate-reducing rates in this zone (Canfield & DesMarais 1991), and questions the dogma that sulphate reducers are strictly anaerobes.

Purdy *et al.* (1997) used oligonucleotide probes for sulphate reducing bacteria to detect population changes in slurries of marine and freshwater sediments supplemented with short-chain fatty acids, such as acetate, butyrate, lactate and propionate. They found an increasing number of *Desulfobulbus* spp. in freshwater and marine slurries amended with propionate, while an increasing number of *Desulfobacter* spp. was found after addition of acetate to slurries of the marine site, indicating the different niches of these organisms.

One of the main advantages of the rRNA-SBH approach is that no additional amplification step is needed to increase the amount of molecular marker for detection. Cells are lysed, and the purified rRNA is used directly in the hybridization assay. Of course, the reliable and reproducible extraction of rRNA from bacterial cells in natural samples might pose difficulties. However, the extraction protocol developed by Stahl and co-workers (Stahl *et al.* 1988), which includes bead beating of environmental samples in the presence of hot phenol, has been shown to be an efficient and reliable extraction procedure. A more important problem is the rapid degradation of RNA, which requires special precautions, such as baking of glassware, working with gloves, etc., to prevent this. An advantage is the internal consistency in the hybridization assay; the summation of signals obtained with specific probes (*e.g.* probes specific for the domains *Archaea, Bacteria,* and *Eukarya*) must equal the signal obtained with a general probe (*e.g.* the universal probe), although, discrepancies can arise from differential rRNA degradation (Raskin *et al.* 1997), lack of probe specificity, and the presence of unknown bacterial populations, which do not hybridize to one of the probes (Lin *et al.* 1997). A limitation of the method is that it only estimates the relative abundance of ribosomes. Percentages of total rRNA cannot be readily translated into cell numbers, because the total amount of rRNA relies on the number of cells and the amount of rRNA per cell, which in turn depends on the growth rate; actively growing cells have more rRNA than quiescent cells (Poulsen *et al.* 1993). Thus, for an absolute quantification of specific bacterial populations in natural samples, enumeration of cells is still essential.

4. *In situ* hybridization

In situ or whole cell hybridization is the method of choice to enumerate specific bacterial populations, and to determine their spatial distribution in microbial communities, such as biofilms. Bacterial cells are fixed in paraformaldehyde, spotted onto microscope slides or filters, and dehydrated. The specimens are then incubated with a specific fluorescently-labelled oligonucleotide probe, and observed with an epifluorescence microscope (a detailed protocol is given by Amann (1995). Table 2 gives an overview of different whole cell hybridization studies on mixed bacterial populations. The use of confocal laser scanning microscopy (CLSM) makes it possible to visualize the spatial distribution of specific bacterial populations in 3 dimensions. Harmsen and coworkers (Harmsen *et al.* 1997) used whole cell hybridization and CLSM to detect and localize syntrophic propionate-oxidizing bacteria in anaerobic granular sludge. By using fluorescently-labelled oligonucleotide probes for *Bacteria, Archaea,* different groups of methanogens, and for two syntrophic propionate-oxidising microorganisms, they found that the propionate-oxidising bacteria were intertwined with hydrogen- or formate-consuming methanogens, indicating their synthrophic growth. An interesting paper by Schramm *et al.* (1996) describes the study of structure and function of a nitrifying biofilm by the combination of *in situ* hybridization and microelectrodes. Microelectrode measurements of oxygen and nitrate showed that nitrification was restricted to the outer layer of the biofilm. *In situ* hybridization analysis with probes specific for ammonium-oxidising *Nitrosomonas* species and for nitrite-oxidising *Nitrobacter* species was used to determine their spatial distribution. *Nitrosomonas* was found in dense clusters, with *Nitrobacter* in their vicinity, indicating the metabolic dependency upon each other. Whole cell hybridization has also been combined with flow cytometry to analyse complex mixtures of bacteria (Amann *et al.* 1990; Wallner *et al.* 1995, 1996). An interesting new development is the possibility of sorting specific bacterial populations for subsequent molecular characterization (Wallner *et al.* 1997). By using this approach less abundant populations could be enriched up to 280-fold.

Difficulties with whole cell hybridization include obtaining effective probe penetration into the cells, especially when the larger polynucleotide probes or oligonucleotides labelled with enzymes are used. Furthermore, background fluorescence of inorganic particles, and autofluorescence of phototrophic microorganisms may be a problem. Possibly, the most important limitation of the whole cell hybridization approach is the low signal intensity caused by small numbers of ribosomes, or by inaccessibility of the rRNA for the oligonucleotide probes. The hybridization signal can, however, be increased up to 8-fold by using a combination of 2-hydroxy-3-naphthoic acid-2'-phenylanilide and Fast Red TR (Yamaguchi *et al.* 1996) or even up to 20-fold by the tyramide signal amplification

Table 2: Overview of whole cell hybridization studies on mixed microbial populations

Habitat	Probe specificity[a]	Citation[a]
activated sludge	α, β, γ, Acinetobacter, ammonia-oxidizing bacteria, Bacteria, CFB, Eucarya, filamentous bacteria, sulfate-reducing bacteria, Zoogloea ramigera,	Manz et al. 1994, 1996, 1998; Mobarry et al. 1996; Rossello-Mora et al. 1995; Snaidr et al. 1997; Wagner et al. 1993, 1994a,b,c; Wallner et al. 1995;
upflow anaerobic sludge bed reactors	Archaea, Bacteria, methanogens, propionate-oxidizing bacteria	Harmsen et al. 1996a,b
bacterial biofilms	ammonia-oxidizing bacteria, Bacteria, E. coli, Legionellacaea, sulfate-reducing bacteria	Amann et al. 1992; Kalmbach et al. 1997; Ramsing et al. 1993; Schramm et al. 1997; Szewzyk et al. 1994; Wagner et al. 1995
bacterioplankton	α, β, γ, Bacteria, CFB	Alfreider et al. 1996; Pernthaler et al. 1997;
freshwater sediment	magnetotactic bacterium	Spring et al. 1993
stratified water column	Bacteria, sulfate -reducing bacteria	Ramsing et al. 1996
marine hydrothermal vents	thermophylic bacteria	Harmsen et al. 1997a,b
lake snow	α, β, γ,	Weiss et al. 1996
rhizoshere	Azospirillum brasilense	Assmus et al. 1995
soil	Bacillus megaterium	Fischer et al. 1995; Zardra et al. 1997
root nodules	Frankia spp.	Hahn et al. 1993; Hahn et al. 1997
endosymbionts		Poltz et al. 1994; Springer et al. 1993 1996
worm gut	α, β, γ, Bacteria,	Fischer et al. 1995
parasites	Sarcobium lyticum	Springer et al. 1992

[a]Alphabetically ordered.

(Schönhuber *et al.* 1997; LeBaron *et al.* 1997). An important problem with hybridization techniques in general is that only bacteria for which probes exist can be studied.

5. *In situ* PCR

An intriguing approach is *in situ* PCR amplification of specific gene sequences inside intact bacterial cells, described first by Hodson *et al.* (1995). Bacterial cells are fixed in paraformaldehyde, permeabilized by a lysozyme and proteinase K treatment, and subjected to PCR, either as suspension or coated on microscope slides. The amplification products can be visualized by epifluorescence microscopy directly after incorporation of fluorescently labelled nucleotides in the PCR product, or indirectly by epifluorescence or bright-field microscopy after incorporation of digoxigenin (DIG)-labelled nucleotides and the use of an enzyme or fluorescent-labelled anti-DIG antibody (see Chen *et al.* (1997) for a detailed description of the method). Tani *et al.* (1998) used an alkaline phosphatase-labelled antidigoxigenin antibody and the substrates HNPP and Fast Red TR for the detection of DIG-labelled PCR products resulting in bright red fluorescent cells. In addition, generated amplicons can be detected by *in situ* hybridization with specific fluorescent oligonucleotide probes. Hodson and co-workers used this approach to detect the *nahA* gene and transcripts in *Pseudomonas putida* cells, which were mixed with other bacterial strains to mimic a marine community. In a subsequent paper (Cheng *et al.* 1998) the authors used *in situ* reverse transcription of 16S rRNA to detect and enumerate two lignin-degrading bacteria in mixed cultures and enrichments, and of mRNA to detect the expression of the *todC1* gene in *Pseudomonas putida* cells. Although still in its infancy, *in situ* PCR may become one of the most powerful techniques in microbial ecology. Problems are, however, encountered with the transfer of Taq DNA polymerase, and the fluorescent-labelled or enzyme-labelled antidigoxigenin antibody into the cell, with the leakage of PCR products out of the cell, and with non-specific amplification.

6. Genetic fingerprinting of microbial communities

Genetic fingerprinting techniques provide a pattern or profile of the community diversity based upon physical separation of unique nucleic acid species (Stahl & Capman 1994). The increasing interest in the application of these techniques in microbial ecological studies is due to the fact that they are rapid and relatively easy to perform, but more importantly that they allow the simultaneous analysis of multiple samples, which makes it possible to compare microbial communities from different habitats readily, or to study the behaviour of individual microbial communities over time. I have described the application of 6 different fingerprinting techniques, (1) LMW RNA fingerprinting, (2) DGGE/TGGE, (3) Bb-PEG electrophoresis, (4) SSCP, (5) RAPD and DAF, and (6) RFLP/ARDRA, which are used in microbial ecological studies.

6.1. LMW RNA fingerprinting

A genetic fingerprinting technique that has been used for more than a decade is profiling of low-molecular-weight (LMW) RNA (5S ribosomal RNA (rRNA) and transfer RNA (tRNA)) (Höfle 1988). The technique (see Höfle (1998) for a technical description) is straightforward; total RNA (23S, 16S, and 5S rRNA, as well as tRNA) is extracted from an environmental sample, and separated by high resolution polyacrylamide gel electrophoresis. The separation profiles of the 5S rRNA and tRNA (the 23S and 16S rRNA are too big to enter the gel) can be visualized by silver staining, or by autoradiography if the

RNA was radioactively labelled. Subsequently, the profiles are scanned, and stored in an electronic database for comparison.

LMW RNA profiling was used to monitor bacterial population dynamics in a set of freshwater mesocosms after addition of nonindigenous bacteria and culture medium (Höfle 1992). The addition of the bacteria had no effect on the indigenous bacterioplankton. However, the added culture medium caused an increase of two of the natural bacterial populations, namely, a member related to *Aeromonas hydrophila,* and bacteria related to *Cytophaga johnsonae.* In another study, LMW RNA fingerprinting was used to investigate the diversity and activity of bacterial populations in a stratified water column of the central Baltic Sea (Höfle & Brettar 1996). Analysis of samples taken at different depths from the same site showed a limited number of bacterial taxa throughout the water column. Comparative sequence analysis of a 5S rRNA band obtained from the oxic-anoxic interface revealed the presence of bacteria related to *Thiobacillus denitrificans.* The latter is a chemolithoautotrophic bacterium, the presence of which had been postulated from the chemical gradient and its metabolism, indicated by the oxidation of reduced sulphur compounds and reduction of nitrate and nitrite to nitrogen gas under anaerobic conditions. In a subsequent study, the authors (Höfle & Brettar 1996) used LMW RNA fingerprinting to classify and identify 123 strains of heterotrophic bacteria isolated from the same site, the Gotland Deep in the central Baltic Sea. 76% of the isolated bacterial strains could be identified to the species level, with representatives of the families *Vibrionaceae, Enterobacteriaceae,* and *Pseudomonadaceae.* The most abundant isolates were related to *Shewanella putrefaciens* and a *Pseudomonas* species. Bidle and Fletcher (1995) used LMW RNA fingerprinting to compare free-living and particle-associated bacterial communities from different depths and different sites in an estuary bay. They found that (i) free-living and particle-attached microbial communities from the same site were different in species composition, that (ii) communities taken from different depths at the same site were similar, but that (iii) free-living communities from different sites were different, while particle-associated communities were similar. Furthermore, comparative analysis of bacterial isolates and environmental samples revealed that the isolates were not representative of the dominant community members.

Stoner *et al.* (1996) used a combination of LMW rRNA fingerprinting and denaturing gradient gel electrophoresis (DGGE). Mixtures of 5S rRNA molecules directly extracted from acidic mining environments were separated on gels containing a gradient of acrylamide and urea.

The advantages and problems of LMW RNA fingerprinting are similar to some of those described for the rRNA slot blot hybridization assay. Working with RNA does not require an additional amplification step, but it may be difficult, because it rapidly degrades, forming additional bands in the profiles. Furthermore, the small size of the different LMW RNAs (5S rRNA maximal 131 nucleotides, and tRNA maximal 96 nucleotides) limits their phylogenetic information.

6.2. DGGE and TGGE

In 1993, Muyzer and co-workers introduced another genetic fingerprinting technique in microbial ecology, that of denaturing gradient gel electrophoresis (DGGE; Myers *et al.* 1985) of PCR-amplified 16S rRNA fragments (Muyzer *et al.* 1993). Within a short time this technique has attracted the attention of many environmental microbiologists, and is now used routinely in many laboratories. The technique (see Muyzer *et al.* (1998) for a technical description) is rapid, and straightforward, and does not depend on extensive expensive equipment. Mixtures of PCR products obtained after enzymatic amplification of genomic DNA extracted from a complex assemblage of microbes are separated in polyacrylamide gels containing a linear gradient of DNA denaturants (urea and formamide). Sequence variation among the different DNA molecules influences the melting behaviour, and therefore molecules with different sequences will stop migrating at different positions in the gel. Another technique based on the same principle is temperature gradient gel electrophoresis (TGGE; Riesner et al. 1991), which was also applied to separate 16S rDNA fragments.

DGGE of PCR-amplified 16S rDNA fragments was first used to profile community complexity of a microbial mat and bacterial biofilms (Muyzer et al. 1993). For this purpose, bacterial genomic DNA was extracted from natural samples, and segments of the 16S rRNA genes were amplified in the PCR. This resulted in a mixture of PCR products obtained from the different bacteria present in the sample. The individual PCR products were subsequently separated by DGGE. The result was a pattern of bands, for which the number of bands corresponded to the number of predominant members in the microbial communities. To obtain more detailed information about some of the community members, DGGE profiles were blotted onto nylon membranes and hybridized with a radioactively-labelled oligonucleotide probe specific for sulphate-reducing bacteria. In a subsequent study, Muyzer and de Waal (1994) were able to identify community members by sequencing of DNA eluted from excised DGGE bands. Table 3 gives an overview of the different applications of DGGE and TGGE in microbial ecology. A few of these studies are highlighted here, but for the other studies the reader is referred to Muyzer and Smalla (1998), or to the original articles. Fig. 4 demonstrates the power of fingerprinting techniques in microbial ecological studies, through the comparative analysis of many different samples simultaneously on one gel. DNA extracted from 18 different water samples taken from a 300 litre mesocosm, was used in the PCR to amplify 16S rDNA fragments. Simultaneous DGGE analysis of the PCR products showed similar banding patterns for each of the 18 samples. This demonstrates the efficient mixing of water in the mesocosm, which was necessary for reproducible sampling during a 10 day investigation on the effects of eutrophication on bacterial diversity and activity. In addition, it showed the reproducibility of DNA extraction, amplification, and DGGE analysis.

6.2.1. Studying the genetic diversity of microbial communities

DGGE analysis of 16S rDNA fragments has been used to study the presence and activity of sulphate-reducing bacteria in a stratified water column of Mariager Fjord in Denmark (Teske et al. 1996a). The concept behind this was that PCR products obtained from environmental DNA would demonstrate the presence of different bacterial populations, a measure of biodiversity, and that PCR products obtained after amplification of ribosomal copy DNA (rcDNA) would indicate which of these bacterial populations were active. DGGE comparison of products obtained by PCR and those obtained by reverse transcriptase (RT)-PCR with nucleic acids from different depths showed the presence of two bands in the DGGE patterns for rRNA, which were not visible in the pattern for DNA. From this result the authors concluded that these bands represent two active bacterial populations that are present in low numbers.

DGGE of PCR-amplified 16S rRNA gene fragments has been applied to profile the distribution of microbial populations inhabiting different temperature regions in a hot spring cyanobacterial community (Ferris et al. 1996). DGGE profiles of samples taken from sites with the same temperature were similar, indicating the reproducibility of DNA extraction, PCR amplification, and DGGE analysis. However, different profiles were found for samples from sites with different temperatures. Sequencing of individual bands from the different profiles revealed known but also some new bacterial phylotypes.

Table 3: Overview of the applications of DGGE and TGGE in microbial ecology

Application	Additional information	Citation
to study the genetic diversity of microbial communities	bacterial biofilms, microbial mats	Muyzer et al. 1993; 1994
	deep-sea hydrothermal vents	Muyzer et al. 1995
	bacterial biofilms	Wawer & Muyzer 1995
	cyanobacteria in microbial mats, coastal seawater, and lichens	Nübel et al. 1997
	hot spring cyanobacterial mats	Ferris et al. 1996
	cyanobacteria in microbial mats	Nübel et al. 1998
	biodegraded wall painting	Rolleke et al. 1996
	stratified water column	Teske et al. 1996a; Øvreas et al. 1997
	estuaries	Murray et al. 1996
	freshwater lake	Zwart et al. 1998
	soil, rhizosphere	Felske et al. 1996, 1997, 1998; Führ 1996; Heuer et al. 1995 1997; Heuer & Smalla 1997
	bacteria in coastal sand dunes	Kowalchuk et al. 1997a
	fungi in coastal sand dunes	Kowalchuk et al. 1997b
to study population dynamics in microbial communities	marine mesocosm	Donner et al. 1996; Schäfer and Muyzer 1998
	hot spring cyanobacterial mats	Ferris et al. 1997; Ferris & Ward 1997
	hypersaline microbial mat	Teske 1995
	bacterial biofilm	Santegoeds et al. 1998
	coastal seawater mesocosm	Schäfer & Muyzer 1998
	freshwater aquarium	Hovanec et al. 1998
to study gene expression in mixed populations	[NiFe] hydrogenase gene in Desulfovibrio spp.	Wawer et al. 1997
to monitor enrichment cultures, and to characterize bacterial strains	enrichments of chemoorganotrophic bacteria from a hot spring cyanobacterial mat	Santegoeds et al. 1996; Ward et al. 1996
	coculture of Desulfovibrio and Arcobacter	Teske et al. 1996b
	enrichments of sulfur-oxidizing bacteria from a coastal mud flat and a hydrothermal vent	Brinkhoff & Muyzer 1997; Brinkhoff et al. 1998
	enrichments of methanotrophic bacteria in soil	Jensen et al. 1998
	electrophoretic separation of bacteria	Jaspers & Overmann 1997
	marine bacteria	Wichels 1996
	cyanobacterium Microcoleus chthonoplastes	Garcia-Pichel et al. 1996
	iron-oxidizing bacteria	Buchholz-Cleven et al. 1997
	rhizobia and methanotrophs	Vallaeys et al. 1997
	green sulfur bacteria	Overmann & Tuschak 1997
	Hyphomicrobium spp. (mxaF gene)	Fesefeldt & Gliesche 1997
	BIOLOG plates	Smalla et al. 1998
to compare DNA extraction protocols	e.g., extraction of DNA with or without a bead beating step	Führ 1996; Heuer and Smalla 1997; Liesack et al. 1997
to screen clone libraries for redundancy, and to determine clone representation in the natural environment	nested PCR of cloned inserts of the complete 16S rRNA gene	Kowalchuk et al. 1997; Felske et al. 1997; Hovanec et al. 1998; Nüsslein & Tiedje 1998; Schäfer & Muyzer 1998
to determine rRNA operon microheterogeneity	Paenibacillus polymyxa	Nübel et al. 1996

A   B

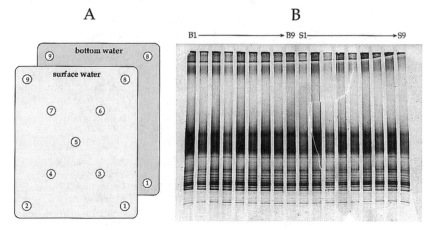

Figure 4: Homogeneity test of a 300 litre seawater mesocosm. (A) Sampling scheme; a total of eighteen 100 ml water samples were taken; 9 from the surface (S) layer, and 9 from the bottom (B) layer of the mesocosm. (B) DGGE analysis of 16S rDNA fragments obtained after enzymatic amplification of genomic DNA extracted from bacterial cells collected by filtration of the water samples (B1-9, S1-9). Note the similar banding patters for each sample, indicating the presence of identical bacteria in the different water samples, and the efficient mixing of the water mass.

Zwart *et al.* (1998) used DGGE to determine the presence of different members belonging to the *Verrucomicrobiales* in a temperate freshwater lake in the Netherlands. Comparative DGGE analysis of DNA fragments obtained from water samples, and by a so-called *nested* PCR from full length cloned rDNA fragments obtained from the same water samples, demonstrated the presence of these bacteria in the lake throughout the year.

Heuer *et al.* (1997) used DGGE and TGGE to study the genetic diversity of actinomycetes in different soils, and to monitor shifts in their abundances in the potato rhizosphere. In this study, the authors used two amplification strategies, first, a direct amplification of the actinomycetes 16S rDNA using group-specific primers, and second an indirect amplification approach, whereby actinomycetes-specific DNA fragments were generated with a forward group-specific primer and a reverse bacterial primer, followed by a second, so-called *nested* PCR with two bacterial primers. By using the direct PCR, the genetic diversity of the actinomycetes could be investigated rapidly by gradient gel electrophoresis (DGGE or TGGE). Simultaneous gradient gel electrophoresis of products obtained with the nested PCR and those obtained after amplification of the environmental DNA with the bacterial primers directly, allowed estimation of the abundance of the actinomycetes populations relative to the abundance of the other bacteria present in the soil. DGGE analysis of PCR products generated by this strategy showed that the actinomycetes were present only in low numbers, and that their template DNAs were therefore outcompeted in the amplification process with bacterial primers by template DNAs of other bacteria representing the bulk of the biomass.

PCR-DGGE and sequencing of cloned 16S rDNA molecules were used to study ammonia-oxidizing bacteria in Dutch coastal sand dunes (Kowalchuk *et al.* 1997a). Comparative DGGE analysis of PCR products from environmental DNA and from cloned inserts demonstrated the presence of sequences affiliated to the genus *Nitrosomonas* in dunes relatively close to the sea, while sequences affiliated to the genus *Nitrosospira* were detected in samples from all sites, although different *Nitrosospira* sequence types were detected in dune soils with different pH. In a subsequent study, Kowalchuk *et al.* (1997b) used DGGE to characterize fungal pathogens responsible for the infection of roots of marram grass, a plant important in sand-stabilization of coastal dunes. DGGE analysis of

18S rDNA fragments obtained from the root samples showed a similar diversity as was found with cultivation methods, but their identities were different.

So far, most studies applying genetic fingerprinting techniques have focused on the analysis of 16S rRNA or its encoding gene, but PCR products obtained from functional genes can also be used. Wawer and Muyzer (1995) designed PCR primers to amplify the [NiFe] hydrogenase gene from *Desulfovibrio* species. PCR products obtained from different *Desulfovibrio* strains could be separated easily by DGGE. In addition, PCR products obtained with bacterial DNA extracted from a microbial mat and from different bacterial biofilms demonstrated a greater genetic diversity of *Desulfovibrio* species in the natural microbial mat than in the bacterial biofilms from the man-controlled bioreactors (Wawer & Muyzer 1995; Wawer 1997).

6.2.2. Studying population dynamics in microbial communities

Microbial ecological studies often require the sampling at different time points over a long period. As mentioned in the introduction, cloning techniques are not suited for the analysis of many different samples. By using DGGE or TGGE, many samples taken at different time intervals during the study can be analysed simultaneously. This makes the techniques powerful tools for monitoring community behaviour after environmental changes. Santegoeds *et al.* (1997) have combined microsensor measurements and PCR-DGGE to monitor successional changes both of environmental parameters and bacterial diversity, involving the development of anoxic zones, the start of sulphate reduction and concomitant population changes, in a growing bacterial biofilm. Over time an increasing number of bands was observed in the DGGE profiles, indicating an increase in species richness of bacteria. Recently, Ferris *et al.* (1997) used PCR-DGGE to study the re-establishment of a microbial mat after removal of the entire cyanobacterial layer. The results showed that previously undetected cyanobacteria colonized the remaining part of the mat, and that other cyanobacteria which were present before the disturbance remained undetected for up to 40 days. In a subsequent study, DGGE was used to evaluate seasonal distributions of bacterial populations along a thermal gradient in a hot spring microbial mat (Ferris & Ward 1997). Similar DGGE patterns were found for samples collected at the same site and for sites with the same temperature, regardless of the season. However, different profiles were seen for samples from sites with different temperatures. In a recent study, Hovanec *et al.* (1998) used cloning, rRNA slot-blot hybridization and DGGE to identify and quantify the bacteria responsible for nitrite oxidation in freshwater aquaria. They found that nitrite-oxidation was performed by bacteria affiliated to *Nitrospira marina,* and *N. moscoviensis,* which represented nearly 5% of the total rRNA extracted. DGGE analysis of samples taken at different time points over a total period of 101 days, showed that the *Nitrospira*-like sequences appeared during the onset of nitrite oxidation, became more intense over time, and disappeared after a switch from freshwater to seawater.

6.2.3. Studying gene expression in mixed populations

An exciting new direction within the field of molecular microbial ecology is the use of functional genes as molecular markers to monitor metabolic activity. Recently, Wawer *et al.* (1997) extended the application of DGGE to determine the differential expression of the [NiFe] hydrogenase gene by different *Desulfovibrio* populations in experimental bioreactors. By comparative DGGE analysis of PCR products obtained from both genomic DNA and mRNA, they demonstrated the presence of several different *Desulfovibrio* populations in the bioreactor, but the differential expression of the [NiFe] hydrogenase gene by only one of these populations. The conclusion was that this population might be better adapted to growth on hydrogen than the other *Desulfovibrio* populations, which indicates a niche differentiation of closely related bacterial populations in one community.

6.2.4. Monitoring the enrichment and isolation of bacteria

Brinkhoff and Muyzer (1997) used DGGE to monitor the successful isolation of the sulphur-oxidising bacteria of the genus *Thiomicrospira* from different habitats. By using a specific PCR the authors first screened several habitats for the presence of *Thiomicrospira* species and than attempted to isolate these species by enrichment cultures and selective plating. The success of isolation of different *Thiomicrospira* spp. in pure cultures was monitored by hybridization analysis of DGGE patterns of 16S rDNA PCR products generated with bacterial primers, followed by hybridization analysis of the profiles with a *Thiomicrospira*-specific oligonucleotide probe for which the target site was located within the amplified fragment. By using this combined molecular and microbiological approach the authors were able to isolate and identify in a short period of time seven new *Thiomicrospira* strains from several different habitats. Smalla *et al.* (1998) used TGGE and DGGE of 16S rDNA fragments to analyse BIOLOG GN substrate utilization patterns by microbial communities from the potato rhizosphere and an activated sludge reactor. TGGE analysis of cells from the BIOLOG plates inoculated with cell suspensions from the rhizosphere showed a marked decrease in the number of bands as compared to the number of bands for the original inoculum, as well as a shift in the dominant bacterial populations. The new dominant populations were assigned to the γ subdivision of the Proteobacteria by hybridization analysis of the TGGE profiles. Although, a similar decrease in diversity was found for the BIOLOG plates inoculated with cells from the bioreactor, no shift was found in the dominance of the community members.

6.2.5. Limitations of DGGE and TGGE

One of the limitations of DGGE and TGGE is the separation of only relatively small fragments, up to 500 basepairs (Myers *et al.* 1985), which limits the amount of sequence information for phylogenetic inferences as well as for probe design. Furthermore, it has been demonstrated that it is not always possible to separate DNA fragments which have a certain amount of sequence variation (Vallaeys *et al.* 1997; Buchholz-Cleven *et al.* 1997). Co-migration of DNA fragments can be a problem for retrieving clean sequences from individual bands. Another problem in the study of community diversity on the basis of 16S rRNA genes, using DGGE, TGGE or cloning strategies is the presence in some bacteria of multiple *rrN* operons with sequence microheterogeneity. DGGE and TGGE can visualize this sequence heterogeneity (Nübel *et al.* 1996) which may lead to an overestimation of the number of bacteria within natural communities. The same is true for the double bands in the DGGE or TGGE patterns which may appear when degenerate primers are used in the PCR reactions. Furthermore, the formation of heteroduplex molecules, molecules consisting of strands from two different PCR products, which can be formed under suboptimal amplification conditions (Jensen & Straus 1993), might contribute to difficulties in the interpretation of community complexity from DGGE patterns (Myers *et al.* 1985; Ferris & Ward 1997).

6.3. Bb-PEG electrophoresis

Wawer and co-workers developed a simple and rapid electrophoresis method to detect sequence variation in [NiFe] hydrogenase gene fragments obtained after enzymatic amplification of bacterial DNA from pure cultures (Wawer *et al.* 1995) and environmental samples (Wawer 1997). Electrophoresis is performed in agarose gels containing the DNA ligand bisbenzimide to which long chains chains of polyethylene glycol (PEG) are covalently coupled. Bisbenzimide binds to adenine and thymin (A+T) sequence motifs in the DNA. Therefore, being loaded with the Bb-PEG conjugate, the A+T-rich DNA molecules are more retarded in the gel than the molecules which are low in A+T, and so separation is archieved. Comparative analysis of mixtures of [NiFe] hydrogenase fragments with DGGE and Bb-PEG electrophorese gave a similar number of bands, that is one or two bands for bioreactor samples, and 5 bands for a microbial mat sample (Wawer 1997).

6.4. SSCP

Another fingerprinting technique which is used in microbial ecological studies is Single-Strand-Conformation Polymorphism (SSCP; Orita *et al.* 1989). In this technique, PCR products are denatured, and directly electrophoresed on a non-denaturing gel. Separation is based on differences in the folded conformation of single-stranded DNA, which influences the electrophoretic mobility. Lee and co-workers (1996) used this technique to study the structure and diversity of natural bacterial communities. SSCP of the PCR-amplified 16S-23S rRNA spacer region has also been used to analyse mixtures of bacteria (Scheinert *et al.* 1996). To reduce the complexity of the pattern created by the separation of both single-stranded DNA strands from many different organisms, the authors used one biotinylated, and one unlabelled primer in the PCR to perform magnetic strand separation before the electrophoresis. SSCP analysis of only one single-stranded DNA strand simplified the electrophoretic pattern drastically. Electrophoretic conditions, such as gel matrix, the addition of glycerol to the gel, and temperature, can influence the separation. In addition, only very short fragments (ca. 150 bp) can be optimally separated.

6.5. RAPD and DAF

Randomly Amplified Polymorphic DNA (RAPD; Williams *et al.* 1990) has been used to follow the response of different soil microbial communities to the application of 2,4-D (Xia *et al.* 1995). Breen *et al.* (1995) used a similar approach, namely DNA Amplification Fingerprinting (DAF; Caetano-Anolles *et al.* 1991), to compare microbial communities of different bioreactors, and to monitor population changes within one bioreactor. Both techniques make use of short random primers (5-8 bp in DAF, and 10 bp in RAPD), which anneal at different places of the genomic DNA, generating PCR products of various lengths. The products are separated on agarose or acrylamide gels, and visualized by ethidium bromide or silver staining. RAPD and DAF are commonly used in molecular ecology to study population genetics (Hadrys *et al.* 1992). However, their utility to analyse complex mixtures of bacteria is questionable. Reproducibility is a main problem of these techniques; differences in quality and quantity of template DNA, and in the concentration of $MgCl_2$, and primer may easily result in different patterns (Hadrys *et al.* 1992). In addition, no phylogenetic information can be obtained from the separated bands.

6.6. RFLP and ARDRA

Restriction Fragment Length Polymorphism (RFLP) of PCR-amplified rDNA fragments, otherwise known as Amplified Ribosomal DNA Restriction Analysis (ARDRA) has also been used to characterize microbial communities (see Massol-Deya *et al.* 1995) for a technical description of the method). 16S rDNA fragments are generated using general primers, digested with restriction enzymes with 4-bp recognition sites, electrophoresed in agarose or acrylamide gels, and stained with ethidium bromide or silver. Martinez-Murcia *et al.* (1995) used RFLP analysis of PCR-amplified 16S rDNA fragments to estimate the prokaryotic diversity in hypersaline ponds. Bacterial diversity was found to decrease with increasing salinity, while the reverse was true for archaeal diversity, the higher the salinity the greater the number of bands. Smit *et al.* (1997) used ARDRA to monitor community shifts after copper contamination. ARDRA was also used to follow the succession of microbial communities in an aquifer that was amended with phenol, toluene, and chlorinated aliphatic hydrocarbons. The results showed a low number of bands indicating a low microbial diversity. Similar patterns were found for the original community and those which received different carbon sources, indicating a stable community. Furthermore, simultaneous analysis of bacterial strains isolated from the community with environmental samples indicated the presence of these isolates in the environment.

A problem of estimating microbial diversity by ARDRA is that the number of fragments is not related to the number of different amplified DNA fragments, nor to the number of predominant community members. The number of restriction fragments produced from the different PCR products may differ. Recently, this problem was overcome by the use of fluorescent PCR products in the RFLP analysis. Briefly, PCR products are terminally labelled during the amplification process by the use of a fluorescent primer in the PCR reagent mixture. The PCR products are digested with a restriction enzyme as usual and subsequently assayed on an automatic DNA sequencer. Only those bands carrying the fluorescent label, the terminal restriction fragments, are detected. Liu *et al.* (1997) used Terminal Restriction Fragment Length Polymorphism (T-RFLP) to determine the genetic diversity of microbial communities from activated and bioreactor sludge, aquifer sand, and termite guts. Thirty six bands could be detected in the termite guts, but as many as 72 bands were detected in the community profiles obtained from the 3 other environments. Bruce (1997) used the same approach, but under a different name, fluorescent-PCR-restriction fragment length polymorphism (FluRFLP), to analyse bacterial communities in mercury-polluted and pristine soil and sediment samples. Instead of using 16S rRNA, the *mer* (mercury resistance) gene was used as a molecular marker. Advantages of the technique are (i) the high resolution electrophoretic separation on an automatic DNA sequencer, (ii) the use of intra-lane markers, which facilitates gel-to-gel comparison, and (iii) the possibility to quantify bands directly. Unfortunately, hybridization analysis or sequencing of excised bands for a further identification of the community members are not possible. Furthermore, the automatic DNA sequencer needed to perform T-RFLP is outrageously expensive.

7. Limitations of molecular techniques in microbial ecological studies

It must be emphasized that as with every method, molecular biological techniques are not free from limitations and biases. These may already be introduced by sample handling. For instance, Rochelle *et al.* (1994) found that different sample handling procedures, such as aerobic or anaerobic storage, or direct freezing of the samples, greatly affected the species composition found by 16S rRNA sequence analysis. Also, the extraction of nucleic acids from bacterial cells is not free from biases. Problems are encountered with the reliable and reproducible lysis of all bacterial cell as well as with the extraction of intact nucleic acid, and the removal of substances, such as humic acids and bacterial exopolysaccharides, which may inhibit DNA digestion with restriction enzymes and PCR amplification (*e.g.* Wheeler & Stahl 1996). PCR itself can be an important source of errors and biases. Amplification efficiency of genes using whole bacterial cells as template instead of extracted DNA could be affected by the physiological state of the cells (Silva & Batt 1995). Differential or preferential amplification of rRNA genes by PCR has been described by Reysenbach *et al.* (1992). Addition of acetamide to the PCR reaction was used to facilitate template denaturation and to prevent preferential amplification (Reysenbach *et al.* 1992). Recently, Suzuki and Giovannoni (1996) found that preferential amplification might be caused by reannealing of the template DNA, thereby inhibiting primer binding. Farrelly *et al.* (1995) demonstrated the effect of genome size and the copy number of 16S rRNA genes on the quantities of PCR products. Another problem in the use of PCR to amplify mixed target DNAs is the formation of so-called chimeric molecules (Liesack *et al.* 1991; Kopczynski *et al.* 1994). Also the cloning approach is not free from biases. Rainey *et al.* (1994) described different cloning efficiencies for different cloning vectors and with different primer pairs.

8. Retrieval of useful information from complex mixtures of microorganisms

One of the problems with the study of microbial communities with molecular microbiological methods, such as PCR, is the enormous diversity of microorganisms typically present. By using DNA-DNA reannealing experiments, Torsvik *et al.* (1990a,b) found that there might be as many as 10^4 different bacterial genomes present in soil samples. It will be obvious that all of these different genomes cannot easily be retrieved by the cloning approach or by genetic fingerprinting. Nevertheless, substantial information about the species composition from very complex microbial communities can be obtained. For instance, bacterial cells can be dislodged from soil (*e.g.* Priemé *et al.* 1996) and fractionated by electrophoresis (Jaspers & Overmann 1997) or by filtration (Rappé *et al.* 1998), prior to the amplification process. Community DNA can be fractionated according to its mol% G+C content using bisbenzimide/CsCl centrifugation (Holben *et al.* 1993; Holben & Harris 1995). Øvreas *et al.* (1995) used this approach to fractionate complex mixtures of DNA extracted from soil samples prior to PCR amplification and DGGE analysis. Recently, Nüsslein and Tiedje (1998) used the same approach to characterize dominant and rare bacterial populations in Hawaiian soil. To lower the bacterial diversity, total extracted DNA was fractionated by bisbenzimide equilibrium centrifugation into a DNA fraction with a mol% G+C content of 63, and a fraction with a mol% G+C content of 35. Comparative sequence analysis of the cloned 16S rDNA PCR products from the 63% G+C fraction revealed phylotypes affiliated to microorganisms, such as *Pseudomonas, Rhizobium-Agrobacterium,* and *Rhodospirillum,* while sequences of the 35% G+C fraction were related to *Clostridia.* The phylogenetic affiliation of the phylotypes from the two G+C fractions, was found to be consistent with the mol% G+C of their most related cultivated counterparts.

Hybridization analysis of fingerprinting profiles with group-specific probes can reveal the presence of certain groups of organisms, even if individual bands are hidden in a smear of ethidium bromide stained bands (*e.g.* Teske *et al.* 1996a). Heuer *et al.* (1995) used digoxigenin-labelled polynucleotide probes under stringent hybridization conditions to detect particular microorganisms, such as *Agrobacterium tumefaciens,* in DGGE or TGGE patterns. These probes were produced by enzymatic amplification of the hypervariable V6 region (Neefs *et al.* 1990) (from position 971 to position 1057 in *E. coli*) of the 16S rRNA of particular bacterial strains using universal primers flanking this region. The advantage of this strategy is that no sequence information is required to produce the probes.

Particular bacterial groups, which are rare members of complex assemblages, can also be studied by the analysis of PCR products obtained with group-specific primers, such as those for cyanobacteria (Nübel *et al.* 1997), beta-ammonium oxidizers (Kowalchuk *et al.* 1997a), or actinomycetes (Heuer *et al.* 1997). An interesting strategy is the amplification of DNA fragments obtained with group-specific primers, such as those for the beta-ammonium oxidizers (McCaig *et al.* 1994; Voytek & Ward 1995) followed by a reamplification of these PCR products with nested DGGE primers. This approach makes it possible to determine the ecological importance of particular bacteria within microbial communities. Furthermore, the complexity can be reduced by using PCR primers for functional genes, which are only present in particular bacterial populations (Wawer & Muyzer 1995).

9. Concluding remarks and future directions

The use of molecular biological techniques has provided an unparalleled opportunity to study microbial communities *in situ*, without the need for isolation. The cloning approach shows us who is there, while the application of specific probes in whole cell hybridization reveals how many of them are present, and where they are located in a microbial community. Genetic fingerprinting makes it possible to monitor the behaviour of microbial assemblages over time, through monitoring of population shifts after environmental stress. However, none of these techniques is all-encompassing, or perfect. Apart from the technical limitations, the use of rRNA as a molecular marker may limit the quest for describing microbial diversity. It may be too conserved to reveal differences between closely related, but ecologically different microorganisms. An example is the phylogenetic affiliation of several bacterial species belonging to the alpha-2 group of Protebacteria (Fig. 5). The 16S rRNA sequences of some of these microorganisms have similarity values of 97% or more and might therefore be regarded as strains of the same species by the criteria described by Stackebrandt and Goebel (1994). However, their physiology, and ecological roles are completely different. For instance, *Nitrobacter winogradskyi* is a chemolithotrophic nitrifyer, *Rhodopseudomonas palustris* a phototrophic microorganism, and *Afipia felis* a human pathogen. In this respect, Cohan and coworkers (Palys *et al.* 1997) argue for the use of protein-encoding genes to discover and classify ecological diversity among closely related bacteria, because the sequences of these genes might be more discriminative then those encoding rRNA. Moreover, the use of protein-encoding genes opens up the exciting possibility of catching active bacteria red-handed, and to study niche differentiation (Wawer *et al.* 1997).

Regarding the biases and limitations of the individual techniques, only a combined application of different molecular biological techniques will reveal the real dimension of microbial diversity in nature. In addition, the application of microbiological techniques to isolate bacteria in pure cultures will also be needed, for example to create phylogenetic frameworks of protein-encoding gene sequences, as well as for the classification and identification of closely related bacteria.

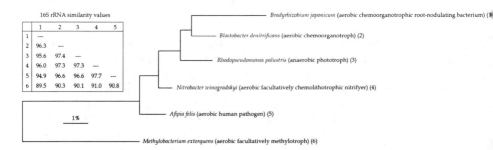

Figure 5: 16S rRNA similarity values and phylogentic tree of bacteria belonging to the alpha-2 group of the Proteobacteria. The tree is based on complete 16S rRNA sequences, and created with the maximum likelihood method as implemented in the software programme ARB. The bar represent 1% sequence divergence. Note the close phylogenetic affiliation of species with different physiologies and ecological roles.

For that purpose, new isolation strategies need to be applied, such as the dilution culture strategy (Button et al. 1993; Schut et al. 1993) or the cultivation of organisms in gradients of nutrients (Emerson & Moyer 1997). Molecular biological methods, such as DGGE or whole cell hybridization, can then be used as tools to monitor enrichment cultures and to follow the successful isolation of ecologically relevant bacteria in pure cultures (e.g. Brinkhoff & Muyzer 1997). Furthermore, a detailed investigation of the environmental parameters is necessary to unravel the role of microorganisms, and to help to establish the appropriate culture conditions to isolate these organisms in pure cultures. In this respect, future studies in microbial ecology must be of a polyphasic nature combining molecular biological techniques with microbiological methods, and methods to determine environmental parameters. Only then may we understand the relationship between microorganisms and their living and non-living environment, which is the goal of microbial ecology.

Acknowledgements

I want to thank Hendrik Schäfer, Gary Carvalho, and two anonymous reviewers for careful reading and helpful suggestions to improve the manuscript.

References

Alfreider A, Pernthaler J, Amann R et al. (1996) Community analysis of the bacterial assemblages in the winter cover and pelagic layers of a high mountain lake by in situ hybridization. Applied and Environmental Microbiology, 62, 2138-2144.

Amann RI, Binder BJ, Olson RJ, Chisholm SW, Devereux R, Stahl DA (1990) Combination of 16S rRNA-targeted oligonucleotide probes with flow cytometry for analyzing mixed microbial populations. Applied and Environmental Microbiology, 56, 1919-1925.

Amann RI, Stromley J, Devereux R, Key R, Stahl DA (1992) Molecular and microscopical identification of sulfate-reducing bacteria in multispecies biofilms. Applied and Environmental Microbiology, 58, 614-623.

Amann RI, Ludwig W, Schleifer K-H (1995) Phylogenetic identification and in situ detection of individual microbial cells without cultivation. Microbiology Reviews, 59, 143-169.

Amann RI (1995) In situ identification of micro-organisms by whole cell hybridization with rRNA-targeted nucleic acid probes. Molecular Microbial Ecology Manual 3.3.6, 1-15.

Atlas RM, Bartha R (1987) Microbial Ecology - Fundamentals and Applications. Benjamin/Cummings Publishing Company, Inc., Menlo Park.

Assmus B, Hutzler P, Kirchhof G, Amann R, Lawrence JR, Hartmann A (1995) In situ localization of Azospirillum brasilense in the rhizosphere of wheat with fluorescently labeled rRNA-targeted oligonucleotide probes and scanning laser microscopy. Applied and Environmental Microbiology, 61, 1013-1019.

Barns SM, Fundyga RE, Jeffries MW, Pace NR (1994) Remarkable archaeal diversity detected in a Yellowstone National Park hot spring environment. Proceedings of the National Academy of Sciences USA, 91, 1609-1613.

Barns SM, Delwiche CF, Palmer JD, Pace NR (1996) Perspectives on archaeal diversity, thermophily, and monophylly from environmental rRNA sequences. Proceedings of the National Academy of Sciences USA, 93, 9188-9193.

Benson DA, Boguski MS, Lipman DJ, Ostell J (1997) GenBank. Nucleic Acids Research, 25, 1-6.

Bidle KD, Fletcher M (1995) Comparison of free-living and particle-associated bacterial communities in the Chesapeake Bay by stable Low-Molecular-Weight RNA analysis. Applied and Environmental Microbiology, 61, 944-952.

Borneman J, Skroch PW, O'Sullivan KM et al. (1996) Molecular microbial diversity of an agricultural soil in Wisconsin. Applied and Environmental Microbiology, 62, 1935-1943.

Borneman J, Triplett EW (1997) Molecular microbial diversity in soils from eastern Amazonia evidence for unusual microorganisms and microbial population shifts associated with deforestation. Applied and Environmental Microbiology, 63, 2647-2653.

Bowman JP, McCammon SA, Brown MV, Nichols DS, McMeekin TA (1997) Diversity and association of psychrophilic bacteria in Antartic sea ice. *Applied and Environmental Microbiology,* **63**, 3068-3078.

Breen A, Rope AF, Taylor D, Loper JC, Sferra PR (1995) Application of DNA amplification fingerprinting (DAF) to mixed culture bioreactors. *Journal of Industrial Microbiology,* **14**, 10-16.

Brinkhoff T, Muyzer G (1997) Increased species diversity and extended habitat range of sulfur-oxidizing *Thiomicrospira* spp. *Applied and Environmental Microbiology,* **63**, 3789-3796.

Britschgi TB and Giovannoni SJ (1991) Phylogenetic analysis of a natural marine bacterioplankton population by rRNA gene cloning and sequencing. *Applied and Environmental Microbiology,* **57**, 1707-1713.

Brock TD (1987) The study of microorganisms *in situ*: progress and problems. In: *Ecology of Microbial Communities,* (eds. Fletcher M, Gray TRG, and Jones JG) Cambridge University Press, Cambridge. p. 1-18.

Bruce KD (1997) Analysis of *mer* gene subclasses within bacterial communities in soils and sediments resolved by fluorescent-PCR-restriction fragment length polymorphism profiling. *Applied and Environmental Microbiology,* **63**, 4914-4919.

Buchholz-Cleven BEE; Rattunde B, Straub KL (1997) Screening for genetic diversity of isolates of anaerobic Fe(II)-oxidizing bacteria using DGGE and whole-cell hybridization. *Systematic and Applied Microbiology,* **20**, 301-309.

Button DK, Schut F, Quang P, Martin R, Robertson BR (1993) Viability and isolation of marine bacteria by dilution culture: theory, procedure, and initial results. *Applied and Environmental Microbiology,* **59**, 881-891.

Byers HK, Stackebrandt E, Hayward C, Blackall LL (1998) Molecular investigation of a microbial mat associated with the Great Artesian Basin. *FEMS Microbiology Ecology,* **25**, 391-403.

Caetano-Anolles G, Bassam GJ, Gresshof PM (1991) High resolution DNA amplification fingerprinting using very short arbitrary oligonucleotide primers. *Biotechnology,* **9**, 553-556.

Canfield DE, DesMarais DJ (1991) Aerobic sulfate reduction in microbial mats. *Science,* **251**, 1471-1473.

Chen F, Dustman W, Moran MA, Hodson RE (1998) *In situ* PCR methodologies for visualization of microscale genetic and taxonomic diversities of prokaryotic communities. *Molecular Microbial Ecology Manual,* **3.3.9**, 1-17.

Chen F, González JM, Dustman WA, Moran MA, Hodson RE (1997) *In situ* reverse transcription, an approach to characterize genetic diversity and activities of prokaryotes. *Applied and Environmental Microbiology,* **63**, 4907-4913.

DeLong EF, Franks DG, Alldredge AL (1993) Phylogenetic diversity of aggregate-attached vs. free-living marine bacterial assemblages. *Limnology and Oceanography,* **38**, 924-934.

DeLong EF, Wu KY, Prézelin BB, Jovine RVM (1994) High abundance of Arcaea in Antartic marine picoplankton. *Nature,* **371**, 695-697.

De los Reyes FL, Ritter W, Raskin L. (1997) Group-specific small-subunit rRNA hybridization probes to characterize filamentous foaming in activated sludge systems. *Applied and Environmental Microbiology,* **63**, 1107-1117.

Donner G, Schwarz K, Hoppe H-G, Muyzer G (1996) Profiling the succession of bacterial populations in pelagic chemoclines. *Archiv furHydrobiologie: Special Issues in Advanced Limnology,* **48**, 7-14.

Emerson D, Moyer C (1997) Isolation and characterization of novel iron-oxidizing bacteria that grow at circumneutral pH. *Applied and Environmental Microbiology,* **63**, 4784-4792.

Farrelly V, Rainey FA, Stackebrandt E (1995) Effect of genome size and rrn gene copy number on PCR amplification of 16S rRNA genes from a mixture of bacterial species. *Applied and Environmental Microbiology,* **61**, 2798-2801.

Felske A, Engelen B, Nübel U, Backhaus H (1996) Direct ribosomal isolation from soil to extract bacterial rRNA for community analysis. *Applied and Environmental Microbiology,* **62**, 4162-4167.

Felske A, Rheims H, Wolterink A, Stackebrandt E, Akkermans ADL (1997) Ribosome analysis reveals prominant activity of an uncultured member of the class Actinobacteria in grassland soils. *Microbiology,* **143**, 2983-2989.

Felske A, Wolterink A, van Lis R, Akkermans ADL (1998) Phylogeny of the main bacterial 16S rRNA sequences in Dentse A grassland soils (The Netherlands). *Applied and Environmental Microbiology,* **64**, 871-879.

Ferris MJ, Muyzer G, Ward DM (1996) Denaturing gradient gel electrophoresis profiles of 16S rRNA-defined populations inhabiting a hot spring microbial mat community. *Applied and Environmental Microbiology,* **62**, 340-346.

Ferris MJ, Nold SC, Revsbech NP, Ward DM (1997) Population structure and physiological changes within a hot spring microbial mat community following disturbance. *Applied and Environmental Microbiology,* **63**, 1367-1374.

Ferris MJ, Ward DM (1997) Seasonal distributions of dominant 16S rRNA-defined populations in a hot spring microbial mat examined by denaturing gradient gel electrophoresis. *Applied and Environmental Microbiology*, **63**, 1375-1381.

Fesefeldt A, Gliesche CG (1997) Identification of *Hyphomicrobium* spp. using PCR-amplified fragments of the *mxaF* gene as a molecular marker. *Systematic and Applied Microbiology*, **20**, 387-396.

Fischer K, Hahn D, Amann RI, Daniel O, Zeyer J (1995) *In situ* analysis of the bacterial community in the gut of the earthworm *Lumbricus terrestris* L. by whole-cell hybridization. *Canadian. Journal of Microbiology*, **41**, 666-673.

Führ A (1996) Untersuchungen zu der Biodiversität natürlicher Bakterienpopulationen im Boden mit der denaturierenden Gradientengelelectrophorese (DGGE) von 16S rDNA-Sequenzen. PhD-thesis Universitat Kaiserslautern, Germany.

Fuhrman JA, McCallum K, Davis AA (1993) Phylogenetic diversity of subsurface marine microbial communities from the Atlantic and Pacific Oceans. *Applied and Environmental Microbiology*, **59**, 1294-1302.

Garcia-Pichel F, Prufert-Bebout L, Muyzer G (1996) Phenotypic and phylogenetic analyses show Microcoleus chtonoplastes to be a cosmopolitan cyanobacterium. *Applied and Environmental Microbiology*, **62**, 3284-3291.

Giovannoni SJ, Britschgi TB, Moyer CL, Field KG (1990) Genetic diversity in Sargasso Sea bacterioplankton. *Nature*, **345**, 61-62.

Godon J-J, Zumstein E, Dabert P, Habouzit F, Moletta R (1997) Molecular microbial diversity of an anaerobic digestor as determined by small-subunit rDNA sequence analysis. *Applied and Environmental Microbiology*, **63**, 2802-2813.

Gordon DA, Giovannoni SJ (1996) Detection of stratified microbial populations related to *Chlorobium* and *Fibrobacter* species in the Atlantic and Pacific Oceans. *Applied and Environmental Microbiology*, **62**, 1171-1177.

Grey JP, Herwig RP (1996) Phylogenetic analysis of the bacterial communities in marine sediments. *Applied and Environmental Microbiology*, **62**, 4049-4059.

Gwynfryn Jones J (1996) Modern molecular techniques and environmental microbiology. In: *Molecular Approaches to Environmental Microbiology,* (eds. Pickup RW, and JR Saunders), pp.1-17 Ellis Horwood, London.

Hammond PM (1995) Described and Estimated species numbers: an objective assessment of current knowledge. In: *Microbial Diversity and Ecosystem Functioning* (eds. Allsopp, D, Colwell RR, Hawksworth DL), pp. 29-71. Cab International, Oxford.

Hadrys H, Balick M, Schierwater B (1992) Applications of random amplified polymorphic DNA (RAPD) in molecular ecology. *Molecular Ecology*, **1**, 55-63.

Hahn D, Amann RI, Zeyer J (1993a) Whole-cell hybridization of Frankia strains with fluorescence or digoxygenin-labeled 16S rRNA-targeted oligonucleotide probes. *Applied and Environmental Microbiology*, **59**, 1709-1716.

Hahn D, Amann RI, Zeyer J (1993b) Detection of mRNA in *Streptomyces* cells by whole-cell hybridization with digoxigenin-labeled probes. *Applied and Environmental Microbiology*, **59**, 2753-2757.

Hahn D, Zepp K, Zeyer J (1997) Whole cell hybridization as a tool to study *Frankia* populations in root nodules. *Physiologia Plantarum*, **99(4)**, 696-706.

Harmsen HJM, Kengen HM, Akkermans ADL, Stams AJM, de Vos WM (1996a) Detection and localization of synthrophic propionate-oxidizing bacteria in granular sludge by *in situ* hybridization using 16S rRNA-based oligonucleotide probes. *Applied and Environmental Microbiology*, **62**, 1656-1663.

Harmsen HJM, Akkermans ADL, Stams AJM, de Vos WM (1996b) Population dynamics of propionate-oxidizing bacteria under methanogenic and sulfidogenic conditions in anaerobic granular sludge. *Applied and Environmental Microbiology*, **62**, 2163-2168.

Harmsen HJM, Prieur D, Jeanthon C (1997) Group-specific 16S rRNA-targeted oligoncleotide probes to identify thermophilic bacteria in marine hydrothermal vents. *Applied and Environmental Microbiology*, **63**, 4061-4068.

Heuer H, Hartung Engelen B, Smalla K (1995) Studies on microbial communities associated with potato plants by BIOLOG and TGGE patterns. *Medische Faculteit Landbouw Universiteit Gent*, **60/4b**, 2639-2645.

Heuer H, Smalla K (1997) Application of denaturing gradient gel electrophoresis (DGGE) and temperature gradient gel electrophoresis (TGGE) for studying soil microbial communities. In: *Modern Soil Microbiology* (eds. van Elseas JD, Trevors JT, and Wellington EMH), pp. 353-373. Marcel Dekker, New York.

Heuer H, Krsek M, Baker P, Smalla K, Wellington EMH (1997) Analysis of actinomycete communities by specific amplification of genes encoding 16S rRNA and gel electrophoretic separation in denaturing gradient. *Applied and Environmental Microbiology*, **63**, 3233-3241.

Hiorns WD, Methé BA, Nierzwicki-Bauer, Zehr JP (1997) Bacterial diversity in Adirondack montain lakes as revealed by 16S rRNA gene sequences. *Applied and Environmental Microbiology,* **63**, 2957-2960.

Hodson RE, Dustman WA, Garg RP, Moran MA (1995) *In situ* PCR for visualization of microscale distribution of specific gene products in prokaryotic communities. *Applied and Environmental Microbiology,* **61**, 4047-4082.

Höfle M (1988) Identification of bacteria by low molecular weight RNA profiles: a new chemotaxonomic approach. *Journal of Microbiology Methods,* **8**, 235-248.

Höfle M (1992) Bacterioplankton community structure and dynamics after large-scale release of nonindigenous bacteria as revealed by low-molecular-weight RNA analysis. *Applied and Environmental Microbiology,* **58**, 3387-3394.

Höfle MG, Brettar I (1996) Genotyping of heterotrophic bacteria from the central Baltic Sea by use of low-molecular-weight RNA profiles. *Applied and Environmental Microbiology,* **62**, 1383-1390.

Höfle MG (1998) Genotyping of bacterial isolates from the environment using Low-Molecular-Weight RNA fingerprints. *Molecular Microbial Ecology Manual,* **3.3.7**, 1-23.

Holben WE, Calabrese VGM, Harris D, Ka JO, Tiedje JM (1993) Analysis of structure and selection in microbial communities by molecular methods. In: *Trends in microbial ecology,* (eds. Guerrero R, Pedrós-Alió, C), pp. 367-370. Spanish Society for Microbiology, Barcelona, Spain.

Holben WE, Harris D (1995) DNA-based monitoring of total bacterial community structure in environmental samples. *Molecular Ecology,* **4**, 627-631.

Holt JG, Krieg NR, Sneath PHA, Staley JT, Williams ST (1994) *Bergey's Manual of Determinative Bacteriology.* Williams & Wilkins, Baltimore.

Hovanec TA, Taylor LT, Blakis A, deLong EF (1998) Nitrospira-like bacteria associated with nitrite oxidation in freshwater aquaria. *Applied and Environmental Microbiology,* **64**, 258-264.

Hugenholz P, Pitulle C, Hershberger Kl, Pace NR (1998) Novel division level bacterial diversity in a Yellowstone hot spring. *Journal of Bacteriology,* **180**, 366-376.

Jaspers E, Overmann J (1997) Separation of bacterial cells by isoelectric focusing, a new method for analysis of complex microbial communities. *Applied and Environmental Microbiology,* **63**, 3176-3181.

Jensen MA, Straus N (1993) Effect of PCR conditions on the formation of heteroduplex and single-stranded DNA products in the amplification of bacterial ribosomal DNA spacer regions. *PCR Methods Application,* **3**, 186-194.

Jensen S, Øvreas L, Daae FL, Torsvik V (1998) Diversity in methane enrichments from agricultural soil revealed by DGGE separation of PCR amplified 16S rDNA fragments. FEMS Microbiology Ecology, 26, 17-26.

Kalmbach S, Manz W, Szewzyk U (1997) Dynamics of biofilm formation in drinking water: phylogenetic affiliation and metabolic potential of single cells assessed by formazan reduction and *in situ* hybridization. *FEMS Microbiology Ecology,* **22**, 265-279.

Kopczynski ED, Bateson M, Ward DM (1994) Recognition of chimeric small-subunit ribisomal DNAs composed from genes from uncultivated microorganisms. *Applied and Environmental Microbiology,* **60**, 746-748.

Kowalchuk GA, Stephen JR, De Boer W, Prosser JI, Embley TM, Woldendorp JW (1997a) Analysis of proteobacteria ammonia-oxidizing bacteria in coastal sand dunes using denaturing gradient gel electrophoresis and sequencing of PCR amplified 16S rDNA fragments. *Applied and Environmental Microbiology,* **63**, 1489-1497.

Kowalchuk GA, Gerards S, Woldendorp JW (1997b) Detection and characterization of fungal infections of *Ammophila arenaria* (Marram grass) roots by denaturing gradient gel electrophoresis of specifically amplifed 18S rDNA. *Applied and Environmental Microbiology,* **63**, 3858-3865.

LeBaron P, Catala P, Fajon C, Joux F, Baudart J, Bernard L (1997) A new sensitive, whole-cell hybridization technique for detection of bacteria involving a biotinylated oligonucleotide probe targetting rRNA and tyramide signal amplifcation. *Applied and Environmental Microbiology,* **63**, 327-3278.

Lee D-H, Zo Y-G, Kim S-J (1996) Nonradioactive method to study genetic profiles of natural bacterial communities bz PCR-Single-Stranded-Conformation Polymorphism. *Applied and Environmental Microbiology,* **62**, 3112-3120.

Liesack W, Weyland H, Stackebrandt E (1991) Potential risks of gene amplification by PCR as determined by 16S rRNA analysis of a mixed culture of strictly barophilic bacteria. *Microbial Ecology,* **21**, 191-198.

Liesack W, Janssen PH, Rainey FA, Ward-Rainey NL, Stackebrandt E (1997) Microbial diversity in soil: the need for a combined approach using molecular and cultivation techniques. In: *Modern Soil Microbiology* (eds. van Elsas JD, Trevors JT, Wellington EMH), pp. 375-439. Marcel Dekker, New York.

Lin C, Stahl DA (1995) Taxon-specific probes for the cellulolytic genus *Fibrobacter* reveal abundant and novel equine-associated populations. *Applied and Environmental Microbiology,* **61**, 1348-1351.

Lin C, Raskin L, Stahl DA (1997) Microbial community structure in gastrointestinal tracts of domestic animals: comparative study using rRNA-targeted oligonucleotide probes. *FEMS Microbiology Ecology*, **22**, 281-294.

Liu W-T, Marsh TL, Cheng H, Forney LJ (1997) Characterization of microbial diversity by determining terminal restriction fragment length polymorphisms of genes encoding 16S rRNA. *Applied and Environmental Microbiology*, **63**, 4516-4522.

Ludwig W, Strunk O, Klugbauer S, Klugbauer N, Weizenegger M, Neumaier J, Bachleitner M, Schleifer K.-H. (1998) Bacterial phylogeny based on comparative sequence analysis. *Electrophoresis*, **19**, 554-568.

Maidak BL, Olsen GJ, Larsen N, Overbeek R, McCaughey MJ, Woese CR (1997) The RDP (Ribosomal Database Project). *Nucleic Acids Research*, **25**, 109-110.

Manz W, Wagner M, Amann R, Schleifer K-H (1994) *In situ* characterization of the microbial consortia active in two wastewater treatment plants. *Water Research*, **28**, 1715-1723.

Manz W, Amann R, Ludwig W, Vancanneyt M, Schleifer K-H (1996) Application of a suite of 16S rRNA-specific oligonucleotide probes designed to investigate bacteria of the phylum Cytophaga-Flavobacter-Bacteroides in the natural environment. *Microbiology*, **142**, 1097-1106.

Manz W, Eisenbrecher M, Neu TR, Szewzyk U (1998) Abundance and spatial organization of Gram-negative sulfate-reducing bacteria in activated sludge investigated by *in situ* probing with specific 16S rRNA targeted oligonucleotides. *FEMS Microbiology Ecology*, **25**, 33-41.

Martinez-Murcia AJ, Acinas SG, Rodriguez-Valera F (1995) Evaluation of prokaryotic diversity by restrictase digestion of 16S rDNA directly amplified from hypersaline environments. FEMS *Microbiology Ecology*, **17**, 247-256.

Massol-Deya AA, Odelson DA, Hickey RF, Tiedje JM (1995) Bacterial community fingerprinting of amplified 16S and 16-23S ribosomal DNA gene sequences and restriction endonuclease analysis (ARDRA). *Molecular Microbial Ecology Manual*, **3.3.2**, 1-18.

McCaig AE, Embley TM, Prosser JI (1994) Molecular analysis of enrichment cultures of marine ammonia oxidisers. *FEMS Microbiology Letters*, **120**, 363-368.

McInerney JO, Wolkinson M, Patching JW, Embley TM, Powell R (1995) Recovery and phylogenetic analysis of novel archaeal rRNA sequences from a deep-sea deposit feeder. *Applied and Environmental Microbiology*, **61**, 1646-1648.

Mobarry BK, Wagner M, Urbain V, Rittmann BE, Stahl DA (1996) Phylogenetic probes for analyzing abundance and spatial organization of nitrifying bacteria. *Applied and Environmental Microbiology*, **62**, 2156-2162.

Moyer Cl, Dobbs FC, Karl DM (1995) Phylogenetic diversity of the bacterial community from a microbial mat at an active, hydrothermal vent system, Loihi Seamount, Hawaii. *Applied and Environmental Microbiology*, **61**, 1555-1562.

Mullins TD, Britschgi TB, Krest RL, Giovannoni SJ (1995) Genetic comparison reveal the same unknown bacterial lineages in Atlantic and Pacific bacterioplankton communities. *Limnology and Oceanography*, **40**, 148-158.

Munson MA, Nedwell DB, Embley TM (1997) Phylogenetic diversity of *Archaea* in sediment samples from a coastal salt marsh. *Applied and Environmental Microbiology*, **63**, 4729-4733.

Murray AE, Hollibaugh JT, Orrego C (1996) Phylogenetic comparisons of bacterioplankton from two California estuaries compared by denaturing gradient gel electrophoresis of 16S rDNA fragments. *Applied and Environmental Microbiology*, **62**, 2676-2680.

Muyzer G, de Waal EC, Uitterlinden AG (1993) Profiling of complex microbial populations by denaturing gradient gel electrophoresis analysis of polymerase chain reaction-amplified genes encoding for 16S rRNA. *Applied and Environmental Microbiology*, **59**, 695-700.

Muyzer G and de Waal EC (1994) Determination of the genetic diversity of microbial communities using DGGE analysis of PCR-amplified 16S rRNA. *NATO ASI Series*, **G35**, 207-214.

Muyzer G, Teske A, Wirsen CO, Jannasch HW (1995) Phylogenetic relationships of *Thiomicrospira* species and their identification in deep-sea hydrothermal vent samples by denaturing gradient gel electrophoresis of 16S rDNA fragments. *Archives of Microbiology*, **164**, 165-171.

Muyzer G, Smalla K (1998) Application of denaturing gradient gel electrophoresis (DGGE) and temperature gradient gel electrophoresis (TGGE) in microbiol ecology. *Antonie van Leeuwenhoek*, **73**, 127-141.

Muyzer G, Brinkhoff T, Nübel U, Santegoeds C, Schäfer H, Wawer C (1998) Denaturing gradient gel electrophoresis (DGGE) in microbial ecology. *Molecular Microbial Ecology Manual*, **3.4.4**, 1-27.

Myers RM, Fischer SG, Lerman LS, Maniatis T (1985) Nearly all single base substitutions in DNA fragments joined to a GC-clamp can be detected by denaturing gradient gel electrophoresis. *Nucleic Acids Research*, **13**, 3131-3145.

Myers RM, Maniatis T, Lerman LS (1987) Detection and localization of single base changes by denaturing gradient gel electrophoresis. *Methods in Enzymology*, **155**, 501-527.

Neefs J, van de Peer Y, Hendriks L, de Wachter R (1990) Compilation of small ribosomal subunit RNA sequences. *Nucleic Acid Research,* **18**, 2237-2242.

Nübel U, Engelen B, Felske A *et al.* (1996) Sequence heterogeneities of genes encoding 16S rRNAs in *Paenibacillus polymyxa* detected by temperature gradient gel electrophoresis. *Journal of Bacteriology,* **178**, 5636-5643.

Nübel U, Garcia-Pichel F, Muyzer G (1997) PCR primers to amplify 16S rRNA genes from cyanobacteria. *Applied and Environmental Microbiology,* **63**, 3327-3332.

Nüsslein K, Tiedje JM (1998) Characterization of the dominant and rare members of a young Hawaiian soil bacterial community with small-subunit ribosomal DNA amplified from DNA fractionated on the basis of its guanine and cytosine composition. *Applied and Environmental Microbiology,* **64**, 1283-1289.

Ohkuma M, Kudo T (1996) Phylogenetic diversity of the intestinal bacterial community in the termite *Reticulitermes speratus. Applied and Environmental Microbiology,* **62**, 461-468.

Olsen GJ, Lane DJ, Giovannoni SJ, Pace NR (1986) Microbial ecology and evolution: a ribosomal approach. *Annual Review of Microbiology,* **40**, 337-365.

Orita M, Iwahana H, Kanazawa H, Hayashi K, Sekiya T (1989) Detection of polymorphisms of human DNA by gel electrophoresis as single-strand conformation polymorphisms. *Proceedings of the National Academy of Sciences USA,* **86**, 2766-2770.

Overmann J, Tuschak C (1997) Phylogeny and molecular fingerprinting of green-sulfur bacteria. *Archives of Microbiology,* **167**, 302-309.

Øvreas L, Castberg T, Torsvik V (1995) Analysis of natural microbial communities using reassociation of total DNA in combination with bisbenzimide density gradients and DGGE. In: *Proceedings of the Workshop on Application of DGGE and TGGE in Microbial Ecology* (eds. Smalla K and Muyzer G). BBA, Braunschweig, Germany.

Øvreas L, Forney L, Daae FL, Torsvik V (1997) Distribution of bacterioplankton in meromictic lake Saelenvannet, as determined by denaturing gradient gel electrophoresis of PCR-amplified gene fragments coding for 16S rRNA. *Applied and Environmental Microbiology,* **63**, 3367-3373.

Pace NA, Stahl DA, Lane DJ, Olsen G (1986) The analysis of natural microbial communities by ribosomal RNA sequences. *Advances in Microbial Ecology,* **9**, 1-55.

Pace NR (1997) A molecular view of microbial diversity and the biophere. *Science,* **276**, 734-740.

Palys T, Nakamura LK, Cohan FM (1997) Discovery and classification of ecological diversity in the bacterial world: the role of DNA sequence data. *Internatioal Journal of Systematic Bacteriology,* **47**, 1145-1156.

Pedrós Alió C, Guerrero R (1994) Prokaryotology for the limnologist. In: *Limnology Now: A Paradigm of Planetary Problems,* (ed. Margalef R). pp. 37-57.

Pernthaler J, Posch T, Simek K, Vrba J, Amann R, Psenner R (1997) Contrasting bacterial strategies to coexist with a flagellate predator in an experimental microbial assemblage. *Applied and Environmental Microbiology,* **63**, 596-601.

Polz MF, Distel DL, Zarda B *et al.* (1994) Phylogenetic analysis of a highly specific association between endosymbiotic sulfur-oxidizing bacteria and a marine nematode. *Applied and Environmental Microbiology,* **60**, 4461-4467.

Poulsen LK, Ballard G, Stahl DA (1993) Use of rRNA fluorescence *in situ* hybridization for measuring the activity of single cells in young and established biofilms. *Applied and Environmental Microbiology,* **59**, 1354-1360.

Priemé A, Sitaula JIB, Klemedtsson AK, Bakken LR (1996) Extraction of methane-oxidizing bacteria from soil. *FEMS Miocrobiology Ecology,* **21**, 59-68.

Purdy KJ, Nedwell DB, Embley M, Takii S (1997) Use of 16S rRNA-targeted oligonucleotide probes to investigate the occurrence and selection of sulfate-reducing bacteria in response to nutrient addition to sediment slurry microcosms from a Japanese estuary. *FEMS Microbiology Ecology,* **24**, 221-234.

Ramsing NB, Kühl M, Jørgensen BB (1993) Distribution of sulfate-reducing bacteria, O_2, and H_2S in photosynthetic biofilms determined by oligonucleotide probes and microelelectrodes. *Applied and Environmental Microbiology,* **59**, 3840-3849.

Ramsing NB, Fossing H, Ferdelman TG, Andersen F, Thamdrup B (1996) Distribution of bacterial populations in a stratified fjord (Mariager Fjord, Denmark) quantified by *in situ* hybridization and related to chemical gradients in the water column. *Applied and Environmental Microbiology,* **62**, 1391-1404.

Rainey FA, Ward N, Sly LI, Stackebrandt E (1994) Dependence on taxon composition of clone libraries for PCR amplified, naturally occurring 16S rDNA, on the primer pair and the cloning system. *Experientia,* **50**, 796-797.

Rappé MS, Suzuki MT, Vergin KL, Giovannoni SJ (1998) Phylogenetic diversity of ultraplankton plastid small-subunit rRNA genes recovered in environmental nucleic acid samples from the Pacific and Atlantic Coasts of the United States. *Applied and Environmental Microbiology,* **64**, 294-303.

Raskin L, Stromley JM, Rittmann BE, Stahl DA (1994a) Group-specific 16S rRNA hybridization probes to describe natural communities of methanogens. *Applied and Environmental Microbiology,* **60**, 1232-1240.

Raskin L, Poulsen LK, Noguera DR, Rittmann BE, Stahl DA (1994b) Quantification of methanogenic groups in anaerobic biological reactors by oligonucleotide probe hybridization. *Applied and Environmental Microbiology*, **60**, 1241-1248.

Raskin L, Zheng D, Griffin ME, Stroot PG, Misra P (1995) Characterization of microbial communities in anaerobic bioreactors using molecular probes. *Antonie van Leeuwenhoek*, **68**, 297-308.

Raskin L, Rittmann BE, Stahl DA (1996) Competition and coexistence of sulfate-reducing and methanogenic populations in anaerobic biofilms. *Applied and Environmental Microbiology*, **62**, 3847-3857.

Raskin L, Capman WC, Sharp R, Stahl DA (1997) Molecular ecology of gastrointestinal ecosystems. In: *Gastrointestinal Microbiology and Host Interactions*, vol. 2, (eds. Mackie RI, White BA, Isaacson RE). Chapman and Hall, London.

Rath J, Wu KY, Herndl GJ, DeLong EF (1998) High phylogenetic diversity in a marine-snow-associated bacterial assemblage. *Aquatic Microbial Ecology*, **14**, 261-269.

Reysenbach A-L, Giver, LJ, Wickham GS, Pace NR (1992) Differential amplification of rRNA genes by polymerase chain reaction. *Applied and Environmental Microbiology*, **58**, 3417-3418.

Riesner D, Henco K, and Steger G (1991) Temperature-gradient gel electrophoresis: a method for the analysis of conformational transitions and mutations in nucleic acids and proteins. *Advances in Electrophoresis*, **4**, 169-250.

Risatti JB, Capman WC, Stahl DA (1994) Community structure of a microbial mat: The phylogenetic dimension. *Proceedings of the National Academy of Sciences USA*, **91**, 10173-10177.

Rochelle PA, Cragg BA, Fry JC, Parkes RJ, Weightman AJ (1994) Effect of sample handling on estimation of bacterial diversity in marine sediments by 16S rRNA gene sequence analysis. *FEMS Microbiology Ecology*, **15**, 215-226.

Rölleke S, Muyzer G, Wawer C, Wanner, G, Lubitz W (1995) Identification of bacteria in a biodegraded wall painting by denaturing gradient gel electrophoresis of PCR-amplified 16S rDNA fragments. *Applied and Environmental Microbiology*, **62**, 2059-2065.

Rossello-Mora RA, Wagner M, Amann R, Schleifer K-H (1995) The abundance of Zoogloea ramigera in sewage treatment plants. *Applied and Environmental Microbiology*, **61**, 702-707.

Saiki RK, Gelfand DH, Stoffel S *et al.* (1988) Primer-directed enzymatic amplification of DNA with a thermostable DNA polymerase. *Science*, **239**, 487-491.

Santegoeds CM, Nold SC, Ward DM (1996) Denaturing gradient gel electrophoresis used to monitor the enrichment culture of aerobic chemoorganotrophic bacteria from a hot spring cyanobacterial mat. *Applied and Environmental Microbiology*, **62**, 3922-3928.

Santegoeds CM, Muyzer G, and de Beer D (1998) Biofilm dynamics studied with microsensors and molecular techniques *Water Science Techchnology*, **37**, 125-129.

Scheinert P, Krausse R, Ullman U, Söller R, Krupp G (1996) Molecular differentiation of bacteria by PCR amplification of the 16S-23S rRNA spacer. *Journal of Microbiology Methods*, **26**, 103-117.

Schmidt TM, DeLong EF, Pace, NR (1991) Analysis of marine picoplankton community by 16S rRNA gene cloning and sequencing. *Journal of Bacteriology*, **173**, 4371-4378.

Schönhuber W, Fuchs B, Juretschko S, Amann R (1997) Improved sensitivity of whole-cell hybridization by the combination of horseradish peroxidase-labeled oligonucleotides and tyramide signal amplification. *Applied and Environmental Microbiology*, **63**, 3268-3273.

Schramm A, Larsen LH, Revsbech NP, Ramsing NB, Amann R, Schleifer K-H (1996) Structure and function of a nitrifying biofilm as determined by *in situ* hybridization and the use of microelectrodes. *Applied and Environmental Microbiology*, **62**, 4641-4647.

Schut F, de Vries EJ, Gottschal JC, Robertson BR, Harder W, Prins RA, Button DK (1993) Isolation of typical marine bacteria by dilution culture: growth, maintenance, and characteristics of isolates under laboratory conditions. *Applied and Environmental Microbiology*, **59**, 2150-2160.

Sharp R, Ziemer CJ, Stern MD, Stahl DA (1998) Taxon-specific associations between proteozoal and methanogen populations in the rumen and a rumen system. *FEMS Microbiology Ecology*, **26**, 71-78.

Silvia MC, Batt CA (1995) Effect of cellular physiology on PCR amplification efficiency. *Molecular Ecology*, **4**, 11-16.

Smalla K, Wachterdorf U, Heuer H, Liu W-T, Forney L (1998) Analysis of BIOLOG GN substrate utilization patterns by microbial communities. *Applied and Environmental Microbiology*, **64**, 1220-1225.

Smit E, Leeflang P, Wernars K (1997) Detection of shifts in microbial community structure and diversity in soil caused by coppet contamination using amplified ribosomal DNA restriction analysis. *FEMS Microbiology Ecology*, **23**, 249-261.

Snaidr J, Amann R, Huber I, Ludwig W, Schleifer K-H (1997) Phylogenetic analysis and *in situ* identification of bacteria in activated sludge. *Applied and Environmental Microbiology*, **63**, 2884-2896.

Spring S, Amann R, Ludwig W, Schleifer K-H, van Gemerden H, Petersen N (1993) Dominating role of an unusal magnetotactic bacterium in the microaerobic zone of a freshwater sediment. *Applied and Environmental Microbiology*, **59**, 2397-2403.

Springer N, Ludwig W, Drozanski W, Amann R, Schleifer K-H (1992) The phylogenetic status of *Sarcobium lyticum*, an obligate intracellular bacterial parasite of small amoebae. *FEMS Microbiology Letters*, **96**, 199-202.

Springer N, Ludwig W, Amann R, Schmidt HJ, Goertz H-D, Schleifer K-H (1993) Occurrence of fragmented 16S rRNA in an obligate bacterial endosymbiont of *Paramecium caudatum*. *Proceedings of the National Academy of Sciences USA*, **90**, 9892-9895.

Springer N, Amann, Ludwig W, Schleifer K-H, Schmidt H (1996) *Polynucleobacter necessarius*, an obligate bacterial endosymbiont of the hypothrychous ciliate *Euplotes aediculatus*, is a member of the beta-subclass of Proteobacteria. *FEMS Microbiology Letters*, **135**, 333-336.

Stackebrandt E, Goebel BM (1994) Taxonomic note: a place for DNA-DNA reassociation and 16S rRNA sequence analysis in the present species definition in bacteriology. *International Journal of Systematic Bacteriology*, **44**, 846-849.

Stahl DA, Flesher B, Mansfield HR, Montgomery L (1988) Use of phylogenetically based hybridization probes for studies of ruminal ecology. *Applied and Environmental Microbiology*, **54**, 1079-1984.

Stahl DA and Capman WC (1994) Application of molecular genetics to the study of microbial communities. *NATO ASI Series*, **G35**, 193- 206.

Stoner DL, Browning CK, Bulmer DK, Ward TE, MacDonell MT (1996) Direct 5S rRNA assay for monitoring mixed-culture bioprocesses. *Applied and Environmental Microbiology*, **62**, 1969-1976.

Strunk O, Gross O, Reichel B *et al*. Arb: a software environment for sequence data. *Nucleic Acids Research*, in press.

Suzuki MT, Giovannoni SJ (1996) Bias caused by template annealing in the amplification of mixtures of 16S rRNA genes by PCR. *Applied and Environmental Microbiology*, **62**, 625-630.

Szewzyk U, Manz W, Amann R, Schleifer K-H, Stenstrom T-A (1994) Growth and *in situ* detection of a pathogenic *Escherichia coli* in biofilms of a heterotrophic water-bacterium by use of 16S- and 23S-rRNA-directed fluorescent oligonucleotide probes. *FEMS Microbiology Ecology*, **13**, 169-175.

Teske A (1995) Phylogenetische und Ökologische Untersuchungen an Bakterien des oxidativen und reductiven marinen Schwefelkreislaufs mittels ribosomaler RNA. PhD-thesis. University Bremen, Bremen, Germany.

Teske A, Wawer C, Muyzer G, Ramsing N (1996a) Distribution of sulfate-reducing bacteria in a stratified fjord (Mariager Fjord, Denmark) as evaluated by most-probable-number counts and denaturing gradient gel electrophoresis of PCR-amplified ribosomal DNA fragments. *Applied and Environmental Microbiology*, **62**, 1405-1415.

Teske A, Sigalevich P, Cohen Y, Muyzer G (1996b) Molecular identification of bacteria from a coculture by denaturing gradient gel electrophoresis of 16S ribosomal DNA fragments as a tool for isolation in pure cultures. *Applied and Environmental Microbiology*, **62**, 4210-4215.

Torsvik V, Goksoyr J, and Daale FL (1990a) High diversity in DNA of soil bacteria. *Applied and Environmental Microbiology*, **56**, 782-787.

Torsvik V, Salte K, Sorkeim R, Goksoyr J (1990b) Comparison of phenotypic diversity and DNA heterogeneity in a population of soil bacteria. *Applied and Environmental Microbiology*, **56**, 776-781.

Vallaeys T, Topp E, Muyzer G *et al*. (1997) Evaluation of denaturing gradient gel electrophoresis in the detection of 16S rDNA sequence variation in rhizobia and methanotrophs. *FEMS Microbiology Ecology*, **24**, 279-285.

Voytek MA, Ward BB (1995) Detection of ammonium-oxidizing bacteria of the beta-subclass of the class *Proteobacteria* in aquatic samples with the PCR. *Applied and Environmental Microbiology*, **61**, 1444-1450.

Wagner M, Amann R, Lemmer H, Schleifer K-H (1993) Probing activated sludge with oligonucleotides specific for Proteobacteria: Inadequacy of culture-dependent methods for describing microbial community structure. *Applied and Environmental Microbiology*, **59**, 1520-1525.

Wagner M, Amann R, Kämpfer P *et al.*(1994a) Identification and *in situ* detection of gram-negative filamentous bacteria in activated sludge. *Systematic and Applied Microbiology Microbiology*, **17**, 405-417.

Wagner M, Assmus B, Hartmann A, Hutzler P, Amann R (1994b) *In situ* analysis of microbial consortia in activating sludge using fluorescently labelled, rRNA-targeted oligonucleotide probes and confocal scanning laser microscopy. *Journal of Microscopy*, **176**, 181-187.

Wagner M, Rath G, Amann R, Koops H-P, Schleifer K-H (1995) *In situ* identification of ammonia-oxidizing bacteria. *Systematic and Applied Microbiology Microbiology*, **18**, 251-264.

Wallner G, Erhart R, Amann R (1995) Flow cytometric analysis of activated sludge with rRNA-targeted probes. *Applied and Environmental Microbiology*, **61**, 1859-1866.

Wallner G, Steinmetz I, Bitter-Suermann D, Amann R (1996) Combination of rRNA-targeted hybridization probes and immuno-probes for the identification of bacteria by flow cytometry. *Systematic and Applied Microbiology*, **19**, 569-576.

Wallner G, Fuchs B, Spring S, Beisker W, Amann R (1997) Flow sorting of microorganisms for molecular analysis. *Applied Environmental Microbiology*, **63**, 4223-4231.

Ward DM, Weller R, Bateson MM (1990a) 16S rRNA sequences reveal numerous uncultivated microorganisms in a natural environment. *Nature*, **345**, 63-65.

Ward DM, Weller R, Bateson MM (1990b) 16S rRNA sequences reveal uncultured inhabitants of a well-studied thermal community. *FEMS Microbiology Reviews*, **75**, 105-116.

Ward DM, Ferris Mj, Nold SC, Bateson MM, Kopczynski ED, Ruff-Roberts AL (1994) Species diversity in hot spring microbial mats as revealed by both molecular and enrichment culture approaches - relationship between biodiversity and community structure. *NATO/ASI Series*, **G35**, 33-44.

Ward DM, Ruff-Roberts, AL, Weller R (1995) Methods for extracting RNA or ribosomes from microbial mats and cultivated microorganisms. *Molecular Microbial Ecology Manual*, **1.2.3**, 1-14.

Ward DM, Santegoeds CM, Nold SC, Ramsing NB, Ferris MJ, Bateson Mm (1996) Biodiversity within hot spring microbial mat communities: molecular monitoring of enrichment cultures. *Antonie van Leeuwenhoek*, **71**, 143-150.

Wawer C (1997) Molekularbiologische Charakterisierung von sulfat-reduzierenden Bakterien in Umweltproben unter den Aspekten Diversität und Aktivität. PhD-thesis, University of Bremen, Germany.

Wawer C, Muyzer G (1995) Genetic diversity of *Desulfovibrio* spp. in environmental samples analyzed by denaturing gradient gel electrophoresis of [NiFe] hydrogenase gene fragments. *Applied and Environmental Microbiology*, **61**, 2203-2210.

Wawer C, Rüggeberg H, Meyer G, Muyzer G (1995) A simple and rapid electrophoresis method to detect sequence variation in PCR-amplified DNA fragments. *Nucleic Acids Research*, **23**, 4928-4929.

Wawer C, Jetten MSM, Muyzer G (1997) Genetic diversity and expression of the [NiFe] hydrogenase large subunit gene of *Desulfovibrio* spp. in environmental samples. *Applied and Environmental Microbiology*, **63**, 4360-4369.

Weiss P, Schweitzer B, Amann R, Simon M (1996) Identification *in situ* and dynamics of bacteria on limnetic organic aggregates (Lake Snow). *Applied and Environmental Microbiology*, **62**, 1998-2005.

Weller R, Ward DM (1989) Selective recovery of 16S rRNA sequences from natural microbial communities in the form of cDNA. *Applied and Environmental Microbiology*, **55**, 1818-1822.

Weller R, Walsh Weller J, Ward DM (1991) 16S rRNA sequences of uncultivated hot spring cyanobacterial mat inhabitants retrieved as randomly primed cDNA. *Applied and Environmental Microbiology*, **57**, 1146-1151.

Wheeler Alm, E, Stahl DA (1996) Extraction of microbial DNA from aquatic sediments. *Molecular Microbial Ecology Manual*, **1.1.5**, 1-29.

Wichels A (1996) Untersuchungen zur Diversität mariner Bakteriophagen und zu ihrer Verbreitung in der Nordsee. PhD-thesis, University Hamburg, Germany.

Wise MG, McArthur JV, Shimkets LJ (1997) Bacterial diversity of a Carolina bay as determined by 16S rRNA gene analysis: confirmation of novel taxa. *Applied and Environmental Microbiology*, **63**, 1505-1514.

Williams JGK, Kubelik AR, Livak KJ, Rafalski JA, Tingey SV (1990) DNA polymorphisms amplified by arbitrary primers are useful as genetic markers. *Nucleic Acids Research*, **18**, 6531-6535.

Woese CR (1987) Bacterial evolution. *Microbiology Reviews*, **51**, 221-271.

Yamaguchi N, Inaoka S, Tani K, Kenzaka T, Nasu M (1996) Detection of specific bacterial cells with 2-hydroxy-3-naphthoic acid-2-phenylanilide phosphate and Fast Red TR *in situ* hybridization. *Applied and Environmental Microbiology*, **62**, 275-278.

Yamamoto H, Hiraishi A, Kato K, Chiura HX, Maki Y, Shimizu A (1998) Phylogenetic evidence for the existence of novel thermophilic bacteria in hot spring sulfur-turf microbial mats in Japan. *Applied and Environmental Microbiology*, **64**, 1680-1687.

Xia X, Bollinger J, Ogram A (1995) Molecular genetic analysis of the response of three soil microbial communities to the application of 2,4-D. *Molecular Ecology*, **4**, 17-28.

Zarda B, Hahn D, Chatzinotas A (1997) Analysis of bacterial community structure in bulk soil by *in situ* hybridization. *Archives of Microbiology*, **168(3),**185-192.

Zwart G, Huismans R, van Agterveld MP *et al.* (1998) Divergent members of the bacterial division Verrucomicrobiales in a temperate freshwater lake. *FEMS Microbiology Ecology*, **25**, 159-169.

Advances in Molecular Ecology
G.R. Carvalho (Ed.)
IOS Press, 1998

Bacterial Evolution and the Nature of Species

J. Peter W. Young

Department of Biology, University of York, PO Box 373, York YO10 5YW, U.K.
e-mail: jpy1@york.ac.uk

Taxonomists classify bacteria into species, even though the genetic systems and ecology of bacteria are very different from those of higher organisms. Do bacteria have species in the conventional sense? This chapter considers the likely impact of the various recombination mechanisms available to bacteria, and reviews some of the relevant evidence based on genetic variation at the molecular level. It is clear that bacterial species vary widely in their degree of intraspecific recombination, and that in some groups there is also considerable genetic exchange between related species. There appear to be clearly separated species even in some bacteria which are strongly clonal. It is likely that gene exchange is a major cohesive mechanism in some species, but that for others the main force is periodic selection, which depends on ecological equivalence. A consideration of the question of species in bacteria can offer a new perspective on the general issues surrounding the nature of species.

1. Who needs species?

Ever since the system was formalized by Linnaeus, systematists have bestowed Latin binomials on every form of life. The fundamental unit of systematics is the species and, while certain schools of systematists have argued bitterly about the nature and even the existence of species (see Otte & Endler 1989), the rest of biological science has, by and large, taken them for granted. Indeed, ecologists and geneticists would find it hard to go about their separate businesses without a strong concept of species identity. To a crude approximation, ecologists deal with the success of different species but assume that all individuals within a species are equivalent, while population geneticists deal with the relative success of different genes within one species at a time. Of course, there have been efforts by ecologists to take into account genetic diversity and by population geneticists to include population dynamics, but theory that can handle "leaky" species is rare. Given our dependence on the species concept as an intellectual prop, it would be comforting to find that all life was neatly and unambiguously divided into species in the field as well as the in the book. Of course *Homo sapiens* does indeed describe a very clearly circumscribed and biologically distinct class of organisms, a fact that must have influenced the thinking of Linnaeus, the type specimen of our species. What causes this distinctness?

2. Why are there species?

There are many different ideas about what species are and how they are created and maintained. Probably the most enduring and widely accepted are based on the so-called "biological species concept" encapsulated in Mayr's (1963) definition of species: "groups of interbreeding natural populations that are reproductively isolated from other such groups". This is a genetic definition and has two complementary parts: recombination between individuals in the species maintains coherence, while barriers to recombination between species keep the species distinct. The vision may be clear, but it is readily apparent that it cannot describe all organisms. Purely clonal organisms, for example, cannot have species of this kind because they have no recombination to bind them together. In an attempt to encompass such organisms, Mayr later (1982) extended the definition by asserting that a species also "occupies a specific niche in nature". Niche is an ecological concept that does not depend on any particular genetic system. The problem, of course, is that this last, ecological, part of the definition has no logical relation to the earlier, genetic, criteria. It is not hard to find examples of organisms that conform to the genetic but not the ecological definition, or vice versa, or both, or neither. It is true that among familiar eukaryotes there are many organisms that, like primates, form species that are both genetically and ecologically coherent, but what about organisms as alien as bacteria?

3. Why are bacteria interesting?

Bacteria are the most important organisms on earth. They carry out many vital processes that eukaryotes are not capable of: recycling nitrogen gas from the air into forms that plants and animals can use, for example. Bacteria are also a rich source of biotechnological products, such as antibiotics, and may be deliberately released to enhance crop growth, reduce environmental pollution, and so on. Bacteria are very poorly known: we have described only a minute fraction of the diversity in the bacterial world. One problem here is to know how to divide up and name the different bacteria. Since the biology of bacteria is very different from that of birds or trees, it is not clear whether our usual concept of a species is directly applicable. Do bacteria have clearly defined species, or is there too much genetic exchange between widely different bacteria, or too much clonal growth without recombination, or too much physiological flexibility?

The rise of molecular ecology has spawned a whole new way of looking at the diversity of microbial communities by examining the diversity of certain key molecules, notably the small subunit ribosomal RNA (SSU rRNA). Taxonomic (and hence ecological) inferences based on a single gene will be reliable only if there is little recombination.

Gene transfer has been shown to be important in the evolution of pathogenic bacteria in response to drug treatments (Bennett 1995) and of degrading bacteria in response to novel pollutants (Vandermeer *et al.* 1992). This process could also cause the spread of genes from genetically modified organisms that we might introduce into the environment: it is important to have a clearer picture of where they might go and how fast.

This chapter explores bacterial gene exchange: how they do it, how often they do it, and the consequences for population genetics, taxonomy and phylogeny.

4. How do bacteriologists define bacterial species?

In practice, bacteriologists do not normally define species on the basis of reproductive isolation, as the relevant biology is seldom sufficiently well understood. Instead, the criteria for species are based on cross-hybridization of total genomic DNA: there is often a more or less clear gap between intraspecific hybridizations, which show more than 70% relatedness, and the considerably lower values found between species. This bimodality in the distribution of pairwise genetic distances is evidence for the reality of bacterial species but, as we shall discuss later, does not tell us whether the species are maintained by genetic or by ecological forces. DNA:DNA hybridization has numerous problems: there are many technical variants and results are not directly comparable between laboratories; multiple pairwise comparisons are required so large studies are laborious and full distance matrices are seldom obtained; hybridization declines to background levels at quite moderate levels of DNA sequence divergence; and the contributions of plasmid and chromosomal DNA cannot be distinguished. The advantage over DNA sequencing is that the whole genome is examined, not just a single gene. However, as sequencing becomes easier the possibility of sampling a representative range of genes, as suggested by Young *et al.* (1991), becomes more attractive as an alternative. The current trend in bacterial taxonomy is to place less weight on DNA hybridization and to consider data from as many different techniques as possible, the so-called "polyphasic" approach (Vandamme *et al.* 1996). This does not lead to any very clear theoretical basis for the concept of species.

5. What do we know about the phylogeny of bacteria?

Over the last two decades, SSU rRNA has emerged as the undisputed standard for determining phylogenetic relationships (*e.g.* Figure 1). The numerous reasons for this have been discussed many times (*e.g.* Woese 1987; Young 1992; Olsen *et al.* 1994); the most important are that rRNA is universal, is conserved in function, and has both highly conserved and rather rapidly evolving sections. Papers that describe new species of bacteria now routinely include 16S rRNA sequences; this allows the species to be attached confidently to the right branch of the phylogenetic tree, confirms its distinctness, and also provides information that can be used to develop identification tools. Thousands of bacterial 16S sequences are available in the public databases and through specialist services (Maidak *et al.* 1997; van der Peer *et al.* 1998). There is a temptation to rely on this approach almost to the exclusion of other information. Furthermore, recent major advances in microbial ecology have been based on the sequences of 16S genes cloned from environmental samples; these represent a host of organisms that have not yet been cultured (*e.g.* Giovanonni *et al.* 1990; Ward *et al.* 1990). Some of the advances in this field are discussed in the chapter by Muyzer elsewhere in this book. The assumption (usually unstated) is that there is almost no exchange of chromosomal genes between bacterial species, so that the phylogeny of 16S is representative of the phylogeny of the genome as a whole. Are we right to place such heavy weight on the evidence from just one gene?

It is usually assumed that ribosomal rRNA genes are not transferred between species, and that their evolution in different lineages is therefore independent. This is a necessary condition for constructing valid phylogenies. However, Sneath (1993) presented a detailed analysis of a set of sequences that showed clear evidence for recombination between SSU genes in different lineages of the genus *Aeromonas*, and similar phenomena are apparent in the data for rhizobia (Young & Haukka 1996).

On the large phylogenetic scale, 16S rRNA trees are supported by analysis of other genes (Ludwig *et al.* 1993). Figure 2 shows a tree based on the amino acid sequences encoded by a number of bacterial *recA* genes. It is striking that the major bacterial "kingdoms" defined on the basis of 16S comparisons (Fig. 1) are also apparent when RecA is studied: Gram-positives, the alpha, gamma and beta groups of the *Proteobacteria*, and the cyanobacteria. A detailed comparison of RecA and 16S phylogenies has been published (Eisen 1995), demonstrating remarkable congruence on the large and medium phylogenetic scales.

However, 16S sequences are now frequently being used to support phylogenetic inferences at the generic and even species level. At this level, 16S is often too conserved to give clear conclusions, and also the potential for gene exchange may be much greater. We

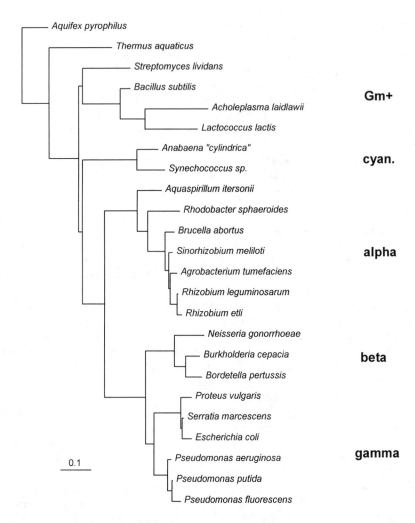

Figure 1: Phylogeny of bacteria based on the sequence of small subunit ribosomal RNA. A maximum likelihood tree of similar taxa to those in Fig. 2, extracted from the Ribosomal Database Project (Maidak 1997). Scale bar indicates 0.1 substitutions per site.

really do not have convincing evidence that within a genus, and between closely related genera, the 16S phylogeny is representative of the whole chromosomal genome. We do know, however, that within some bacterial species there may be substantial recombination, so that different chromosomal segments have different phylogenies (Milkman & McKane 1995). In sexually-reproducing eukaryotes this is, of course, the normal situation, so we can ask whether the recombination within bacterial species is evidence that bacteria, too, are sexual organisms.

6. Do bacteria have sex?

In the "conventional sex" of higher eukaryotes, genetic recombination is inextricably associated with reproduction. The fusion of two independent cells to form a diploid carrying both sets of genetic information is followed (sometimes many cell generations later) by a

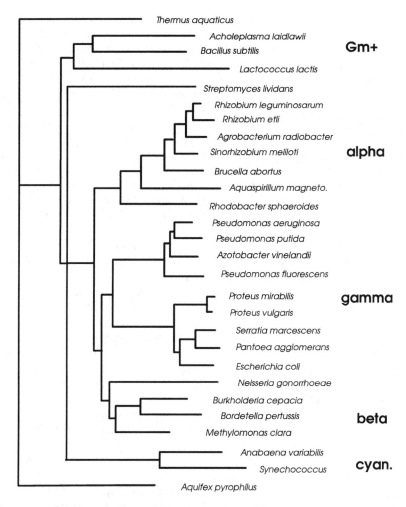

Figure 2: Phylogeny of bacteria based on the amino acid sequence of the RecA protein (by Neighbor-Joining method, Saitou & Nei 1987).

meiotic process that regenerates the haploid state. The independent segregation of chromosomes at meiosis and the crossing-over between homologous chromosomes ensure that each daughter cell has a roughly equal genetic contribution from each of the original parents. Two important evolutionary effects of recombination are to prevent the inexorable accumulation of deleterious mutations that afflicts clonal populations of finite size ('Muller's ratchet', Muller 1964), and to increase the rate at which a population can adapt to changing circumstances (Muller 1932). While more rapid adaptation and the purging of deleterious mutations may be the selective forces that have led to the evolution of sex in eukaryotes, the most obvious consequence is probably the maintenance of discrete species.

Bacteria have several processes that bring together genetic material from different lineages. The three most widespread are (i) conjugation encoded by plasmids or transposons, (ii) transduction via phage particles and (iii) transformation by the uptake of DNA from the environment.

To explore the evolutionary consequences we need to distinguish between incoming DNA that is homologous to recipient DNA, on the one hand, and novel incoming DNA on the other. Homologous DNA creates a transient partial diploid, and may replace the resident version by homologous recombination. Novel DNA, on the other hand, may survive if it can be stabilized (by transposition or plasmid establishment) and is beneficial, or at least not too deleterious to the recipient. The well-known spread of antibiotic-resistance genes has largely resulted from transfer of novel DNA, but it is the transfer of homologous DNA that is comparable with eukaryotic sex. If it is sufficiently frequent it could stop Muller's ratchet, speed adaptation by bringing together independent beneficial mutations, and provide the 'genetic cohesion' that maintains the identity of species.

In each of the three main mechanisms for bacterial gene exchange, only a part of the donor's genome is introduced into the recipient, and none of the processes is directly coupled to the reproductive cycle. For these reasons, the rate of recombination is likely to be much more variable in bacteria than in sexual eukaryotes, and is not predictable *a priori*. It may be relatively low, perhaps too low to be effective. Indeed, it can be argued that none of the processes evolved "for" chromosomal recombination, as in each case there are other explanations for their evolution.

This is most obvious for transduction by bacteriophages, which are viruses that infect bacteria. The phage takes over the metabolism of its host bacterial cell and uses it to produce many copies of its own genome and package these into protein coats. These infectious particles then escape, usually by bursting the host cell. If they encounter another suitable host cell, they will bind to it and release their genetic material into the cell, starting another infectious cycle. Occasionally a suitable length of host DNA becomes packaged in a phage coat in place of the phage genome. Since the phage proteins are programmed to deliver their cargo of DNA to another bacterial cell, the recipient will in this case acquire part of the donor bacterial genome, some of which may be incorporated by recombination. This process is called "generalized transduction", since any part of the host genome may be transferred in this way. From the point of view of the phage, it is of no benefit because the phage genome is not propagated. Since it is the phage genome that encodes the machinery, it is reasonable to regard generalized transduction as a "mistake" made by that machinery rather than a process "designed for" bacterial gene transfer.

Certain phage can also transfer bacterial genes by "specialized transduction". These phage can insert themselves into the bacterial genome where they may be inherited as part of the genome for many generations, a state called "lysogeny". Eventually, something triggers them to excise themselves and produce a mass of phage particles in the usual way (the "lytic" phase). Excision from the genome is often imprecise, so that genes adjacent to the insertion site may also be incorporated in the phage particles and delivered to a recipient. In this case, too, there is no direct benefit to the phage genome so the transfer of host DNA is probably accidental.

Conjugation is a complex process involving special cell surface structures (pili) made by donor cells and used to anchor the donor to suitable recipients so that DNA can be transferred. The transfer process involves replication, so both partners have copies of the transferred DNA. The conjugative apparatus is encoded by a large suite of genes, and these are usually carried on a plasmid, although conjugative transposons are also known. The origin of transfer, a specific DNA sequence that leads the movement into the recipient, is normally on the same genetic element, so conjugation is a process whereby the selfish plasmid can spread through the bacterial population. Transfer of chromosomal DNA can occur if the plasmid becomes integrated into the chromosome, as in the Hfr (high-frequency recombination) strains of *Escherichia coli* that were such a valuable tool in the early days of bacterial genetics, or the plasmid acquires a short segment of the bacterial chromosome, as in F′ strains. As with transduction, the transfer of chromosomal DNA by conjugation seems to be a by-product of a process that exists primarily to promote the spread of a selfish DNA element.

The evolution of transformation, the third bacterial gene transfer mechanism, is more controversial. It is ironic, therefore, that studies of bacterial transformation laid the foundation for modern molecular biology, including molecular ecology, by demonstrating that DNA was the hereditary material. In 1928, Griffith demonstrated that an avirulent strain of *Streptococcus pneumoniae* could acquire virulence from a heat-killed virulent strain, and in 1944 Avery *et al.* proved that the transforming principle was DNA. Three roles that have been suggested for bacterial transformation are nutrient uptake, recombinational repair of DNA damage, and genetic exchange.

Redfield (1993a,b) showed that competence (the ability to take up DNA) in *Bacillus subtilis* or *Haemophilus influenzae* is induced by nutrient limitation but not by DNA damage, suggesting that transformation may be primarily a form of feeding. Theoretical arguments also suggest that the conditions necessary for transformation to evolve as an error repair system are restrictive, since there are risks that a competent cell will pick up less-favoured alleles from its dead conspecifics, and may even be transformed to a nontransformable state (Redfield *et al.* 1997).

7. How effective is bacterial sex?

Since all the bacterial recombination processes are "optional", in that bacteria can reproduce and thrive without invoking them, it is important to establish whether they actually have a significant influence on bacterial evolution or are merely laboratory curiosities. This can be done by examining the distribution of molecular genetic variation: if sex is ineffective, the population structure will be clonal and different genes will share the same phylogeny. This will be true both above and below the species boundary.

The first extensive evidence came from studies of enzyme polymorphism. All such studies showed that bacterial species were highly polymorphic, and most revealed some disequilibrium between loci, but Maynard Smith *et al.* (1993) showed how to analyse the data in a more informative way. Their statistic I_A (index of association) assesses the deviation of the population from the panmictic situation in which there is no correlation between alleles at different loci. Their calculations showed that bacteria varied widely. Some bacterial species, such as *Escherichia coli*, *Salmonella enterica* and *Haemophilus influenzae* appear to be more or less clonal. Others, such as *Neisseria gonorrhoeae* and *N. meningitidis* have little or no linkage disequilibrium, suggesting that recombination is very effective. *Sinorhizobium meliloti* and *S. medicae* are also panmictic when treated separately. If the data for these two species are combined, a significant disequilibrium appears, suggesting that these are "good" species, each panmictic but well differentiated from each other. These two species are closely related, and in fact at the time of the analysis by Maynard Smith *et al.* (1993) they were still named as two subgroups of the same species: *Rhizobium meliloti* A and B. They are somewhat separated ecologically and perhaps geographically, since *S. meliloti* is the normal symbiont of perennial alfalfa, which is widely cultivated, whereas *S. medicae* has been isolated from annual medics in the Mediterranean region, but they do occur together on some host species so opportunities for gene exchange would presumably occur. The role of geographic and ecological isolation in bacterial population genetics has scarcely been explored.

In the past decade, several bacterial groups have been investigated in more detail by comparative sequencing of various genes. By and large the data for *E. coli* and *S. enterica* have confirmed their clonal status: the phylogenies of different genes are congruent within species and the two species are well separated (Nelson *et al.* 1991; Nelson & Selander 1992; Boyd *et al.* 1994), although some recombination could be detected (Dykhuizen & Green 1991; Guttman & Dykhuizen 1994). A major exception is the *E. coli gnd* gene, which may have experienced strong hitchhiking because it is adjacent to a strongly selected and highly polymorphic O-antigen determinant gene (Dykhuizen & Green 1991; Nelson & Selander 1994). The pattern of variation in a 10kb region around the *trp* operon of *E. coli* showed that distinct sequence types were distributed in mosaic stretches or "clonal frames" (Milkman & McKane 1995). The most likely recombination mechanisms in *E. coli* are conjugation and transduction, and McKane & Milkman (1995) demonstrated experimentally that transformation using phage P1 could produce mosaic recombination patterns resembling those found naturally. Interestingly, a single transduction event often led to the incorporation of several nonadjacent segments of donor DNA, perhaps because the incoming DNA was being fragmented by restriction enzymes. Hence one recombination event at the cell level becomes several at the chromosome level, further complicating any attempt to define recombination rates. Milkman and McKane (1995) have characterized the evolution of *E. coli* as "clonal descent compromised by recombination".

Extensive comparative sequence data are also available for *Neisseria* species. In contrast to *E. coli*, the dominant mechanism of gene exchange in this genus is transformation. It seems to be very effective, since data for a number of different genes generate incongruent phylogenies, indicating an extensive history of recombination both within and between species (Spratt *et al.* 1995; Zhou *et al.* 1997). This is true not only for genes under strong selection, such as those for penicillin-binding proteins, but also for "housekeeping" genes. One exception is the *recA* gene, which gives a strongly-supported phylogeny consistent with the data from total DNA-DNA hybridization and with phenotypic analysis (Feil *et al.* 1996). Why should this gene behave differently? Feil *et al.* compare *recA* with *adk*, and conclude that selection at *recA* may be relatively relaxed since nonsynonymous substitutions are relatively more frequent. They argue that this may have allowed *recA* sequences to diverge to the point that they became poor substrates for recombination and hence could escape from the homogenization process and evolve independently in each lineage. Differences in transformation uptake rates and selection acting on the recombinants will also contribute to differences in the behaviour of genes.

The relationship between sequence divergence and recombination is interesting as it is potentially reciprocal: recombination prevents divergence, but divergence also prevents recombination. Genes that arrive in a recipient will only be able to replace their resident homologues if they are sufficiently similar in sequence to undergo homologous recombination. This similarity is assessed by the mismatch repair system (which involves, ironically, the product of the *recA* gene). Homologous genes from *E. coli* cannot usually be incorporated into *S. enterica* by homologous recombination, as these genomes are about 20% diverged and heteroduplexes are rejected by the mismatch system encoded by *mutL*, *mutS* and *mutH*. If this system is disrupted by mutation, however, recombination can occur (Rayssiguier *et al.* 1989). This finding offers the intriguing prospect of an "adjustable" species barrier, which normally keeps two species isolated but could occasionally be lowered for long enough to allow genes to slip across. Recent data from *Bacillus*, however, indicate that the primary barrier is not the mismatch repair system but the initiation of a heteroduplex, which requires a region of perfect identity (Majewski & Cohan 1998). If this is generally true, it may mean that the susceptibility of the recipient is predictable on the basis of sequence similarity alone, and less subject to the vagaries of mutation and physiological state. Nevertheless, the requirement for matching sequence means that the barrier to recombination will depend on the gene under consideration. Genes that are more

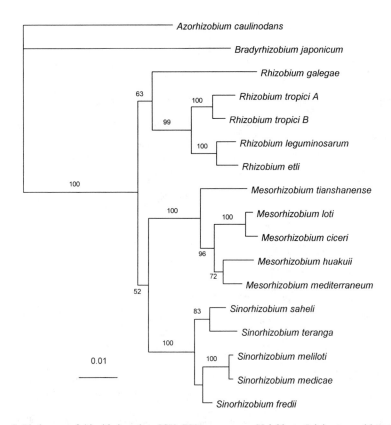

Figure 3: Phylogeny of rhizobia based on SSU rRNA sequences. Neighbour-Joining tree with percent bootstrap support (1000 replicates) indicated where this exceeds 50%.

conserved may recombine successfully over a wider taxonomic range than those that evolve rapidly.

New information on the range of interspecific transfers is emerging from our studies of rhizobia (unpublished data of SA Lloyd-McGilp, L Rigottier-Gois, SL Turner). These bacteria are probably more like enterics than like *Neisseria*, in that conjugation and transduction are likely to be important rather than transformation. On the whole the species are "well-behaved", with different genes giving the same phylogeny, but occasionally a gene seems to have come in from another genus, judging by its unexpected placement in the phylogeny. For example, the *recA* tree (not shown) is closely similar to that for SSU rRNA (Figure 3), but the *glnII* tree (Figure 4) shows considerable rearrangement in the genus *Mesorhizobium*, an anomalous placement of *Rhizobium galegae* (which, for other genes, is external to the rest of the genus *Rhizobium*) and a surprisingly short branch for the gene from *Bradyrhizobium japonicum*, which is a distantly related organism. It remains to be established whether these genes have been acquired by homologous replacement, but the tree suggests that the transfers occurred a long time ago, when the divergence between the corresponding genes was much less than it is today.

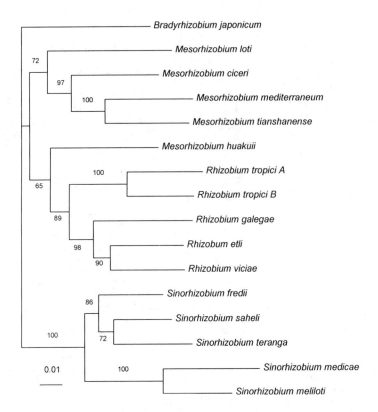

Figure 4: Phylogeny of rhizobia based on the amino acid sequence of glutamine synthetase II. Neighbour-Joining tree with percent bootstrap support (1000 replicates) indicated where this exceeds 50%.

8. Are bacterial species maintained by genetics or by ecology?

As I indicated at the beginning, Mayr's (1982) definition offers two alternative explanations for species, one genetic and one ecological. This distinction was made explicit by Templeton (1989), who discusses "genetic cohesion mechanisms" (i.e. recombination and barriers to recombination) and "demographic cohesion mechanisms" (i.e. ecological equivalence, a common niche). Templeton points out that these are not mutually exclusive: there is a broad middle ground within which both are effective, but at one extreme lie purely asexual organisms, which have no genetic cohesion, and at the other lie syngameons, which are ecologically differentiated populations that still experience significant gene flow.

Cohan (1994, 1995) has espoused the ecological species concept for bacteria (though he does not describe it in exactly those terms). He has developed the idea that discrete species can be maintained even if gene flow within species is no greater than gene flow between species. The homogenising force in this case is not recombination but periodic selection, that is, selective sweeps through the species as new advantageous genes arise and spread. The consequences of periodic selection for quasi-asexual species were described by Muller (1932), and were invoked early in the study of bacterial enzyme polymorphism as an explanation for the finding that the level of heterozygosity, though high, was much less than predicted by neutral theory given the vast size of bacterial populations (Milkman 1973,

Levin 1981). Implicit in these ideas is the concept of an ecologically-defined species, because a new advantageous variant will only replace those individuals that are otherwise ecologically equivalent, or "demographically exchangeable" in Templeton's (1989) parlance. Under this model, each bacterial species should correspond to a discrete ecological niche, and the number and nature of species will be determined by the underlying niche structure. In some instances, for example in the case of host-specific pathogens, the niches may be very clear cut, but in other circumstances there may be more of a continuum. Taking into account this diversity as well as the great range in the levels of genetic recombination, it seems unlikely that the nature of species will be uniform across all bacteria.

Maynard Smith (1995), after discussing the correlated features of a typical eukaryote species, concludes that "in bacteria, no species concept could be devised that would carry this heavy load of meanings and theoretical implications". Before bacteriologists hang their heads in shame, it is as well to remember that the concept of species has not been universally successful in the eukaryote world either. Maynard Smith asserts that "a bird-watcher expects to be able to identify every bird seen", which is doubtless true. A watcher in Northern Europe would have no trouble distinguishing a herring gull (*Larus argentatus*) from a lesser black-backed gull (*L. fuscus*). If they could see further they might become confused, however, because these are in fact the two overlapping ends of a ring species that spreads right around the arctic through a number of graded intermediates. Mitochondrial DNA studies suggest that there is now little gene flow, but the components are still closely related (Wink *et al.* 1994). To take another example, Darwin's finches on the Galapagos, famous for their ecological distinctness, have recently been shown to hybridize extensively (Grant & Grant 1997). The fact that even "well behaved" eukaryotes have problems does not improve our understanding of bacterial species, of course, though it suggests that the gulf between eukaryotes and prokaryotes is not so wide. Nevertheless, Maynard Smith is no doubt right to suspect that most bacteria lie further from the conventional concept of species. Our main task at this stage should be to describe clearly what is actually happening, at both the genetic and the ecological levels, rather than to fret over the precise application of a poorly-fitting paradigm.

References

Avery OT, MacLeod CM, McCarty M (1944) Studies on the chemical nature of the substance inducing transformation of pneumococcal types. Induction of transformation by a deoxyribonucleic acid fraction isolated from pneumococcus type III. *Journal of Experimental Medicine*, **79**, 137-158.

Bennett PM (1995) The spread of drug resistance. In: *Population Genetics of BacteriaSymposium of the Society for General Microbiology*, (eds. Baumberg S, Young JPW, Wellington EMH, Saunders JR), 52, pp. 317-344. Cambridge University Press, Cambridge.

Boyd EF, Nelson K, Wand FS, Whittam TS, Selander RK (1994) Molecular genetic basis of allelic polymorphism in malate dehydrogenase (MDH) in natural populations of *Escherichia coli* and *Salmonella enterica*. *Proceedings of the National Academy of Sciences, USA*, **91**, 1280-1284.

Cohan FM (1994) Genetic exchange and evolutionary divergence in prokaryotes. *Trends in Ecology and Evolution*, **9**, 175-180.

Cohan FM (1995) Does recombination constrain neutral divergence among bacterial taxa? *Evolution*, **49**, 164-175.

Dykhuizen DE, Green L (1991) Recombination in *Escherichia coli* and the definition of biological species. *Journal of Bacteriology*, **173**, 7253-7268.

Eisen JA (1995) The RecA protein as a model for molecular systematic studies of bacteria - comparison of trees of RecAs and 16S ribosomal-RNAs from the same species. *Journal of Molecular Evolution*, **41**, 1105-1123.

Feil E, Zhou J, Maynard Smith J, Spratt BG (1996) A comparison of the nucleotide sequences of the *adk* and *recA* genes of pathogenic and commensal *Neisseria* species: evidence for extensive interspecies recombination within *adk*. *Journal of Molecular Evolution*, **43**, 631-640.

Giovannoni SJ, Britschgi TB, Moyer CL, Field KG (1990) Genetic diversity in Sargasso sea bacterioplankton. *Nature*, **345**, 60-63.

Grant PR, Grant BR (1997) Mating patterns of Darwin's finch hybrids determined by song and morphology. *Biological Journal of the Linnean Society*, **60**, 317-343.

Griffith F (1928) The significance of pneumococcal types. *Journal of Hygiene*, **27**, 113-159.

Guttman DS, Dykhuizen DE (1994) Clonal divergence in *Escherichia coli* as a result of recombination, not mutation. *Science*, **266**, 1380-1383.

Levin BR (1981) Periodic selection, infectious gene exchange and the genetic structure of *E. coli* populations. *Genetics*, **99**, 1-23.

Ludwig W, Neumaier J, Klugbauer N *et al.* (1993) Phylogenetic relationships of bacteria based on comparative sequence analysis of elongation-factor TU and ATP-synthase beta-subunit genes. *Antonie van Leeuwenhoek*, **64**, 285-305.

Maidak BL, Olsen GJ, Larsen N, Overbeek R, McCaughey MJ, Woese CR (1997) The RDP (Ribosomal Database Project). *Nucleic Acids Research*, **25**, 109-111.

Majewski J, Cohan FM (1998) The effect of mismatch repair and heteroduplex formation on sexual isolation in *Bacillus*. *Genetics*, **148**, 13-18.

Maynard Smith J (1995) Do bacteria have population genetics? In: *Population Genetics of Bacteria. Symposium of the Society for General Microbiology 52*, (eds. Baumberg S, Young JPW, Wellington EMH, Saunders JR), pp. 1-12. Cambridge University Press, Cambridge.

Maynard Smith J, Smith NH, O'Rourke M, Spratt BG (1993) How clonal are bacteria? *Proceedings of the National Academy of Sciences, USA*, **90**, 4384-4388.

Mayr E (1963) *Animal Species and Evolution*. Belknap Press, Cambridge MA.

Mayr E (1982) *The Growth of Biological Thought*. Belknap Press, Cambridge MA.

McKane M, Milkman R (1995) Transduction, restriction and recombination patterns in *Escherichia coli*. *Genetics*, **139**, 35-43.

Milkman (1973) Electrophoretic variation in *Escherichia coli* from natural sources. *Science*, **182**, 1024-1026.

Milkman R, McKane M (1995) DNA sequence variation and recombination in *E. coli*. In: *Population Genetics of Bacteria, Symposium of the Society for General Microbiology*, (eds. Baumberg S, Young JPW, Wellington EMH, Saunders JR), 52, pp. 127-142. Cambridge University Press, Cambridge.

Muller HJ (1932) Some genetic aspects of sex. *American Naturalist*, **66**, 118-138.

Muller HJ (1964) The relation of recombination to mutational advance. *Mutation Research*, **1**, 2-9.

Nelson K, Whittam TS, Selander RK (1991) Nucleotide polymorphism and evolution in the glyceraldehyde-3-phosphate dehydrogenase gene (*gapA*) in natural populations of *Salmonella* and *Escherichia coli*. *Proceedings of the National Academy of Sciences, USA*, **15**, 6667-6671.

Nelson K, Selander RK (1992) Evolutionary genetics of the proline permease (*putP*) and control region of the proline utilization operon in populations of *Salmonella* and *Escherichia coli*. *Journal of Bacteriology*, **174**, 6886-6895.

Nelson K, Selander RK (1994) Intergeneric transfer and recombination of the 6-phosphogluconate gene (*gnd*) in enteric bacteria. *Proceedings of the National Academy of Sciences, USA*, **91**, 10277-10231.

Olsen GJ, Woese CJ, Overbeek R (1994) The winds of (evolutionary) change - breathing new life into microbiology. *Journal of Bacteriology*, **176**, 1.

Otte D, Endler JA (1989) *Speciation and its consequences*: Sinauer, *Sunderland* MA.

Rayssiguier C, Thaler DS, Radman M (1989) The barrier to recombination between *Escherichia coli* and *Salmonella typhimurium* is disrupted in mismatch-repair mutants. *Nature*, **342**, 396-401.

Redfield RJ (1993a) Genes for breakfast - the have-your-cake-and-eat-it-too of bacterial transformation. *Journal of Heredity*, **84**, 400-404.

Redfield RJ (1993b) Evolution of natural transformation - testing the DNA-repair hypothesis in *Bacillus subtilis* and *Haemophilus influenzae*. *Genetics*, **133**, 755-761.

Redfield RJ, Schrag MR, Dean AM (1997) The evolution of bacterial transformation: sex with poor relations. *Genetics*, **146**, 27-38.

Saitou N, Nei M (1987) The neighbor-joining method: a new method for reconstructing phylogenetic trees. *Molecular Biology and Evolution*, **4**, 406-425.

Sneath PHA (1993) Evidence from *Aeromonas* for genetic crossing-over in ribosomal sequences. *International Journal of Systematic Bacteriology*, **43**, 626-629.

Spratt BG, Smith NH, Zhou J, O'Rourke M, Feil E (1995) The population genetics of the pathogenic *Neisseria*. In: *Population Genetics of Bacteria* (eds. Baumberg S, Young JPW, Wellington EMH,

Saunders JR), Symposium of the Society for General Microbiology 52, pp. 143-160. Cambridge University Press, Cambridge.

Templeton A (1989) The meaning of species and speciation: a genetic perspective. In: *Speciation and its consequences* (eds. Otte D, Endler JA). Sinauer, Sunderland MA.

Vandamme P, Pot B, Gillis M, Devos P, Kersters K, Swings J (1996) Polyphasic taxonomy, a consensus approach to bacterial systematics. *Microbiological Reviews,* **60,** 407-438.

Van de Peer Y, Caers A, De Rijk P, De Wachter R (1998) Database on the structure of small ribosomal subunit RNA. *Nucleic Acids Research,* **26,** 179-182.

Vandermeer JR, Devos WM, Harayama S, Zehnder AJB (1992) Molecular mechanisms of genetic adaptation to xenobiotic compounds. *Microbiological Reviews,* **56,** 677-694.

Ward DM, Weller R, Bateson MM. (1990) 16S ribosomal RNA sequences reveal numerous uncultured microorganisms in a natural community. *Nature,* **345,** 63-65.

Wink M, Kahl U, Heidrich P (1994) Genetic distinction of *Larus argentatus, L. fuscus* and *Larus cachinnans. Journal für Ornithologie,* **135,** 73-80.

Woese, CR (1987) Bacterial evolution. *Microbiological Reviews,* **51,** 221-271.

Young JPW (1992) Phylogenetic classification of nitrogen-fixing organisms. In: *Biological Nitrogen Fixation* (eds. Stacey G, Burris RH, Evans HJ), pp. 43-86. Chapman and Hall, New York.

Young JPW, Downer HL, Eardly BD (1991) Phylogeny of the phototrophic *Rhizobium* strain BTAi1 by polymerase chain reaction-based sequencing of a 16S rRNA gene segment. *Journal of Bacteriology,* **173,** 2271-2277.

Young JPW, Haukka K (1996) Diversity and phylogeny of rhizobia. *New Phytologist,* **133,** 87-94

Zhou J, Bowler LD, Spratt BG (1997) Interspecies recombination, and phylogenetic distortions, within the glutamine synthetase and shikimate dehydrogenase genes of *Neisseria meningitidis* and commensal *Neisseria* species. *Molecular Microbiology,* **23,** 799-812.

Advances in Molecular Ecology
G.R. Carvalho (Ed.)
IOS Press, 1998

Ancient DNA: Problems and Perspectives for Molecular Microbial Palaeoecology

Franco Rollo

Dept of Molecular, Cell and Animal Biology,
University of Camerino, I-62032 Camerino, Italy
e-mail: rollo@cambio.unicam.it

DNA can be extracted from a variety of human, animal and plant archaeological, palaeontological, and museum specimens. We can use sequence information from an old or ancient double helix to address questions ranging from the sex determination of a Bronze Age human skeleton to the assignment of a stuffed bird to its proper systematic position. While the methods employed to isolate, replicate and sequence ancient and modern DNA are basically the same, manipulation and analysis of the former requires more stringent approaches. DNA in archaeological deposits is affected by hydrolytic and oxidative damage, resulting in base loss, base modification and strand cleavage. The chances of DNA surviving over long periods is low, unless the environment offers particularly favourable conditions. Theoretical calculations and empirical observations suggest that DNA may not be able to survive for more than 50,000-100,000 years. Because of the tiny amounts of DNA which can be extracted from an archaeological specimen and the sensitivity of the detection methods employed, stringent laboratory precautions and systematic controls are required to avoid contamination. In addition, several criteria of authenticity have to be met. The use of the DNA technology to describe ancient bacterial communities is discussed, including particular problems in their study mainly due to contamination by modern microorganisms. Despite these problems, thanks to an accurate archaeometrical evaluation of the specimens and the application of appropriate criteria ("palaeoecological consistency"), it is possible, at least under some circumstances, to determine the composition of the original microbial flora of an ancient human or animal body.

1. Brief historical background

The development of molecular genetic techniques over the last two decades has made it possible to study the processes of molecular evolution. Phylogenetic inference suffers, however, from limitations posed by the fact that it is obtained through analysis of the present day structure of genes. The possibility of retrieving and studying ancient DNA molecules offers the opportunity to assess the genealogical relationships of extinct species. Moreover, the study of the DNA from ancient communities of organisms can provide a historical perspective to molecular ecology.

The first article describing the analysis of an ancient DNA sequence was published in 1984 (Higuchi *et al.* 1984); it presented the results of an investigation aimed at ascertaining the phylogenetic position of the quagga, an extinct equid. The authors started with an approximately 150-year-old fragment of desiccated muscle tissue which was used for DNA extraction. Subsequently, to assess whether any of the original genetic material of the quagga was left, the DNA was tested by molecular hybridization with the DNA of zebra, the closest living relative. To perform sequence analysis, the quagga DNA was cloned into a lambda phage vector. Clones carrying mitochondrial (mt) DNA inserts were identified by hybridization and the inserts subcloned into an M13 vector to be further used for nucleotide sequencing. The results of this and of a further study published a few years later (Higuchi *et al.* 1987) clearly demonstrated that the quagga mtDNA was actually identical to that of a Burchell zebra.

The year following the "quagga paper", Pääbo (1985a,b) reported the cloning of the DNA of an ancient human. Following the painstaking screening of 23 Egyptian mummies, one 2,400-year-old mummy of a child was found to contain relatively long (3.4 kilobase pair) fragments of DNA that could be cloned in a plasmid vector. Molecular hybridization and sequence analyses showed that a clone contained two human repetitive DNA sequences of the *Alu* family. This achievement is now considered to be probably the result of contamination from modern DNA, nevertheless it gave the ancient DNA field an unprecedented boost at the time.

In the same year, Rollo (1985) showed that short nucleic acid fragments could be isolated from 3300-year-old cress (*Lepidium sativum* L.) seeds found in the tomb of the so-called Architect Kha, from the necropolis of Thebes. When characterized by enzymatic digestion, polyacrylamide gel electrophoresis and molecular hybridization to cloned plant genes, the nucleic acid fragments were shown to be ribonuclease-sensitive, low molecular weight (<150 bp in length) and still capable of binding to modern plant genes for ribosomal RNA (rRNA).

The first attempts to recover the original DNA in archaeological specimens were hampered by serious technical difficulties posed by the state of fragmentation of the ancient double helices, by their rarity and by the problem of distinguishing between the original (ancient) fraction of the DNA and the contaminants. Fortunately, at least some of the major problems have been overcome by the introduction of the polymerase chain reaction (PCR). This technique allows the selective amplification of a rare type of DNA fragment, on the basis of its nucleotide sequence, even if it is mixed with a large number of other fragments. This is precisely the situation found, almost invariably, by archaeomolecular investigators.

At the end of the 1980's, thanks to the introduction of the PCR, the archaeomolecular field expanded considerably (Pääbo *et al.* 1989). However it became clear, that due to the very high sensitivity of this technique, the PCR tended to give misleading results if not employed with great care. At this time, Pääbo *et al.* (1990) provided the first experimental evidence that enzymatic amplification of highly fragmented and modified DNA can produce chimerical sequences. A few years later (Herrmann and Hummel 1994) the ancient DNA experts had become sufficiently confident in their methods to confront issues as arduous as the analysis of DNA isolated from paraffin-embedded clinically-collected human tissues (Greer 1991), the reconstruction of the phylogeny of extinct birds on the basis of museum specimens (Cooper *et al.* 1992), and the genetic history of the domestication of maize, wheat and other crop plants (Rollo *et al.* 1991; Goloubinoff *et al.* 1993; Brown *et al.* 1994).

In recent times (Audic & Béraud-Colomb 1997), DNA tests have been employed for the screening of large samples of archaeological bone for sex determination (Lassen *et al.* 1996) to reconstruct the peopling of the Americas (Lalueza Fox 1996) and to detect globin gene mutations (Béraud-Colomb *et al.* 1995). The most striking result of recent years and, perhaps, of all ancient DNA studies is the unveiling of the genetic relationships between modern and Neanderthal man by sequence analysis of a hypervariable part of the mtDNA control region starting from a palaeoanthropological specimen (Krings *et al.* 1997).

In a (neo)ecological perspective, it is worth mentioning that ancient DNA and palaeontological information can be implemented to design recovery plans for endangered species. The Laysan duck was, historically, common on the small island of Laysan (Hawaii). Presently, however, only a small number of individuals survive. Bones of small ducks, however, can be recovered from Pleistocene and Holocene deposits all over the Hawaiian chain, thus suggesting that the species was once widespread. To test this hypothesis, Cooper *et al.* (1996) extracted DNA from subfossil duck bone, amplified two short fragments from the variable portions of the mitochondrial control region, and compared the palaeontological sequences with the corresponding sequences of Laysan duck, Hawaiian duck (koloa), migratory mallard, and African black duck. The results showed that the subfossil bone DNA perfectly matched that of the Laysan duck, thus providing a justification for the reintroduction of this bird to the islands within its former range.

Finally, a recent investigation on the origin of the human immunodeficiency virus (HIV) highlights the potential of the ancient DNA analysis for studies on microbial evolution. It is known that both of the AIDS viruses (HIV-1 and HIV-2) originated in Africa, possibly from chimpanzee (HIV-1) and sooty mangabey (HIV-2) viruses. Zhu *et al.* (1998) utilized a human blood specimen almost 40 years old from Kinshasa (Democratic Republic of Congo) to amplify short (approximately 300 bp) segments of the RNA viral genome, using reverse transcription followed by polymerase chain reaction. Phylogenetic analysis of the sequence data indicated that HIV-1 was probably introduced into humans shortly before the 1940's or early 1950's, possibly propelled by sanitary and ecologically important factors such as large-scale vaccination campaigns (with multiple use of non-sterilized needles), easier access to transportation, increasing population density and more frequent sexual contacts.

2. Unravelling a specimen's history

The idea that an archaeomolecular investigation is no more than the application of standard molecular genetic techniques to the analysis of aged materials is at best reductive. To fully appreciate the difference between working with recent and ancient specimens we must first become acquainted with concepts and terms rarely encountered in genetics and molecular biology textbooks such as "taphonomy", "taphonomical history" and "diagenesis".

Taphonomy, a Grecian neologism created in the 1940s by the Russian palaeontologist Efremov, literally means "the law of the tomb". Taphonomy is described usually as a subdiscipline of palaeontology, but its methods and data are often applied to more recent, that is archaeological, contexts. The taphonomical history of a specimen can sometimes be relatively well known or, conversely, can be largely obscure. The history of an Egyptian pre-Dynastic mummy, for example, such as the 5300 year-old mummy from Gebelein, now at the British Museum, is rather straightforward. This is a human corpse buried in a shallow pit in the desert that mummified due to a rapid process of sand dehydration. The mummy lay undisturbed in its grave for more than five thousand years until it was exhumed by archaeologists.

Alternatively, an example of how a taphonomical history can be controversial is offered by the so-called Tyrolean iceman, or Ötzi, a mummified human body found in an Alpine glacier on 19 September 1991 at 3270 m above sea level. The most relevant feature of the find, which was later radiocarbon dated to 3350-3100 BC, corresponding to Late Neolithic, is the exceptional state of preservation of the mummy and of the clothing and equipment found on the body and near it. They include, among many other items, extremely perishable ones such as a large fragment of a cloak made of knotted tufts of grass, a fur hat and a wooden bow with arrows and quiver (Spindler 1995).

The iceman lay in a chamber-like depression, below a rocky ledge, sheltered from the shearing flow of glacial ice. Thus trapped, the corpse was not expelled with the regular glacial turnover. Following the discovery, several hypotheses have been proposed regarding the process of mummification. Until 1995, the prevailing one was that the corpse had undergone rapid dehydration by a warm wind (an autumn föhn) and had been covered subsequently by snow. An alternative speculation was that the body and equipment became rapidly frozen, then covered by a porous layer of snow which allowed the body to air desiccate (Spindler 1995). Bahn (1996), on the other hand suggested that the corpse was preserved in the same way as the many frozen carcasses of mammoths and other Ice Age animals in Siberia and Alaska. They were preserved by the build-up of ice in the sediments that enveloped the bodies: the ice layers desiccated the soil and dehydrated the carcasses. Unlike freeze-drying, where the original form remains intact, this process shrivels the body.

None of these hypotheses, however, can entirely account for a number of features which are being progressively revealed by the investigations carried out independently in several laboratories. For example, histological and biochemical analyses (Bereuter et al. 1997) have shown an almost complete loss of the iceman's epidermis, accompanied by profound post-mortem alterations of skin triacylglycerols, which imply a prolonged (up to several months) immersion in water before dry weather and, possibly, warm winds desiccated the corpse. Such a scenario is, to some extent, supported by findings of algal (chrysophicean) cysts on the man's grass clothing and by the fact that the largest fraction of the DNA that can be extracted from the Neolithic grass comes from algae (Rollo et al. 1995a; 1995b; 1997).

3. How long can DNA last?

The fundamental issue "how long does DNA last?" can be re-expressed as "how fast does DNA degrade?". The latter implies a neontological (empirical) approach that can be implemented in the laboratory using ordinary test tubes or, at most, micro- and mesocosms, while the former issue (due to limited human life-span) implies a palaeontological or archaeological approach.

The double helix presents several points of weakness. Bases (purinic bases in particular) tend to be lost as a result of hydrolytic cleavage of the base-sugar bond (N-glycosidic bond) and, in correspondence with the baseless sites, strands break through a reaction of beta-elimination. With time, such mechanisms leads to a progressive fragmentation of the helix into tiny fragments. Hydrolysis is also responsible for base deamination. Both temperature and pH of the medium strongly influence this reaction (Lindahl & Nyberg 1972; 1974).

In addition to hydrolysis, oxidative damage caused by the direct interaction of ionising radiation with the DNA, as well as mediated by free radicals created from water molecules by ionising radiation, will give rise to modification of the bases followed by the destruction of their ring structure. Other mechanisms, such as alkylation or UV irradiation are unlikely to affect buried remains. Also the sugar residues are subject to attack by oxygen with the final result of a strand breakage (Lindahl 1993).

Generally, nucleic acids are hydrolysed at substantial initial rates when introduced into wastewater, seawater, freshwater, sediments, and soils (Table 1). This is mainly due to

Table 1: Half-life of DNA in various environments[a]

Location	Half-life (h)
Aquatic environment	
Wastewater	0.017-0.23
Freshwater	4.2-5.5
Sea water	3.4-83
Marine sediment	140-235
Terrestrial environment	
Soil	9.1-28.2

[a]from Lorenz & Wackernagel (1994) modified

enzymatic activity of DNA-degrading microorganisms (Lorenz & Wackernagel 1994). However, particulate constituents of soils and sediments such as quartz, feldspar, and clay minerals possess sorptive capacities for inorganic and organic material including DNA and proteins. In addition to minerals, organic compounds such as humic acids can form complexes with DNA. Up to 10% of total organic phosphate in soil comes from DNA bound to humic acids. Some experimental observations indicate that DNA half-life may be very long in sediments, in particular if the DNA is inside dead cells.

From this premise, we can predict that a DNA molecule will be very short-lived in a warm environment rich in water, oxygen, and microorganisms. Conversely, the same molecule will have relatively high chances of surviving for years, decades, centuries, and even millennia if kept in a cold, dry, anoxic, and sterile environment.

The question "how long does DNA last?" can be addressed only by comparisons of samples of different age, nature, and origin (archaeological or palaeontological approach). Since the first report describing the identification of quagga DNA, results have accumulated and we currently have much evidence showing that under certain circumstances the original DNA can be reliably identified in plant, animal and human remains dating up to 50,000 years before present (BP). The chances of success, however, differ dramatically among samples.

In the course of an investigation carried out by Höss et al. (1996), DNA was extracted from the remains of 35 ground sloths from various parts of North and South America. Two specimens of *Mylodon darwinii*, a species that became extinct at the end of the last glaciation (approximately 12,000 years BP), yielded amplifiable DNA. However, of the total DNA extracted, only 1/1000 originated from the sloth, as assessed by molecular hybridization using modern sloth DNA; the remaining part was composed of fungal and bacterial DNA. In addition, even in the two cases where amplifiable DNA was found, it was not possible to obtain fragments longer than 140 bp. Despite this, over 1100 bp of mitochondrial 12s and 16s ribosomal DNA sequences from *M. darwinii* could be reconstructed. Phylogenetic analyses using homologous sequences from extant edentate groups suggested the *M. darwinii* was more closely related to the two-toed than the three-toed sloths and thus an arboreal life-style must have evolved at least twice among sloths. Other implications were that the Edentate order contains ancient lineages which diverged before the end of the Cretaceous period.

Attempts to amplify very short (104 bp) portions of the mitochondrial gene for 12s ribosomal RNA in DNA preparations obtained from baboon and other monkey bones from the North Saqqara Baboon Galleries, Egypt (4th to 1st century B.C.) gave puzzling results. Sequence analysis of cloned amplification products actually indicated that the DNA from the bones was either of human, chicken, or unknown origin (van der Kuyl *et al.* 1994) and no original (monkey) sequence could be found. Equally, the screening of more than one hundred human mummified and skeletonized remains, dating to dynastic Egypt, showed that only two samples contained short fragments of the original DNA (Krings, unpublished results).

Rollo et al. (1994a) succeeded in PCR amplification of mitochondrial and nuclear sequences from 1000-year-old maize kernels found in a Peruvian archaeological site (Huari culture). However, the amplification efficiency was shown to correlate strongly with the length of the target sequence. For example, while 80-100% of DNA preparations (from single kernels) produced amplification signals when the length of the target sequence was between 80 and 100 bp, the proportion decreased to 20-30% when the target length was raised to 130 bp. No amplification signal was produced by PCR systems designed to amplify target sequences of 150 and 160 bp in length.

On the other hand, quite interestingly, a relatively high rate of success has been reported for permafrost-preserved Siberian mammoths despite the older age of the specimens. The woolly mammoth, Mammuthus primigenius, was widely distributed across northern Eurasia and North America in the late Pleistocene. Mammuthus is thought to have originated in Africa 5 million years ago, where it shared a common ancestor with the two living species of elephantid, the African elephant (Loxodonta africana) and Asian elephant (Elephas maximus). Studies using protein analysis performed in the past have failed to resolve the trichotomy between the genera Mammuthus, Loxodonta and Elephas. To solve this issue, Hagelberg et al. (1994) extracted DNA from bones of two frozen Siberian mammoths. The first individual, the Khatanga mammoth, consisted of the partial carcass of an adult male excavated in 1977 from alluvial sand in the eastern Taimyr peninsula. Using accelerator mass spectrometry (AMS) radiocarbon dating, the specimen was established to be at least 47,000 years old. The second sample was from a mandible excavated in 1975 from the Allaikha river, north-eastern Siberia. The mandible, dated to more than 46,000-47,000 years BP on autochthonous plant vegetation remains and AMS dating, lay in permafrost at 16 m below the surface. DNA extraction from the mammoth bone samples carried out in parallel with three forensic and three prehistoric human bone samples and an extraction blank (no bone), followed by PCR amplification with the highly conserved mitochondrial primers L14841 and H15149, consistently gave phylogenetically meaningful sequences.

In a similar investigation, Höss et al. (1994) extracted DNA from soft tissues of five different mammoths varying in age from 9,700 to more than 50,000 years. Enzymatic amplification of a 93-base-pair fragment of the mitochondrial 16s ribosomal RNA gene yielded an amplification product from four of the five individuals, specifically from seven of the fifteen extractions performed. More recently, similar results have been obtained in the case of the Enmynveyem mammoth by Derenko et al. (1997). This mammoth was discovered in 1986 in the Enmynveyem River Valley of the Chukotka Peninsula of north-eastern Siberia. The remains, radiocarbon dated to 32,850 +/- 900 years BP, consist of intact portions of the right hind femur, tibia and fibula with articulated muscle and skin.

The above-cited Tyrolean iceman, on the other hand, has been the object of a detailed molecular analysis by research teams in Munich and Oxford (Handt et al. 1994a). To assess whether some of the original DNA of the Neolithic man were left, the copy number of fragments of mtDNA (D-loop region) was estimated by competitive PCR. The PCR amplified mtDNA was subsequently cloned into a plasmid vector and sequenced. The alignment of a number of amplicon sequences showed that the body had been heavily contaminated by modern human DNA, as witnessed by the contemporaneous presence of several different mitochondrial sequences in the same specimen. Nevertheless, by applying the principle that the ancient mtDNA should be low molecular weight (<150 bp in length), the Munich team succeeded in indicating one sequence as the most likely candidate for being the original sequence of the iceman's mtDNA. This result was independently confirmed in the Oxford laboratory. Once compared with the mtDNA of contemporary populations, the iceman's mtDNA was found to correspond to types relatively frequent in northern Italy as well as in central and northern European countries.

In the course of the nineties, several reports have announced the isolation of DNA from palaeontological samples many million of years old, such as dinosaur bone (Woodward *et al.* 1994), plant leaves (Golenberg *et al.* 1990; Golenberg 1991), and amber-preserved insects and plants (Cano *et al.* 1993; 1994; De Salle *et al.* 1993). Although apparently authentic ancient DNA was recovered, these results were later challenged on the basis of empirical and theoretical evidence (Sidow *et al.* 1991; Priest 1995). For example, the mitochondrial cytochrome b sequence of an 80-million-year-old dinosaur from the Upper Cretaceous Blackhawk Formation in Utah (Woodward *et al.* 1994), which was recovered from multiple extractions and PCR amplifications, was later recognized by phylogenetic arguments as being most probably of human origin (Hedges & Schweitzer 1995).

A particularly accurate investigation on amber-entombed insects has recently been performed by Austin *et al.* (1997). Fifteen specimens of fossil insect, representing three species and body sizes and two different localities and ages (Dominican amber and East African copal), were tested for the presence of insect DNA using several primer pairs designed to bind to insect, fungal, and vertebrate mitochondrial DNA. Their results showed that in no case were they able to amplify authentic insect DNA, not even from the relatively recent (a few million years) copal.

At the present state of knowledge, according to theoretical calculations and experimental observations, we can tentatively put the upper temporal threshold for DNA survival somewhere between 50,000 and 100,000 years (Lindahl 1997).

4. The "Archaeometric" approach

An advanced school of thought maintains that no entirely convincing authentication can be performed on the sole basis of a nucleotide sequence retrieved from an ancient sample. Rather, sequence analysis should be the last link in a chain of assays ("archaeometric approach"). An outline of this protocol is given below.

First, the specimen is analysed for cell and tissue preservation using ordinary histological techniques. Then the sample is submitted to molecular tests to verify whether the original DNA has survived. Finally, the target DNA fragments are PCR amplified, cloned, and sequenced, and the sequences examined for phylogenetic consistency with the specimen.

An example is given by a study (Colson *et al.* 1997) in which seventy-two animal and human bones were examined for histological preservation, nitrogen content, and the presence of amplifiable DNA. The success rate in recovering DNA from ancient bone was best correlated with the preservation of the structure of the bone, rather than with the preservation of its nitrogen content. Discriminant analysis suggested that histology was the best discriminant variable and that survival of DNA was not correlated with the age of the sample within the range of 200-12,000 years BP.

Very recently, Vernesi *et al.* (1998) have suggested that the estimation of the bacterial DNA fraction in preparations from archaeological bone might be used as a diagenetic parameter. The principle of this analysis is that if the bone histology is preserved, the compact portion of some bones (e.g. femur) should be relatively bacteria free.

Well-known diagenetic tests are evaluations of the degree of racemization of some amino acids and quantification of a specific template, for example, a mitochondrial or plastidial sequence using quantitative PCR. The principle of the amino acid racemization assay is simple and has long been used by geochemists and palaeontologists. More recently, it has been shown that it can also be employed as a useful tool in the analysis of ancient DNA (Poinar *et al.* 1996). With the exception of the optically-inactive glycine (Gly), all amino acids used in proteins can exist in the form of two optical isomers (enantiomers), the D (*dextro*-rotatory) and the L (*levo*-rotatory) form. Of the two, only the L-enantiomer is used in protein biosynthesis. Upon the death of the cell, the protein L-amino acids turn into D-enantiomers until, after some time, the two forms are present in equal amounts (racemization). The rate at which racemization takes place differs from amino acid to amino acid. The process is influenced by temperature and by the presence of water and certain metal ions. The L-amino acids produced by living organisms on Earth are totally racemized (D/L = 1) in the geological environment on timescales of 10^5 to 10^6 years.

It has been shown that the racemization of aspartic acid (Asp) which has one of the fastest racemization rates, is similar, over a wide temperature range, to DNA depurination (Bada *et al.* 1994; Poinar *et al.* 1996). We can thus use racemization of Asp as an indicator of DNA degradation. In other words, we can use racemization figures for Asp to predict whether or not a certain sample will contain the original DNA (Table 2).

There is also other useful information that can be obtained by checking a sample for amino acid racemization. Because the racemization of Asp is faster than that of other amino acids such as alanine (Ala) and leucine (Leu), one should expect to find a greater D/L ratio for the former and a lower for the latter one if the amino acids are of the same age. In contrast, a D/L ratio for Ala and Leu greater than that for Asp may be taken as evidence of contamination by more recent amino acids. A D/L Asp greater than 0.1 should be taken as a strong argument against the usefulness of a specimen for ancient DNA studies. As a cautionary note on the generalized use of amino acid racemization tests, however, we should note that the values of D/L Asp for amber-entombed insects have been reported to be in the range 0.01-0.08 (Poinar *et al.* 1996). Indeed, the analysis of such specimens is now seen by some specialists as questionable.

In general, contamination of ancient DNA is of two types. The first type will affect all amplifications to the same extent. These contaminations are due to contemporary DNA present in reagents used in tissue extractions or enzymatic amplification. They are generally easily detected by using appropriate controls, such as amplifications from fake extractions and amplifications where no template DNA is added. Of greater concern are contaminations of the second type, which affect individual extractions or amplifications.

Table 2: Extent of aspartic acid racemization in archaeological and palaeontological samples

Sample	Provenance	Age (yr)	D/L Asp
Human soft tissue	Peru	1000	0.035[b]
Papio cynocephalus	Egypt	2300	0.18[a]
Human bone	Egypt	4500	0.30[a]
Human soft tissue	Alps	5300	0.06[c]
Megalonyx sp.	Florida	13,000	0.33[a]
H. neandertalensis	Germany	unknown	0.11[a]
Mammuthus primigenius	Siberia	50,000	0.05[a]

[a]Poinar *et al.* (1996); [b]Cano *et al.* (unpublished data); [c]Ubaldi *et al.* (1998)

They may stem from the handling of archaeological specimens prior to sampling, or from laboratory aerosols or amplification products. The main way to identify this second type of contamination is to repeat experiments from two or more independent samples from each individual studied.

In the case of ancient human and animal remains, the most common subject of investigation is perhaps mitochondrial (mt) DNA. The analysis of this molecule poses particularly serious problems due to the ease of sample contamination by modern mtDNA. Recent work (Handt *et al.* 1994b; Handt *et al.* 1996) suggests that quantitative PCR can be employed to estimate mtDNA copy number in a mummified human tissue and that this estimate can be used as an additional validation criterion for ancient DNA.

A commonly experienced aspect of PCR is the low reproducibility of the amount of product yield, even under the most controlled assay conditions. This variability may depend on different causes, including thermal cycler performance, reaction conditions, presence of inhibitors, and differences in sample preparation and purification of nucleic acids (Clementi *et al.* 1993). A reliable approach to molecular quantitation using PCR amplification is that based on coamplification of two similar templates (the target sequence and the reference template introduced at a known amount) of equal or similar length sharing the primer recognition sequences. During amplification, the two templates compete for the same primer set (competitive PCR), and consequently amplify at the same rate independently of the number of PCR cycles and of any predictable or unpredictable variable influencing the PCR amplification.

Austin *et al.* (1997) have recently established a methodology to deal with most specimens. In brief, this methodology recommends careful selection of specimens (on the basis of evidence for good cellular and /or biomolecular preservation), choices of tissue samples that represent the best possible site for DNA preservation, and careful sample preparation (e.g. surface sterilization) to eliminate surface contamination. The operations should be carried out in a laboratory dedicated exclusively to ancient specimens. Work on ancient DNA should be temporally separated from that on modern DNA. Further, in order to detect any contamination, multiple negative controls should be performed during DNA extraction and PCR set up.

A crucial step is the authentification of the results. Accordingly to Austin *et al.* (1997), putatively ancient DNA sequences should be reproducibly obtained from different extractions from the same sample, and from different tissue samples from different specimens. When the target DNA has a very low copy number, as in the case of mtDNA from Neanderthal bone (Krings *et al.* 1997), the ultimate test of authenticity should be independent replication in two separate laboratories.

5. Perspectives for molecular microbial palaeoecology

A particularly interesting sector in the archaeomolecular field is the study of ancient microorganisms: bacteria, filamentous fungi, yeasts, algae protozoans, and viruses. The analysis of the DNA of ancient microorganisms in ancient human and animal remains can contribute to the understanding of issues as different as the spreading of a new disease (Tautenberg *et al.* 1997), the mummification process (Rollo *et al.* 1997), and the effect of diet on historical human populations (Ubaldi *et al.* 1998).

The majority of studies published so far have considered pathogenic microorganisms ("palaeopathological approach"). These microorganisms include bacteria such as *Mycobacterium tuberculosis* (Salo *et al.* 1994; Dixon *et al.* 1995; Crubezy *et al.* 1997; Faerman *et al.* 1997), *Mycobacterium leprae* (Rafi *et al.* 1994), *Yersina pestis* (Hummel *et al.* 1994) and *Treponema pallidum* (Rogan & Lentz, 1995). In all of these cases, the experimental approach has been DNA extraction from desiccated soft tissue or bone, and PCR amplification using PCR primer pairs (or sets of nested primer pairs) designed on the basis of highly variable regions of the bacterial chromosome. Examples of this approach are given by the work of Salo *et al.* (1994) and of Faerman *et al.* (1997). The former started from a lung lesion of a spontaneously mummified body of an adult (40-45 year-old) female who died 1000 years ago in Southern Peru. The tomb from which the body was exhumed was in a burial site (Chiribaya Alta) used by the Chiribaya, a mostly agricultural population that occupied the Lower Osmore Valley near the coastal community of Ilo. DNA was extracted from lesion tissue and enzymatically amplified using a primer pair designed to bind to a 123-bp fragment of DNA which is part of a repetitive (10-16 copies per bacterial chromosome) insertion sequence- (IS) like element of 1361 bp in length called IS6110. The presence of this element in *M. tuberculosis* has been shown to correlate closely with clinically diagnosed tuberculosis.

In ancient Europe, tuberculosis was one of the most widely prevalent infectious diseases. Incidence in bone pathology in skeletal remains from medieval Lithuania suggests that 18-25% of the population suffered from the disease. Faerman *et al.* (1997) detected the presence of *M. tuberculosis* in skeletal remains from Lithuania, dated to the 15th-17th centuries, by amplifying a part of the IS6110 element and found that a much higher percentage of individuals was infected than previously thought.

In studying ancient pathogenic protozoans, Taylor *et al.* (1997) have developed a nested PCR method for amplifying *Plasmodium* nucleic acid. Their method detects all four malaria-producing *Plasmodium* species pathogenic to humans and was designed to amplify small fragments of DNA likely to remain in archaeological specimens. The method has been applied to two human ribs from separate individuals who had died almost 60 years previously from anaemia thought to be due to malaria. *Plasmodium* DNA was confirmed in one of these cases. Sequencing of the PCR product identified the causative species as *Plasmodium falciparum*. It is important, however, to note that when the test was applied to the Granville mummy, the result was negative. This mummy is of a female aged about 50 years from the site of Gurna (Egypt) (approximately 700 BC) and had previously been reported positive for *Plasmodium falciparum* using immunological methods.

To investigate the origin of the fungal hyphae that cover the grass clothing (cloak, boots) of the Tyrolean iceman, Rollo *et al.* (1994b; 1995a,b) and Ubaldi *et al.* 1996) submitted two radiocarbon-dated samples of grass to DNA extraction. The DNA was then PCR amplified using, respectively, primer pairs specific for the region containing the internal transcribed spacers and the 5.8s rDNA (ITS), and primer pairs specific for an approximately 600-bp long fragment of the nuclear small-subunit ribosomal DNA (SSU rDNA) repeat units of eukaryotes. The amplification products were cloned and sequenced. Sequence analysis of twenty ITS and ten SSU rDNA amplicons indicated that three types of fungal DNA could be extracted from the Neolithic grass. Phylogenetic analyses, using 5.8s and SSU rDNA fungal reference sequences from databases, showed that the DNAs came, respectively, from a basidiomycete, phylogenetically close to *Leucosporidium scottii*, a psychrophilic yeast-like microorganism isolated, among other substrates, from soil, plant material and water in Antarctica and Canada, and from two ascomycetes, one of which is possibly related to the Eurotiales.

The human treponematoses (syphilis, bejel, yaws and pinta) are caused by spiral bacteria of the genus *Treponema*, which belongs to the family of *Treponemataceae* in the order of the *Spirochaetales*. The origin of the treponematoses, syphilis in particular, has been a controversial subject in the history of medicine. According to the so-called

Columbian theory, syphilis was unknown in Europe prior to Columbus' return from his first voyage in 1493. At that time, a disease called guayanaras or bubas was already known to exist among the natives of the West Indies, and the descriptions of this disease point to a treponematosis, either yaws or syphilis (Noordhoek 1991). In attempting to provide a molecular characterization for the Renaissance treponemes, Marota *et al.* (1997) performed a molecular analysis of the matter that stained a bandage found on the mummy of Maria of Aragon (1503-1568), and that covered an ulcer. DNA was extracted from a small amount of desiccated matter and PCR amplified using primer pairs designed to bind to short fragments (respectively, 95, 135, and 207 bp in length) of the 16s ribosomal rRNA gene of *Treponema pallidum*. Amplification products of the expected lengths were cloned into a plasmid vector and sequenced. Sequence comparison of almost thirty amplicons identified bacteria of the genera *Streptofusia, Mycobacterium, Peptostreptococcus, Propionibacterium, Clostridium,* and *Capnocytophaga*. Although no *T. pallidum* were detected, the presence of *Capnocytophaga sputigena* and of other representatives of the oral microbiota, suggested that the patient might have undergone a "salivation cure". This cure was prescribed by Renaissance doctors to patients suffering from "*Morbus gallicus*".

Attempts to identify ancient microorganisms which are not obligate parasites of humans or animals, by molecular methods is hampered by the difficulty of distinguishing between the DNA of truly ancient saprobes or opportunists, and the DNA of soil microorganisms that may have colonized the remains in more recent times. To overcome this problem, the present author proposes the application of a criterion of palaeoecological consistency. Briefly, one should check whether the putative eco-physiology and distribution of the microorganisms identified on the basis of DNA sequencing is consistent with the present characteristics of the site from which the specimen comes or, rather, the inferences from DNA analysis are congruent with the microbial dwellers of a living body. In other words, it is necessary to establish that putatively ancient DNA makes palaeoecological sense. It is important to note that in the case of ubiquitous microorganisms, such as certain species of clostridia, it will be extremely difficult, if not impossible, to determine for each individual sequence whether it comes from an ancient or a modern microorganism. However, the sequences as a whole will provide some information.

It is now recognized that all external body surfaces have a normal resident bacterial flora, and this includes the digestive tract. Because of cell turnover, gut surfaces are coated with dead and desquamating cells, and these provide an excellent basal nutrient source, to which can be added nutrients passing through the lumen and the gut (Hill 1995). The bacterial flora represents a significant component of the complex intestinal ecosystem. Its distribution along the intestinal tract is, however, highly variable in number and composition and can be influenced by diet, interaction among the different groups of microorganisms, drug taking, toxins and carcinogenic substances. Under normal conditions, the upper part of the small bowel (duodenum, jejunum) is considered to have a low microbial content, while its lower portion (ileum) is characterized by higher cell numbers. The highest microbial content is found in the large bowel (colon).

To investigate the possibility of collecting data on the composition of the bacterial flora of the colon for historical human populations, Ubaldi *et al.* (1998) studied a pre-Columbian mummy. The mummy, presently at the National Museum of Anthropology and Ethnology of Florence, Italy, is of a young woman aged 20 +/-3 years and is known to come from Cuzco (Peru), the ancient capital of the Inca kingdom. The archaeological dating of this body has been the object of repeated revisions in the course of time. In the past decade, on the basis of the funerary objects, the date was assumed to be 15th-17th century A.D. This figure was subsequently changed to 14th century A.D. Radiocarbon analyses performed recently on a group of Andean mummies conserved at the "L. Pigorini" Prehistoric and Ethnographic Museum (Rome, Italy) suggest, however, that a more reliable date might be 9th-10th century A.D. (R. Machiarelli, personal communication). A few years ago, the Andean mummy (natural mummy) was the subject of a necropsy performed by Fornaciari et al. (1992). The dissection of the desiccated body showed that the internal organs, stomach, lungs, intestine, liver, heart, etc. are well preserved.

As a first step, DNA was phenol extracted from samples of oesophagus, stomach, pylorus, small intestine, ascending colon, transverse colon, descending colon, liver, (left and right) lung, diaphragm, pericardium, myocardium, and aorta of the mummy (fourteen in total). The DNA fractions were then analysed by agarose gel electrophoresis. All the extracts were shown to contain short DNA fragments ranging in length from a few dozen base pair to approximately 200 bp. Aorta, pericardium, myocardium, oesophagus, and transverse colon gave the maximum DNA yield as estimated densitometrically. The degree of conservation of the original mummy DNA was determined using two experimental approaches: evaluation of the extent of racemization of aspartic acid, and quantification of mtDNA copy number. The former (performed on myocardic and colon tissue samples) provided a value for the D/L ratio fully comparable with the ratio shown by fresh amino acid preparations (0.035). This result is, in principle, compatible with the preservation of the original mummy DNA. Subsequently, to measure mtDNA copy number, a competitive PCR system according to Förster (1994) was employed. This system is based on the amplification of a short (103 bp) tract of the hypervariable region I of the mtDNA control region in the presence of competitor DNA of 81 bp in length. The results showed that all the different tissue samples contained mtDNA in relatively high copy number (Table 3).

At this point, as both tests convincingly indicated that the original mummy DNA was preserved, the quest for bacterial DNA could be initiated. As a first step, the distribution of the bacterial DNA was determined in the different organs and tissues of the mummy. With this in view, all the DNA preparations were PCR amplified using a primer pair (29f/98r) designed to bind to a very short portion (approximately 100 bp) of the bacterial 16s rDNA according to the principle of the so-called "consensus sequence PCR" (Relman, 1993; Maidak et al. 1997). Different samples produced amplification signals of a different intensity. In particular, liver, lungs, and diaphragm produced no signal or very weak signals. On the other hand ascending, transverse, and descending colon produced very strong signals, while weak signals were produced by pylorus and the small intestine. The abundance of bacterial DNA in the large bowel of the mummy compared to the relatively poor content of the small bowel is best explained with the hypothesis that the desiccation process responsible for the mummification of the body has also preserved the

Table 3: Mitochondrial DNA copy number in different tissue samples from a 1000-year-old Andean mummy

Tissue/organ	mtDNA copy number
Oesophagus	100
Colon	100
Myocardium	200
Aorta	600

data from Ubaldi et al. 1998

intestinal flora ("palaeoecological consistency"). The variations in bacterial DNA copy number might be better appreciated by the use of competitive PCR systems designed on the basis of the 16s rDNA sequences. Competitive PCR could also be used to advantage to estimate the relative proportions of intact (*i.e.* modern) and degraded (*i.e.* ancient) bacterial templates in the different organs of the mummy.

To identify the bacteria, the 16s rDNA amplification products of the transverse colon sample were cloned into a pMOSBlue plasmid vector, and the nucleotide sequence of 15 amplicons was determined. The sequences were then used to scan the EMBL and GeneBank data libraries using Blast and FastA programs. Eleven out of fifteen sequences considered were identified as *Clostridium botulinum*, an organism commonly isolated from soil, marine, and lake sediments. *C. botulinum* (Cato *et al.* 1986) is also found in animal, bird, and fish intestines and in food. The remaining sequences belong to *Clostridium* sp. *C. algidicarnis* and *Eubacterium pectinii*. This rather surprising result might be interpreted as an indication that the Andean woman was fed with honey before death, as *C. botulinum* spores are frequently found in natural honey. We can observe, however, that all these identifications should be treated with caution due to the short length (approximately 60 bp) of the sequences compared, and to the low similarity with the reference sequences displayed by several of them.

To obtain a more convincing inference, the DNA preparation from the transverse colon was PCR amplified using a different primer pair (338f/531r) designed to bind to a longer (196 bp long) portion of the 16s rDNA, and the amplification products were cloned and sequenced. This time the taxon composition was very different from the previous one: *C. algidicarnis* was the predominant species, followed in relative abundance by *C. cochlearium*, *C. aurantibutyricum*, and *C. intestinalis*. This demonstrates that the increase of the target 16s rDNA sequence up to 196 bp has allowed an acceptable identification to be performed while keeping within the size range of the DNA fragments extracted from the mummy tissues and, in general, within a size range compatible with most of the ancient DNA investigations.

One may ask why only 16s rDNA sequences from clostridia are found. There are several possible explanations for this phenomenon. The first is that clostridia are extremely abundant representatives of the anaerobic gut flora. Their proportion is most probably underestimated by the traditional cultivation assays. Secondarily, they are endospore-forming bacteria and it is known that the spore offers an excellent protection to the DNA (Setlow 1992). There is the further possibility of amplification bias (Suzuki & Giovannoni 1996; Wang & Wang 1996); this, however, seems unlikely as two different sets of primers have both given consistent results at least for taxon identification at the genus level. Finally, the prevalence of clostridia might reflect a pathological state of the colon in this particular mummy.

The above research principles are being now implemented in the study of the Tyrolean iceman's bacteriology (Cano *et al.*, unpublished data). To check whether over 5000 years of lying under the glacier have totally cancelled the traces of the bacteria that dwelled in the gastro-intestinal tract of the Neolithic herdsman/hunter, or whether some remains of prehistoric bacteria are left, three types of samples were selected. The first one was represented by grass fragments from the boots and the cloak, and the second and third by biopsies from the iceman's stomach and colon, respectively. DNA was extracted from the three groups of samples and PCR amplified using universal primer pairs targeted to portions of the 16s rDNA. Amplification products were cloned and amplicons from the three groups of libraries sequenced, and the sequences used for database scanning. Preliminary results indicate that the bacterial flora associated with the grass clothing include, among others, species belonging to the genera *Zoogloea*, *Curtobacterium*,

Arthrobacter, and *Sphingobacterium*. On the other hand, bacterial sequences obtained from stomach biopsies seem low in diversity and to consist mainly of *Burkholderia* spp. and *Pseudomonas* spp. Finally, the colon shows a wide array of *Clostridium* and *Eubacterium*, most of which are recognized common inhabitants of the human intestines, and, in addition, some representative of the *Enterobacteria* and *Bacilli* (Table 4).

The strong differences found in the composition of the bacterial flora of the grass clothing (possibly representative of the microbiological situation of the glacier), stomach, and colon, clearly show that the body has been colonized by microorganisms from the external environment only to a limited extent during its long taphonomical history. This, in turn, opens the way to the study of Neolithic human gut microbiota, though with the important limitation posed by the uniqueness of this specimen.

6. Future perspectives

There are several areas where ancient DNA research is expected to play a relevant role in the near future. For example, studies on the history of infectious disease using ancient DNA are still at their infancy. The above-quoted detection of HIV DNA in an archived plasma sample from 1959 (Zhu *et al.* 1998) on the other hand, can be taken as an eloquent example of the potential for a diachronic approach to viral evolution. The analysis of the colon microflora in the gut of an Andean mummy (Ubaldi *et al.* 1998) demonstrates the feasibility of studies on the ancient human microbiota which potentially can span from prehistory to the present. The neolithic, for example, is generally considered as a crucial point in the history of the co-existence of humans and microbes, when the transition of life into larger human aggregations and animal domestication

Table 4: DNA identification of remnants of the original colon microbiota in two
natural mummies compared to living man

Living man[a]	Andean mummy[b]	Iceman[c]
Strict anaerobes		
Clostridia	+	+
Eubacteria	+	+
Peptococci	-	-
Bacteroides	-	+
Fusobacteria	-	-
Bifidobacteria	-	-
Veillonella	-	-
Microaerophilic		
Lactobacilli	-	-
Streptococci	-	-
Enterococci	-	-
Facultative & Aerobes		
Enterobacteria	-	+
Micrococci	-	-
Staphylococci	-	-
Bacilli	-	+

[a]Hill (1995); [b]Ubaldi *et al.* (1998); [c]Cano *et al.* (unpublished data)

favoured the spread of disease, including the infections characterized by an oro-fecal transmission of pathogens.

As the quest for microbial DNA can be extended to animal mummies, we may think of the internal organs of permafrost-preserved carcasses as possible candidates for future palaeomicrobiological investigations. In a recent review, Cooper & Wayne (1998) foresee the analysis of entire communities of prehistoric animals using material from permafrost or cave deposits. While the analysis of mitochondrial and nuclear DNA will certainly provide a better understanding of the systematics and population genetics of prehistoric species, the analysis of bacterial and viral DNA will possibly provide a clue to species extinction, genetic bottlenecks, and to pathways of disease transmission from animals to humans.

References

Audic S, Béraud-Colomb E (1997) Ancient DNA is thirteen years old. *Nature Biotechnology*, **15**, 855-858.

Austin JJ, Smith AB, Thomas R (1997) Palaeontology in a molecular world: the search for authentic ancient DNA. *Trends in Ecology and Evolution*, **12**, 303-306.

Bada JL, Wang XS, Poinar HN, Pääbo S, Poinar GO (1994) Amino acid racemization in amber-entombed insects: implications for DNA preservation. *Geochimica et Cosmochimica Acta*, **58**, 3131-3135.

Bahn PG (1996) *Tombs, Graves and Mummies*. Barnes & Noble, New York.

Béraud-Colomb E, Roubin R, Martin J *et al.* (1995) Human β-globin gene polymorphisms characterized in DNA extracted from ancient bones 12,000 years old. *American Journal of Human Genetics*, **57**, 1267-1274.

Bereuter TL, Mikena T, Reiter C (1997) Iceman's mummification-Implications from infrared spectroscopical and histological studies. *Chemistry European Journal*, **3**, 1032-1038.

Brown TA, Allaby RG, Brown KA, O'Donoghue K, Sallares R (1994) DNA in wheat seeds from European archaeological sites. *Experientia*, **50**, 571-575.

Cano RJ, Poinar HN, Pieniazek NJ, Acra A, Poinar GO (1993) Amplification of DNA from a 120-135-million-year-old weevil. *Nature*, **363**, 536-538.

Cano RJ, Borucki MK, Higby-Schweitzer M, Poinar HN, Poinar GO, Pollard KJ (1994) Bacillus DNA in fossil bees: an ancient symbiosis? *Applied and Environmental Microbiology*, **60**, 2164-2167.

Cato EP, Lance GeorgeW, Finegold SM (1986). Genus *Clostridium*. In: *Bergey's Manual of Systematic Bacteriology* (ed. Holt JG), volume 2, pp. 1157-1160. Williams & Wilkins, Baltimore.

Clementi M, Menzo S, Bagnarelli P, Manzin A, Valenza A, Varaldo PE (1993) Quantitative PCR and RT-PCR in virology. *PCR Methods and Applications*, **2**, 191-196.

Colson IB, Bailey JF, Vercauteren M, Sykes BC (1997) The preservation of ancient DNA and bone diagenesis. *Ancient Biomolecules*, **1**, 109-118.

Cooper A, Mourer-Chauviré C, Chambers GK, von Haeseler A, Wilson AC, Pääbo S (1992) Independent origins of New Zealand moas and kiwis. *Proceedings of the National Academy of Sciences USA*, **89**, 8741-8744.

Cooper A, Rhymer J, James HF *et al.* (1996) Ancient DNA and island endemics. *Nature*, **381**, 484.

Cooper A, Wayne R (1998) New uses for old DNA. *Current Opinion in Biotechnology*, **9**, 49-53.

Crubèzy E, Poveda JD, Montagnon D, Ludes B (1997) Identification of *Mycobacterium tuberculosis* or bovis DNA in Egyptian Pott's disease 5400 year old. *Ancient DNA IV* (Conference Abstracts), Gottingen 5-7 June 1997.

Derenko M, Malyarchuk B, Shields GF (1997) Mitochondrial cytochrome b sequence from a 33 000 year-old woolly mammoth (*Mammuthus primigenius*). *Ancient Biomolecules*, **1**, 149-153.

DeSalle R, Barcia M, Wray C (1993) PCR jumping in clones of 30-million-year-old DNA fragments from amber preserved termites (*Mastotermes electrodominicus*). *Experientia* **49**, 906-909.

Dixon RA, Aveling E, Roberts CA (1995) Detection of a *Mycobacterium tuberculosis* specific insertion element from ancient human rib using the polymerase chain reaction (abstract). *Ancient DNA III* (Conference Abstracts) Oxford, 20th-22nd July, 1995.

Faerman M, Jankauskas R, Gorski A, Bercovier H, Greenblatt CL (1997) Prevalence of human tuberculosis in a medieval population of Lithuania studied by ancient DNA analysis. *Ancient Biomolecules*, **1**, 205-214.

Fornaciari G, Castagna M, Viacava P *et al.* (1992) Malattia di Chagas in una mummia peruviana Inca del Museo Nazionale di Antropologia ed Etnologia di Firenze. *Archivio per l'Antropologia e la Etnologia*, **122**, 369-376.

Förster E (1994) An improved general method to generate internal standards for competitive PCR. *Biotecniques*, **16**, 18-20.

Golenberg EM (1991) Amplification and analysis of Miocene plant fossil DNA. *Philosophical Transactions of the Royal Society of London, B*, **333**, 419-427.

Golenberg EM, Giannasi DE, Clegg MT (1990) Chloroplast DNA sequence from a Miocene *Magnolia* species. *Nature*, **344**, 656-658.

Goloubinoff P, Pääbo S, Wilson AC (1993) Evolution of maize inferred from sequence diversity of an adh2 gene sequence from archaeological specimens. *Proceedings of the National Academy of Sciences USA* , **90**, 1997-2001.

Greer CE, Peterson SL, Kiviat NB, Manos MM (1991) PCR amplification from paraffin-embedded tissues: effects of fixative and fixation time. *American Journal of Clinical Pathology*, **95**, 117-124.

Hagelberg E, Thomas MG, Cook CE, Sher AV, Baryshnikov GF, Lister AM (1994) DNA from ancient mammoth bones. *Nature*, **370**, 333-334.

Handt O, Richards M, Trommsdorff M, Kilger C *et al.* (1994a) Molecular genetic analyses of the Tyrolean Ice Man. *Science*, **264**, 1775-1778.

Handt O, Höss M, Krings M, Pääbo S (1994b) Ancient DNA: methodological challenges. *Experientia*, **50**, 524-529.

Handt O, Krings M, Ward RH Pääbo S (1996) The retrieval of ancient human DNA sequences. *American Journal of Human Genetics*, **59**, 368-376.

Hedges SB, Schweitzer MH (1995) Detecting dinosaur DNA. *Science*, **268**, 1191.

Herrmann B, Hummel S (1994) *Ancient DNA*. Springer-Verlag, New York, Berlin.

Higuchi R, Bowman B, Freiberger M, Ryder O, Wilson AC (1984) DNA sequences from a quagga, an extinct member of the horse family. *Nature*, **312**, 282-284.

Higuchi R, Wrischnik LA, Oakes E, George M, Tong B, Wilson AC (1987) Mitochondrial DNA of the extinct quagga: relatedness and extent of postmortem change. *Journal of Molecular Evolution*, **25**, 283-287.

Hill MJ (1995) The normal gut bacterial flora. In: *Role of Gut Bacteria in Human Toxicology and Pharmacology*, (ed. Hill MJ), pp. 3-17. Taylor & Francis, London.

Höss M, Pääbo S, Vereshchagin NK (1994) Mammoth DNA sequences. *Nature*, **370**, 333.

Höss M, Dilling A, Currant A, Pääbo S (1996) Phylogeny of the extinct ground sloth *Mylodon darwinii*. *Proceedings of the National Academy of Sciences USA*, **93**, 181-185.

Hummel S, Menzel A, Uy A *et al.* (1994) DNA analysis of inherited and infectious disease-perspective for palaeopathology. *Xth European Meeting of the Palaeopathology Association*, 29 August-3 September, Göttingen.

Krings M, Stone A, Schmitz RW, Krainitzki H, Stoneking M, Pääbo S (1997) Neandertal DNA sequences and the origin of modern humans. *Cell*, **90**, 19-30.

Lalueza Fox C (1996) Analysis of ancient mitochondrial DNA from extinct aborigines from Tierra del Fuego-Patagonia. *Ancient Biomolecules*, **1**, 43-54.

Lassen C, Hummel S, Herrmann B (1996) PCR based sex identification of ancient human bones by amplification of X- and Y-chromosomal sequences: a comparison. *Ancient Biomolecules*, **1**, 25-34.

Lindahl T (1993) Instability and decay of the primary structure of DNA. *Nature*, **362**, 709-715.

Lindahl T (1997) Facts and artifacts of ancient DNA. *Cell*, **90**, 1-3.

Lindahl T & Nyberg B (1972) Rate of depurination of native deoxyribonucleic acid. *Biochemistry*, **11**, 3610-3618.

Lindahl T, Nyberg B (1974) Heat induced deamination of cytosine residues in deoxyribonucleic acid. *Biochemistry*, **13**, 3405-3410.

Lorenz MG, Wackernagel W (1994) Bacterial transfer by natural genetic transformation in the environment. *Microbiological Reviews*, **58**, 563-602.

Maidak, BL, Olsen GJ, Larsen N, Overbeek R, McCaughey M, Woese CR (1997) The RDP Ribosomal Database Project. *Nucleic Acids Research*, **25**, 109-111.

Marota I, Fornaciari G, Rollo F (1997) La sifilide nel rinascimento: identificazione di sequenze ribosomali batteriche nel DNA isolato dalla mummia di Maria d' Aragona (XVI secolo). *Antropologia Contemporanea*, in press.

Noordhoek GT (1991) *Syphilis and yaws. A Molecular Study to Detect and Differentiate Pathogenic Treponemes*. PhD thesis, University of Utrecht.

Pääbo S (1985a) Preservation of DNA in ancient Egyptian mummies. *Journal of Archaeological Science*, **12**, 411-417.

Pääbo S (1985b) Molecular cloning of ancient Egyptian mummy DNA. *Nature*, **314**, 644-645.

Pääbo S, Higuchi RG, Wilson AC (1989) Ancient DNA and the polymerase chain reaction. *Journal of Biological Chemistry*, **264**, 9709-9712.

Pääbo S, Irwin DM, Wilson AC (1990) DNA damage promotes jumping between templates during enzymatic amplification. *Journal of Biological Chemistry*, **265**, 4718-4721.

Poinar HN, Höss M, Bada JL, Pääbo S (1996) Amino acid racemization and the preservation of ancient DNA. *Science*, **272**, 864-866.

Priest FG (1995) Age of bacteria from amber. *Science*, **270**, 2015.

Rafi A, Spigelman M, Stanford J, Lemma E, Donoghue H, Zias J (1994) *Mycobacterium leprae* DNA from ancient bone detected by PCR. *Lancet*, **343**, 1360-1361.

Relman DA (1993) The identification of uncultured microbial pathogens. *Journal of Infectious Diseases*, **168**, 1-8.

Rogan PK, Lentz S (1995) Molecular genetics evidence suggesting treponematosis in pre-Columbian Chilean mummies (Conference Abstract). *II World Congress on Mummy Studies*, Universidad di los Andes, Instituto Colombiano di Antropologia.

Rollo F (1985) Characterisation by molecular hybridization of RNA fragments isolated from ancient (1400 B.C.) seeds. *Theoretical and Applied Genetics*, **71**, 330-333.

Rollo F, Venanzi FM, Amici A (1991) Nucleic acids in mummified plant seeds: biochemistry and molecular genetics of pre-Columbian maize. *Genetical Research Cambridge*, **58**, 193-201.

Rollo F, Venanzi FM, Amici A (1994a) DNA and RNA from ancient plant seeds. In: *Ancient DNA* (eds. Herrmann B, Hummel S) Springer-Verlag, New York, Berlin.

Rollo F, Asci W, Antonini S, Ubaldi M (1994b) Molecular ecology of a neolithic meadow, the DNA of the grass remains from the archaeological site of the Tyrolean Iceman. *Experientia*, **50**, 576-584.

Rollo F, Asci W, Marota I, Sassaroli S (1995a) DNA analysis of grass remains found at the iceman's archaeological site. In: *Der Mann im Eis* (eds. Spindler K, Rastbichler-Zissernig E, Wilfing H, zur Nedden D, Nothdurfter H), pp. 91-105. Springer-Verlag, Wien, New York.

Rollo F, Sassaroli S, Ubaldi M (1995b) Molecular phylogeny of the fungi of the Iceman's grass clothing. *Current Genetics*, **28**, 289-297.

Rollo F, Luciani S, Ubaldi M (1997) Ancient microorganisms offer new clues to the Iceman's mummification. *Human Evolution*, **12**, 197-208.

Salo WM, Aufderheide AC, Buikstra J, Holcomb TA (1994) Identification of *Mycobacterium tuberculosis* DNA in a pre-Columbian Peruvian mummy. *Proceedings of the National Academy of Sciences USA*, **91**, 2091-2094.

Setlow P (1992) I will survive: protecting and repairing spore DNA. *Journal of Bacteriology*, **174**, 2737-2741.

Sidow A, Wilson AC, Pääbo S (1991) Bacterial DNA in *Clarkia* fossils. *Philosophical Transactions of the Royal Society of London B*, **333**, 429-433.

Spindler K (1995) *The Man in the Ice*. Phoenix, London.

Suzuki MT, Giovannoni SJ (1996) Bias caused by template annealing in the amplification of mixture of 16S rRNA genes by PCR. *Applied and Environmental Microbiology*, **62**, 625-630.

Tautenberger JK, Reid AH, Krafft AE, Bijwaard KE, Fanning TG (1997) Initial genetic characterization of the 1918 "Spanish" influenza virus. *Science*, **275**, 1793-1796.

Taylor GM, Rutland P, Molleson T (1997) A sensitive polymerase chain reaction method for the detection of *Plasmodium* species DNA in ancient human remains. *Ancient Biomolecules*, **1**, 193-203.

Ubaldi M, Sassaroli S, Rollo F (1996) Ribosomal DNA analysis of culturable deuteromycetes from the iceman's hay: comparison of living and mummified fungi. *Ancient Biomolecules*, **1**, 35-42.

Ubaldi M, Luciani S, Marota I, Fornaciari G, Cano RJ, Rollo F (1998) Sequence analysis of bacterial DNA in the colon of an Andean mummy. *American Journal of Physical Anthropology*, in press.

van der Kuyl A, Dekker J, Attia M, Iskander N, Perizonius W, Goudsmit J(1994) DNA from ancient Egyptian monkey bones. *Ancient DNA Newsletter*, **2**, 19-21.

Vernesi C, Caramelli D, Carbonell i Sala S, Ubaldi M, Rollo F, Chiarelli B (1998) Application of DNA sex tests to bone specimens from three Etruscan (VII-III century BC) archaeological sites. *Ancient Biomolecules*, in press.

Wang GC, Wang Y (1996) The frequency of chimeric molecules as a consequence of PCR co-amplification of 16s rRNA genes from different bacterial species. *Microbiology*, **142**, 1107-1114.

Woodward SR, Weyand NJ, Bunnell M (1994) DNA sequence from Cretaceous period bone fragments. *Science*, **266**, 1229-1232.

Zhu T, Korber TB, Nahmias AJ, Hooper E, Sharps PM, Ho DD (1998) An african HIV-1 sequence from 1959 and implications for the origin of the epidemic. *Nature*, **391**, 594-597.

Advances in Molecular Ecology
G.R. Carvalho (Ed.)
IOS Press, 1998

Clonal Organisms and the Benefits of Sex

Robert C. Vrijenhoek

Center for Theoretical & Applied Genetics, Rutgers University
New Brunswick, New Jersey 08901, USA. e-mail: vrijen@ahab.rutgers.edu

Obligately asexual species are very uncommon among multicellular plants and metazoan animals; yet studies of these rare exceptions to the "rule of sex" provide insights into the long- and short-term benefits of sexual reproduction. Lessons to be learned from clones are especially relevant as we enter an era when the artificial cloning of mammals (and potentially humans) is no longer a fantasy. Sexual reproduction is the ancestral condition for multicellular eukaryotes. Some sexual species have genes that control the switch to asexual reproduction, but many asexual lineages arise because of cytogenetic accidents (*e.g.* interspecific hybridization and polyploidization) that disrupt meiosis. Molecular studies reveal that many asexual taxa are composed of multiple clones that arose independently from the sexual progenitors. Are the successful clones ecological generalists or specialists? Some appear to have a wide tolerance of environmental conditions, and many others appear to flourish under a narrower range of conditions. The niche characteristics of clones are a product of the competitive milieu in which asexual lineages arise. Broadly tolerant clones may be favoured in marginal habitats, where they escape from competition with their sexual ancestors. Conversely, specialized clones may be favoured if the asexual population must live and compete with closely related sexual ancestors (*e.g.* sperm-dependent parthenogens). Despite their ecological success, asexual lineages appear to be evolutionary dead ends. Mutational meltdown hastens the demise of individual clones, but some asexual taxa may persist through periodic additions or replacements of nuclear genomes and genes from extant sexual relatives. With few exceptions, molecular studies provide little evidence for ancient clonal lineages or diversified asexual taxa.

1. Introduction

To most biologists, sex equals mixis—the recombining of genes from discrete individuals. A variety of parasexual processes (transformation, transduction, and conjugation) mixes DNA among prokaryotic individuals. Sex, as practiced by multicellular eukaryotes, arose in single-celled protists, and has undergone little modification for perhaps a billion years. The basic sexual cycle involves two steps: meiosis (which produces haploid gametes) and syngamy (the fusion of gametes to restore diploid zygotes). The two steps may occur in rapid sequence (*e.g.* seed plants and animals in which diploid individuals constitute the dominant life stage), or the steps may be separated as distinct life stages (*e.g.* byrophytes, pteridophytes, and fungi in which haploids constitute the dominant life stage). Although various vegetative forms of reproduction (*e.g.* fission, budding, fragmentation, tillering, etc.) are relatively common among protists, fungi, plants, and acoelomate invertebrates, the vast majority of multicellular eukaryotic species (greater than 99%) reproduce sexually (Bell 1982). Some plants (*e.g.* strawberries and corals) may follow an episode of sex with many rounds of vegetative reproduction, and similarly many invertebrates (*e.g.* aphids, monogonont rotifers, and cladocerans) alternate between sexual and asexual phases during different times of the year. Periodic bouts of meiotic sex result in mixis, and thus, such organisms are facultatively asexual.

Despite the overwhelming evolutionary success of sexual species, obligately asexual lineages have arisen secondarily in most plant and animal phyla. Some facultatively asexual organisms (*e.g. Daphnia* and *Artemia*) occasionally produce obligately asexual lineages that completely suppress meiotic sex and enjoy great ecological success (Hebert & Crease 1983; Browne 1988; Moran 1992). Asexual lineages also arise spontaneously in many plant and animal phyla that are not facultatively asexual. For example, unisexual (*i.e.* all-female) vertebrates and many parthenogenetic insects arise as hybrids, and they often outnumber their sexual progenitors. Their ecological success notwithstanding, most biologists believe asexual species are evolutionary dead ends with limited potential for adaptation and diversification. On the tree-of-life, they comprise little more than a few twigs at the ends of branches that are fundamentally sexual (Maynard Smith 1978). Why are asexual species so unsuccessful in the long term? Are there exceptions—ancient clonal lineages? Can studies of these exceptions answer the question—why reproduce sexually— that has been called the "queen of problems in evolutionary biology" (Bell 1982)?

Current space prevents a comprehensive review of theories about the evolutionary costs and benefits of sex (reviewed by Williams 1975; Maynard Smith 1978; Bell 1982; Michod & Levin 1987). To remain consistent with the primary focus of this book, I discuss some molecular and experimental studies that pertain to theories about sex and cloning. My views are coloured by what I have learned from studying the genetics and evolution of sexual and asexual fish during the past 30 years. Very little of this work would have been possible without the use of allozyme, immunological, and DNA markers that allowed us to identify and distinguish among natural clones in the laboratory and the wild. I use these studies to illustrate how the application of genetic markers allows researchers to probe the morphological, physiological, behavioural and ecological characteristics of clones and thereby provide keys to the adaptive benefits of genotypic diversity and sex.

To understand mixis in eukaryotes, we must examine its combinatorial properties. In each generation, meiosis and syngamy produce an enormous variety of zygotes that face the world anew. Imagine a hypothetical fish (Fig. 1A) with a single pair of chromosomes. Segregation of the chromosomes during meiosis produces two types of gametes (or 2^n, where $n =1$ pair of chromosomes). If another species (Fig. 1B) has two pairs of chromosomes, Mendelian segregation assortment produces $2^2 = 4$ types of gametes; and so on. Consequently, a human, with 23 pairs of chromosomes, can produce 2^{23} or 8,388,608 kinds of gametes, but that is not all. If a cross over (*i.e.* reciprocal exchange between homologous chromosomes) occurs during meiosis, each chromosome pair will produce 4 types of gametes (Fig. 2). If each homologous pair of chromosomes has only one cross over per meiosis (the average is closer to two, Jagiello *et al.* 1976), the number of gametic combinations produced by a single meiotic event is 4^{23}, or 7×10^{13}. Consequently, fertilization of a such an egg with an equally unique sperm creates a zygote that is but one out of $(4^{23})^2$ possible kinds of zygotes, or one in 5×10^{27}. The uniqueness of this zygote is

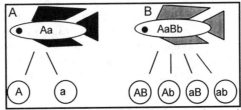

Figure 1: Chromosomal assortment in hypothetical fish with one and two pairs of chromosomes. The number of gametic combinations produced by meiosis is shown below each fish.

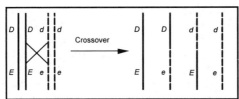

Figure 2: A single cross over between homologous chromosomes carrying the
genes *D* and *E* produces four distinct chromatids.

an underestimate, because we considered only a single meiotic event per parent. Cross overs occur at different positions during independent meiotic events, and give an entirely new set of combinations for the next zygote. In the population at large, we must also consider the number of permutations in which mates can be paired. These gross underestimates notwithstanding, the example clearly illustrates why each sexually produced offspring is unique genetically, with the exception of monozygotic twins. Individuality and diversity are quintessential to mixis.

2. Why have sex?

The previous example illustrates what mixis does, but it fails to explain for what and for whom genotypic diversity is good. The proposed beneficiaries of sex range from species to individuals, and to genes themselves. I consider several of these theories, as they relate to recent empirical studies.

2.1. Sex accelerates evolution

Weismann (1889) promoted the idea that sex provides the variation needed for Darwinian adaptation to changing environments. Fisher (1930) and Muller (1932) restated the hypothesis in genetic terms. If good mutations are rare (*e.g.* $\mu = 10^{-8}$), the probability of two good mutations arising simultaneously in the same asexual lineage is the vanishingly small ($\mu^2 = 10^{-16}$). If the mutations arise in different lineages they will be in competition, and the clone bearing a better mutation will sweep to fixation as the lesser mutation is lost. Both mutations can occur together in the same clone, if one mutation arises first and spreads to near fixation before the second mutation arises in the same lineage. By contrast, mutations occurring simultaneously in different sexual lineages can come together quickly by mixis as each good mutation spreads.

Although intuitively satisfying, this idea suffers fundamental problems. It may provide an adaptive advantage to sexual lineages, but it comes at great expense to individuals (see Why not Clone?). Sexual lineages will not spread at the expense of clones, unless individuals also gain an advantage that compensates for the costs of sex (Williams 1971). Furthermore, it remains unclear whether sex does accelerate adaptive evolution, because mixis also breaks up good gene combinations and may slow their rate of fixation (Eshel & Feldman 1970). Perhaps sex is good because it slows the fixation of narrow specializations that may be beneficial in the short-term but may increase the likelihood of extinction when environments inevitably change (Thompson 1976). Evolving rapidly does not necessarily guarantee evolutionary success. Some "living fossils" like *Limulus,* the horseshoe crab, and *Lingula*, an articulated brachiopod, have changed very little morphologically for hundreds of millions of years.

I know of few experimental studies that directly compare rates of molecular evolution and diversification among sexual and asexual clades (see Ancient Clones). Perhaps that is because we know of so few diversified asexual clades with which to make comparisons. There are reputed to be about 350 species of strictly asexual bdelloid rotifers, but the family is relatively conservative morphologically when compared to monogonont rotifers which are facultatively sexual. Morphological and molecular diversification are not necessarily coupled, however (see Hebert, this volume). For example, an early allozyme study showed that *Limulus polyphemus*, a phylogenetic relic, is essentially as polymorphic as humans, and humans have evolved very rapidly (Selander *et al.* 1971). Perhaps *Limulus* needs sex and genetic diversity just to stay in the same place (see Red Queen, section 2.5.), while humans rapidly exploited a new adaptive realm. Nevertheless, it is unclear if our recent evolutionary burst will guarantee long-term success.

2.2. Sex evades mutational meltdown

Muller (1964) suggested that asexual lineages have a high rate of extinction because slightly deleterious mutations accumulate like a "ratchet mechanism." An asexual population cannot reduce its mutational load below that of the "least loaded" clone. If this clone is lost by chance, the load increases one step, and cannot go back, except for extremely rare back mutations. In contrast, recombination produces offspring with higher and lower loads than the parents, and consequently purifying selection can maintain a low mutational load in a sexual lineage. Muller's ratchet works most effectively in organisms with many genes and a finite population size. Imagine a haploid clone with a genomic mutation rate of $U = 1.0$, one new deleterious mutation per gamete (probably a significant underestimate for vertebrates). Altogether 63% of its eggs (Poisson probability $= 1 - e^{-U}$) would have one or more mutations, and 37% (the "lucky" eggs) would be free of new mutations. Only 13.5% (e^{-2U}) of the eggs produced by a diploid clone would be so lucky, and 5% of a triploid, etc. Most new mutations have slightly deleterious effects even in the heterozygous condition (Simmons & Crow 1977). Although these percentages of lucky eggs may allow clones to escape the ratchet if they have infinitely large populations, the mutational load will ratchet upward in finite populations, as lucky clones are lost by chance (Haigh 1978). Consequently, bacteria with very few genes and effectively infinite population sizes may escape the ratchet, but multicellular eukaryotes with many more genes and finite populations would not be so lucky. Theoretical analyses suggest that "mutational meltdown" will debilitate such populations in 10,000 to 100,000 generations (Lynch *et al.* 1993).

Experimental evidence for mutational meltdown is found in all-female hybridogenetic fish of the genus *Poeciliopsis* (Leslie & Vrijenhoek 1978; 1980). The *P. monacha-lucida* biotype (*ML* for short) arose as an interspecific hybrid of *P. monacha* and *P. lucida*. It reproduces by hybridogenesis (Fig. 3), a process that discards the *L* genome during oogenesis, and transmits only the *M* genome to its ova (Schultz 1969). In nature, this fish mates with males of *P. lucida*, which restores the diploid *ML* complement in each generation. Different degrees of mutational accumulation characterized the distinct *M* genomes (hemiclones) found in *P. monacha-lucida* populations. The hemiclones were distinguished by allozymes and tissue grafting, but not morphology (Vrijenhoek *et al.* 1978; Angus & Schultz 1979). For the most part, these genetic differences were captured (*i.e.* "frozen") from the *P. monacha* gene pool during multiple hybridization events that created new *P. monacha-lucida* lineages.

Some of the hemiclones have persisted long enough to accumulate mutations. These mutations were revealed in the laboratory by artificially inseminating the *ML* strains with sperm from *P. monacha* males (Fig. 3). The presence of a single recessive lethal allele in one of these hemiclonal lineages should result in 50% zygotic mortality of the backcross progeny, compared to the controls. Two independently assorting lethals would cause 75% zygotic mortality; three would cause 88%; etc. Thereby, we estimated "lethal equivalent"

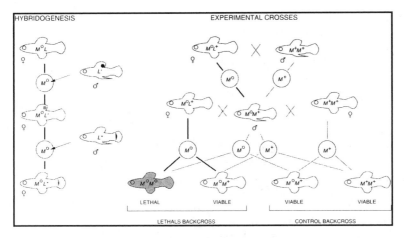

Figure 3: Hybridogenesis and experimental crosses to expose deleterious mutations. During hybridogenesis, only the maternal *M* genome is transmitted to eggs. The paternal genome (*L*) is incorporated; its traits are expressed in the hybrids, but the *L* genome is discarded during oogenesis. Different paternal traits (*e.g.* spots and bars) are substituted in each generation. In the experimental crosses, the *o* and + markers represent a lethal mutant and wild-type allele carried by *M* genomes. If the hemiclonal genome carries one lethal gene, 50% of the progeny of the first backcross will die.

loads of several hemiclonal genomes. Of fourteen hemiclonal strains tested, only two produced males that could be used in the experimental backcrosses. Embryonic mortality in one strain suggested it contained two lethal equivalent mutations, and the second strain probably contained a minimum of four. Of course, we could not exclude the possibility that more numerous semilethal mutations existed in these hemiclones.

Despite uncertainties about the actual number and severity of these mutations, we clearly exposed mutational loads in two hemiclonal strains. Information from other strains supported the hypothesis that these mutations had accumulated within the clonal lineages. Half of the fourteen hemiclonal strains failed to produce any viable M^oM^+ progeny. The M^o genomes of these strains were no longer genetically compatible with a wild-type M^+ genome. Dead and degenerating embryos were found in many of these viviparous females, suggesting the action of developmental lethals. Several hemiclones produced M^oM^+ progeny with significantly elevated postnatal mortality, and other hemiclones produced M^oM^+ progeny with gross developmental abnormalities (vertebral fusions, incomplete cranial caps, and fin creases, etc.). Although the mutations acted as recessives in the M^oL hybrid background, they behaved as dominant lethals and subvitals in the nonhybrid M^oM^+ background. Dominant deleterious mutations would be extremely rare in *P. monacha*, and thus were not likely to be captured during the origins of these hybridogenetic lineages.

Molecular evidence for such mutations exists in a relatively old hemiclonal lineage of *P. monacha-occidentalis*, a hybridogen that relies on *P. occidentalis* males for sperm (Quattro *et al.* 1992a). Hemiclone *MO*/Ia carries a silent allele, *Est-5ᵒ*, for the predominant liver esterase. Instead of expressing two allozymes, as in related *P. monacha-occidentalis* hemiclones, *MO*/Ia expresses only the *Est-5ᵃ* allozyme from *P. occidentalis* (Fig. 4). If crossed with *P. lucida*, the new *ML* hybrids express only the *lucida Est-5ᵈ* allele. Antibodies prepared against normal liver esterase were used in crossed-immunoelectrophoresis to reveal an enzymatically inactive *Est-5ᵒ* protein. We subsequently found a silent alcohol dehydrogenase (*Adh*) allele in a side branch to the *MO*/Ia lineage (Quattro *et al.* 1992a), and a silent lactate dehydrogenase (*Ldh-C*) allele in a

P. monacha-lucida lineage (Vrijenhoek 1984b). The existence of these silent alleles and other deleterious mutations suggests these hemiclones have not arisen recently. Unfortunately, these mutations provide a poor foundation for estimating the evolutionary ages of clones. Notwithstanding, claims for ancient asexual lineages should be accompanied with similar evidence for mutational meltdown (see Ancient Clones, below), unless these clonal organisms have developed extraordinary means for purging such mutations.

To date, these studies of *Poeciliopsis* provide some of the best empirical evidence for mutational meltdown in clonal animals. Independent evidence for similar mutations has been found in similar crosses involving the hybridogenetic frog, *Rana esculenta* (Graf & Polls-Pelaz 1989). Mutational loads also appear to accumulate rapidly in clones of the cyclical parthenogen *Daphnia obtusa* (Innes 1989) and in non-recombining *Drosophila* chromosomes (Rice 1994). Despite their small genome size, the high mutation rates found in some RNA viruses can result in rapid mutational meltdown (Chao 1990; Chao *et al.* 1992). Mitochondria also have very few genes and in some organisms (*e.g.* mammals) have an accelerated mutation rate. Since mtDNA is presumed to be clonal in most organisms, how does it avoid mutational meltdown? Lynch and Gabriel (1990) suggest that a less efficient DNA repair system, as occurs in mitochondria, may facilitate the purging of defective mtDNAs, and hence retard Muller's ratchet. Does less efficient mutation repair also retard the action of Muller's ratchet in the nuclear genomes of successful asexual lineages such as bdelloid rotifers? This fascinating question requires further investigation in corresponding sexual and asexual lineages.

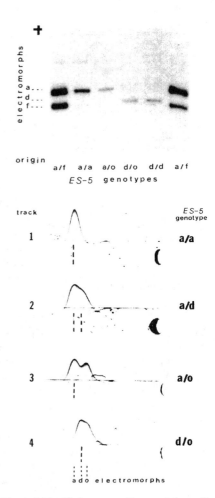

Figure 4: *Est-5⁰* phenotypes. Top panel, lanes: (1 and 6) the two-banded *a/f* genotype from the *P. monacha-occidentalis MO*/IIa strain; (lane 2) *a/a* from *P. occidentalis*; (lane 3) *a/o* from *MO*/Ia; (lane 4) *d/o* from progeny of *MO*/Ia x *P. lucida* male; (5) *d/d/* of the *P. lucida* male. Bottom panel: crossed immunoelectrophoretic patterns produced by each *Est-5⁰* genotype. The dashed line below each peak represents the position of the corresponding *Est-5⁰* electromorph in one-dimensional electrophoresis. From Spinella & Vrijenhoek (1982).

2.3. Sex repairs and rejuvenates damaged DNA

Bernstein *et al.* (1985, 1988) promoted the fascinating theory that mixis is needed to repair and rejuvenate DNA. In this case, DNA damage (double-strand breaks, cross-links, etc.) is distinguished from mutation (nucleotide substitutions). Many of the enzymes involved in repair of DNA are also involved in recombination. Redundancy of DNA (*e.g.* diploidy) provides a back-up copy that can serve as an undamaged template for the repair process. The proponents of this view argue that genotypic diversity is a byproduct of the recombination-repair process, although they may agree that this diversity also provides collateral benefits.

The recombination-repair hypothesis may help to explain the origin of bacterial and eukaryotic sex. Perhaps multicellular eukaryotes are simply stuck with premeiotic repair processes needed to maintain the viability and functionality of DNA, despite the costs of sex. There is merit in this argument, because very few obligately asexual plants and animals are strictly vegetative (mitotic, or agametic parthenogens). Most obligate parthenogens retain aspects of premeiotic chromosome processing during seed or egg production. Are these steps required to repair damaged DNA and restore developmental totipotency? Or is egg production maintained because these organisms need seeds, embryonated eggs, or larvae to disperse? How fast do agametic genomes decay from unrepaired DNA damage? Can plants, which have no discrete germ-cell lines, purge DNA damage with cell deaths during somatic growth (apoptosis). Do animals that have germ-cell lines require premeiotic recombination-repair? What about sponges and coelenterates—do they function developmentally and evolutionarily more like plants or animals? How do rates of molecular evolution differ in organisms with and without discrete germ-cell lines? Is sidereal time or generation time the proper denominator for evolutionary rates in these organisms (see Li 1997 for an edifying discussion of hypotheses regarding molecular rate heterogeneity)? Michod (1995) champions the recombination-repair hypothesis as a general explanation for the origin and maintenance of meiotic sex, and although diligently argued, his book provides little guidance for researchers interested in pursuing this fascinating idea. Comprehensive comparisons of nucleotide substitution rates in closely related gametic vs. agametic lineages are warranted. I suspect that attempts to address the questions posed above will provide considerable fodder for students interested in molecular studies of sexual and asexual organisms.

2.4. Genetic diversity is good in heterogeneous environments

That sex and genotypic diversity may increase the ecological efficiency of species living in heterogeneous environments is an old idea (Weissman 1889; Ghiselin 1974). Although this represents a potential advantage to sexual species, the basic idea was restated by Williams and Mitton (1973) who saw benefits for individuals if diversity decreases competition among the offspring of a single parent. The sib-competition hypothesis was explored by Bell (1982) in his Tangled Bank model, which is essentially similar to the Frozen Niche-Variation (FNV) model, I had developed several years earlier (Vrijenhoek 1979, 1984a). The purpose of the FNV model was to explain the coexistence of multiple clones and their sexual progenitors. Clones are viewed as multi-locus genotypes that were "frozen" from the sexual gene pool. Selection acts on new clones and favors genotypes that minimally overlap the niches of established clones and the sexual progenitors. This produces a diverse assemblage of clones that can coexist with the sexual progenitors, as long as clones do not arise too frequently and completely eclipse the sexual niche (Case & Taper 1986; Weeks 1993).

Studies of niche differences among clones and their sexual relatives provide evidence that genotypic diversity increases ecological efficiency. If individual clones are assumed to have narrower niches than the sexual progenitors, then the FNV model predicts that: (1) a single clone should have limited competitive impact on a variable sexual population (competition is asymmetrical); and (2) a diverse array of specialized clones could eclipse the sexual niche and competitively displace the progenitors. I tested these predictions

(Vrijenhoek 1979) following allozyme and immunological studies that revealed differences in clonal diversity among hybridogenetic populations of *Poeciliopsis* (Angus & Schultz 1979; Angus 1980). The fish populations in some rivers contain a single hemiclone and other rivers contain multiple clones. As predicted, in monoclonal populations the hybridogens comprised only a small fraction (1 to 10%) of the total fish, and provided evidence for asymmetrical competition favoring the sexuals. In contrast, in multiclonal populations the hybridogens were numerically dominant (> 60% of the fish) and they displaced the sexual females from both the mainstream and peripheral stillwater habitats (Vrijenhoek 1979, 1984b). Evidence for asymmetrical competition between individual clones and their sexual counterparts has also been found in lizards and frogs (Case 1990; Semlitsch 1993). Compelling evidence for the competitive superiority of sexual reproducers occurs in lizards (Petren *et al.* 1993). A single gecko clone dominated most south Pacific islands until recently, when a sexual species invaded many islands and competitively displaced the clone. A frozen genotype and niche may be risky when faced with novel sexual invaders.

The FNV model assumes that ecologically relevant phenotypic differences among clones can be frozen from the sexual gene pool. We tested this directly by synthesizing new *Poeciliopsis* clones in the laboratory. Considerable differences in life history traits, behaviour, and morphology existed among more than a dozen synthetic clones (Wetherington *et al.* 1989; Lima 1998). These differences typically encompassed the range of variation observed among natural clones, and thus mutational divergence among clones need not be invoked. How ironic that the success of these all-female fish derives from variation stored in genetically diverse sexual progenitors!

2.5. The Red Queen and a world full of parasites

Phenotypic differences among individuals may be required for species locked into coevolutionary struggles with rapidly evolving biological enemies, particularly microparasites that evolve to exploit the most common host phenotype. This hypothesis is named after the Red Queen in Lewis Carroll's *Through the Looking Glass*, who claimed that "it takes all the running you can do, to keep in the same place" (Van Valen 1973; Bell 1982). Genetic diversity is needed to keep up in the never-ending race with parasites, because rare phenotypes may escape infection and gain a temporary advantage, until they rise in abundance and become the focus of coevolving parasites. This cycle of frequency-dependent fitness preserves genetic diversity in the host and favors the maintenance of sex (Hamilton *et al.* 1981).

Studies of clonally reproducing animals support the Red Queen model. Sexually reproducing *Potamopyrgus* snails appear to be favoured over asexual lineages at localities where helminth parasite infections are more intense (Lively 1987). Applications of allozyme markers to these New Zealand snail populations provided evidence for a rare-clone advantage and time-lagged natural selection, consistent with expectations of the Red Queen model (Dybdahl & Lively 1998). Lively *et al.*(1990) also found evidence for frequency-dependent parasite loads in *Poeciliopsis*. A sexual species living with the fish clones, *P. monacha*, typically had the lowest parasite load and almost twice the variance in parasite load, which is expected if genotypic diversity contributes to variance in susceptibility. An exception to this pattern was found after a local extinction-recolonization event eliminated most variation in a partially isolated *P. monacha* population. The genetically depauperate "founder" population exhibited many signs of inbreeding depression, and the sexual females had a higher parasite load than females of the locally abundant clone. However, restoration of genetic diversity in the founder population was associated with a dramatic drop in the parasite load of the sexuals, while the clone was unaffected. Dealing with this parasite is facilitated by variance in immune response that results from recombinational diversity.

Many biologists now believe the Red Queen model provides one of the most powerful ecological explanations for the maintenance of sex in higher organisms. Several studies have shown that clonal organisms tend to have higher parasite loads than their sexual counterparts, and vice versa (see also, Moritz *et al.* 1991; Ebert 1994; Hanley *et al.* 1995). The Red Queen resembles the Fisher-Muller hypothesis, except that fitness is frequency-dependent in the Red Queen. Rapid decoupling and recoupling of genes involved in disease response appear to be required for the persistence of stable limit cycles between hosts and parasites (Seger & Hamilton 1988).

2.6. Sex arose as an infectious process

Generally, the previous ideas may serve to explain the maintenance of meiotic sex in eukaryotes. The DNA repair hypothesis may also explain its origin if we consider the possibility that recombination arose as a byproduct of DNA repair processes. Nevertheless, parasexual recombinant processes first appeared in prokaryotes. Levin (1987) favors the idea that sex arose as a consequence of purely selfish infectious particles in bacteria. Conjugation and transduction require plasmids and viruses, respectively, to conduct the transfer of genes. It seems difficult to believe, however, that the incorporation of these selfish entities maintains sex in multicellular eukaryotes. Mixis does appear to facilitate the spread of selfish elements (*e.g.* transposons) (Hickey 1982; Hickey & Rose 1987). We occasionally need to be reminded that the physical contact and transfer of fluids between individuals engaged in sex also facilitates the transmission of many infectious agents. Although I doubt our complex sexual behaviour is manipulated by viruses like HIV, it is clear that sex is a double-edged sword. Wouldn't it be curious if the Red Queen turns out to be the simultaneous cause and solution to her own problem! I suspect theories about potential relationships between disease, selfish DNA, and mixis will remain a fertile area for theoretical investigations for many years to come. It is more difficult, however, to see how experiments might be designed to dissect this complicated and ancient cycle. As soon as the primordial soup produced self-replicating and information-bearing molecules, it would surely have produced selfish replicators that could parasitize the process.

3. Why not clone?

Cloning is an efficient mode of reproduction that avoids the costs of sex (reviewed by Lloyd 1988). Clones can faithfully replicate "good" genotypes and avoid the "cost of meiosis" by transmitting 100% of their genes to progeny, rather than the 50% of the genes as in sexual individuals (Williams 1971). All-female (*i.e.* uniparental) species do not pay the "cost of males" (a twofold cost in dioecious species, Maynard Smith 1971) or accept the risks and physiological costs associated with attracting and securing a mate. All-female species have "reproductive assurance," a significant advantage when establishing new colonies, especially when males are rare (Baker 1965). Uniparental reproduction will minimally provide a twofold demographic advantage over sexual females that allocate half their reproductive potential to the production of males. Colonizing parthenogens also have "heterozygosity assurance" (Vrijenhoek 1985), because cloning protects against inbreeding depression associated with severe population bottlenecks and founder events. So why aren't clones more abundant, especially in taxa that are capable of spawning asexual lineages? Perhaps a look at the conditions that favor clones will shed some light on this problem.

3.1. Geographical parthenogenesis, fugitive species, and colonization abilities

It has long been recognized that asexual taxa are more frequent at extreme latitudes, higher altitudes, the margins of a species range, on islands, and in disturbed (e.g. disclimax) communities (Vandel 1928). Several hypotheses attempt to explain this biogeographical pattern commonly known as "geographical parthenogenesis." Vandel and others suggested that parthenogenetic populations expanded more rapidly in the northern latitudes following retreat of the Pleistocene glaciers. Parthenogens should be better colonizers than sexual females because they have reproductive assurance, heterozygosity assurance, and all-female reproduction. At low population densities, they should have at least a twofold advantage over sexual colonists.

Other researchers have argued that parthenogenetic lineages may be inferior competitors in central parts of a species' range where higher species diversity would increase biotic interactions (Glesener & Tilman 1978). Parthenogens are believed to fare better under conditions of low biotic diversity. The proponents of this idea see parthenogens as "fugitives" that escape direct competition with sexual counterparts by favoring ecologically marginal habitats (Wright & Lowe 1968; Moore 1984). Lynch (1984) suggested that "destabilizing hybridization" may prevent some parthenogens from coexisting with their sexual counterparts For example, some parthenogenetic *Cnemidophorus* lizards may be mounted and inseminated by males of a related sexual species. If the eggs of an allotriploid parthenogen *AAB* (the letters represent haploid chromosome sets from sexual progenitors *A* and *B*) are fertilized as a consequence of mating with species *B* and the resulting tetraploid progeny (*AABB*) have a balanced chromosome set, normal meiosis may ensue. Thus, regular matings by sexual males may destabilize an asexual lineage and lead to its local demise.

Unlike true parthenogens, the colonization abilities of sperm-dependent parthenogens is more limited (reviewed by Beukeboom & Vrijenhoek 1998). Apomictic plants and parthenogenetic animals that rely on pollen or sperm to stimulate embryonic development are forced to coexist with a sexually reproducing host. Outcompeting or escaping the host will lead to reproductive failure and extinction. Consequently, hybridogenetic and gynogenetic forms of *Poeciliopsis* have limited distributions encompassed within the ranges of their sexual hosts. In contrast, some true parthenogens have an immense distributions mostly outside the range of their sexual progenitors (e.g. the cockroach *Pycnoscelus surinamensis* and the gecko *Heteronotia binoei*, Parker *et al.* 1977; Moritz 1991).

3.2. General-purpose genotypes

Baker (1965) suggested that many apomictic plants (particularly polyploids and hybrids) have "general-purpose genotypes" and enjoy wider ecological tolerances than their sexual counterparts. He believed that phenotypic plasticity enhanced their abilities to exploit marginal environments. Selection in a varying environment should favor adaptively plastic (general-purpose) clones that fluctuate the least in fitness, because such clones will suffer smaller losses when conditions are poor and should replace specialized clones with more limited tolerance (Lynch 1984). The wide geographical distribution of many asexual plants and animals is cited as support for the General-Purpose Genotype (GPG) hypothesis (Parker *et al.* 1977; Bierzychudek 1985). Molecular markers are needed to test the GPG hypothesis, however, because a widespread asexual taxon may be composed of a single broadly tolerant and phenotypically plastic clone (a general-purpose genotype) or numerous specialized clones with different environmental tolerances, as in the Frozen Niche Variation model (below). Even with adequate genetic markers, the discovery of a widely distributed clone does not by itself provide sufficient evidence for a general-purpose genotype. The clone might occupy a narrow but universally available niche. Some wide-spread apomictic dandelions and parthenogenetic cockroaches depend on human transport and habitat disruption, nowadays a cosmopolitan and abundant niche. This can hardly be taken as evidence that these organisms have general-purpose genotypes.

Nevertheless, the gynogenetic minnow *Phoxinus eos-neogaeus* (Cyprinidae) may have a general-purpose genotype. Allozymes and DNA fingerprints identified a single wide-spread clone in northern Minnesota (Elder & Schlosser 1995). Schlosser and coworkers (1997) compared the ecological and physiological characteristics of this clone with those of its sexual progenitors, *P. eos* and *P. neogaeus*. All the minnows preferred highly oxygenated upland ponds, but the clone was far more abundant in ponds and streams with lower oxygen content. The temporal and spatial unpredictability of the marginal pool and stream environments is believed to favor a general-purpose genotype with a broad intermediate niche. It will be interesting to see if this example withstands further comparative tests involving additional physiological and environmental factors (*cf.* Vrijenhoek 1998).

3.3. Frozen Niche-Variation

When sexual organisms colonize a peripheral habitat or island with low species diversity, they may experience a release from intense interspecific competition. Such "ecological releases" are often associated with phenotypic diversification and niche expansion. Over the short-term, however, recombination acts antagonistically with respect to diversifying selection and retards the stabilization of multimodal phenotypic distributions (Felsenstein 1981). Faithful assortative mating systems, selfing, and limited dispersal may be ways to defeat "antagonistic recombination" (Maynard Smith 1962; Antonovics 1968) and foster diversification. Such processes may have driven diversification of cichlid fishes in African Great Lakes and the polytypic Arctic Charr of Iceland (Vrijenhoek *et al.* 1987). On the other hand, cloning is a highly efficient mechanism for "freezing" ecologically divergent genotypes that can fully exploit an multi-niche environment (Roughgarden 1972). During the past 30 years, my colleagues and I have been investigating frozen phenotypic variation in viviparous topminnows of the genus *Poeciliopsis* (Pisces: Poeciliidae). These small fish live in the desert springs and streams of northwestern Mexico. We have identified numerous differences among clones in food use, predatory efficiency, habitat preference, swimming behaviour, aggressiveness, physiological tolerances, etc. (Schenck & Vrijenhoek 1989; Schultz & Fielding 1989; Weeks *et al.* 1992; Vrijenhoek & Pfeiler 1997).

Ecological-genetic studies of other clonally diverse asexual taxa (*e.g.* lizards, frogs, snails, moths, isopods, brine shrimp, cladocerans, and earthworms) provide abundant evidence for ecological differences among coexisting clones (Hebert 1974; Christensen 1980; Blackman 1981; Futuyma *et al.* 1984; Weider & Hebert 1987; Christensen *et al.* 1988; Browne & Hoopes 1990; Case 1990; Weider 1993; Jokela *et al.* 1997; Semlitsch *et al.* 1997). However, clonal differentiation is not always apparent, if it exists at all (*e.g.* Jaenike *et al.* 1980). Comprehensive ecological-genetic studies require multi-locus genetic markers to confidently identify natural clones and to mark individuals for experimental studies in the field and laboratory. To date, most studies have relied on protein electrophoresis, but allozymes are sometimes too invariant to distinguish among clones. Undetected (*i.e.* cryptic) clonal diversity within composite allozyme genotypes must be considered. For example, tissue grafting studies revealed cryptic variation within several electrophoretically defined clones of *Poeciliopsis* (Moore 1977; Angus & Schultz 1979). However, tissue grafting studies are labor intensive and likely to be conducted in the laboratory, which narrows opportunities to elucidate genotype-by-environment associations. Mitochondrial DNA studies have also revealed cryptic *Poeciliopsis* clones bearing the same composite allozyme genotype, and vice versa (Quattro *et al.* 1991, 1992b). However, the combination of allozyme and mtDNA markers provides a very powerful tool for studying the origin, evolution, and diversity of clonal lineages (Avise *et al.* 1992). Allozymes and DNA fingerprinting have been used together to identify clones of *Phoxinus* minnows (Elder & Schlosser 1995). DNA fingerprints were highly effective at identifying cryptic clones of the self-fertilizing hermaphroditic fish *Rivulus marmoratus* within a single allozyme type (Turner *et al.* 1992). Allozymes, mtDNA, and microsatellite markers have been applied to a bewildering array of sexual and asexual minnows in Iberia that are just beginning to reveal their origins and patterns of clonal diversity (Alves *et al.* 1995, 1997; Carmona *et al.* 1997). Microsatellites have also been used to study the evolution of breeding systems and genetic structure in aphids (Sunnucks *et al.* 1996, 1997). RAPDs may prove to be an effective way to identify plant clones (*e.g.* Huff *et al.* 1993) and they work with aphids (Martínez-Torres *et al.* 1997). Once appropriate genotypic markers are available, it is possible to study the environmental relationships of clonal genotypes. This presupposes that careful ecological studies will be conducted in tandem.

4. Ancient clones?

Although some asexual taxa may flourish ecologically, biologists have long considered them "evolutionary dead ends" with limited potential for adaptation and diversification (Maynard-Smith 1978; White 1978). Consequently, the existence of some putatively ancient asexual taxa represents a "scandal" that contradicts most theories about the adaptive value of sex (Maynard-Smith 1986, 1992; Judson & Normark 1996). Most evidence for ancient clones is weak, however (Little & Hebert 1996). The ostracod family Darwinulidae includes almost 30 species that are presumed to be strictly asexual, including fossil deposits dated at 70 MY or greater (Butlin & Griffiths 1993), but periodic sex probably exists, as rare males are found (cited in Little & Hebert 1996). A careful analysis of molecular diversification in this group is warranted, but even molecular studies are fraught with troublesome assumptions that may lead to misinterpretations about the evolutionary ages of clones. For example, the rate of molecular evolution in Darwinulid ostracods appears to be slow compared with sexual counterparts (Schön *et al.* 1998).

The assumption of equal nucleotide substitution rates in sexual and asexual lineages needs to be tested in each new case study, because accelerated rates may be expected under some circumstances. For example, the obligately asexual brine shrimp *Artemia partheno-genetica* exhibits a high degree of allozyme and mtDNA diversity that corresponds with extensive life-history variation among clones living in species-depauperate salinas of the Mediterranean Basin (Browne & Bowen 1990; Browne 1992; Perez *et al.* 1994). No sexual relatives are known that might have contributed to this allozyme and mtDNA diversity. Taken alone, the mtDNA evidence suggests that diversification arose in a monophyletic clonal lineage that may be 30 MY old. However, allozyme data reported by Browne & Hoopes (1990) for the diploid population at Salin de Giraud in France are consistent with ameiotic recombination. Furthermore, strong selection for salinity tolerance may have accelerated nucleotide substitution rates in these organisms (Hebert, this volume). Molecular substitution rates may vary greatly within and between sexual and asexual lineages, due to their differences in their genetically effective population sizes. A good new mutation will sweep through an asexual population and other variants (neutral and slightly deleterious) will hitchhike along to fixation, because all genes (nuclear and cytoplasmic) are effectively linked in a clone. Because selective sweeps are equivalent to a severe reduction in the effective size of an asexual population, this may result in higher than expected substitution rates of slightly-deleterious substitutions (Ohta 1992;

Charlesworth *et al.* 1993). Mixis decouples good and bad genes and may therefore slow substitution rates.

The diverse family of bdelloid rotifers is believed to be strictly asexual and at least 35 million years (MY) old, based on fossils preserved in amber (Poinar, 1992). Although males have never been seen, it is difficult to rule out cryptic or "covert sex" (Hurst *et al.* 1992) in these organisms. Molecular evidence for ancient bdelloids was first reported by D. Welch & M. Meselson (symposium: "Evolution of Sex" sponsored by the American Genetic Association at Virginia Polytechnic Institute and State University, Blacksburg, Virginia, July 10-11, 1992). They reported highly divergent (and presumably homologous) alleles at a diploid nuclear locus in the bdelloid *Philodina roseola*. In theory, homologous (nonrecombining) alleles should diverge over time and the degree of divergence will reflect clonal age (Birky 1996). However, the present studies of bdelloids can not exclude the possibility that the divergent alleles were of hybrid origin (*i.e.* divergence occurred prior to clone formation). Also, the discovery of three distinct copies of at least one gene in *Philodina roseola* suggests this divergence may represent duplicated gene loci rather than homologous alleles (D. Welch, pers. comm.). Nevertheless, comparative studies of these genes in monogonont rotifers, which are facultatively asexual, have not identified similar duplication or degrees of divergence. The present phylogenetic data on bdelloids are consistent with ancient asexuality, but more work is needed, particularly population genetic studies that look for linkage disequilibrium (an expectation of cloning).

Claims for other putatively ancient asexuals have been contested (Judson & Normark 1996; Little & Hebert 1996). In many cases a cryptic sexual phase was eventually discovered. If the sexual progenitors of an asexual taxon are extinct, or perhaps rare and unsampled, researchers might unknowingly assume the asexuals comprise a monophyletic group. However, clonal diversification may be a consequence of recently frozen variation, and the wrong conclusions will be obtained regarding the age of an asexual taxon. In other cases, putatively asexual organisms may engage in sneaky forms of mixis. For example, mtDNA diversification suggested that a gynogenetic salamander lineage (*Ambystoma*) was 5–6 MY old (Hedges *et al.* 1992; Spolsky *et al.* 1992). However, combined allozyme and mtDNA studies revealed the nuclear genomes of these triploid salamanders may occasionally be replaced by new genomes from the sexual population (Kraus & Miyamoto 1990). Nuclear replacements, losses, and gains are well documented in diploid/triploid complexes of unisexual vertebrates (Schultz & Kallman 1968; Cimino & Schultz 1970; Bogart & Licht 1986; Bogart 1989; Kraus 1989; Goddard & Dawley 1990; Vinogradov *et al.* 1990; Goddard & Schultz 1993; Alves *et al.* 1998). Other cryptic forms of mixis involving transfers of subgenomic amounts of DNA (*e.g.* supernumerary chromosomes) have been described in sperm-dependent unisexual vertebrates (Schartl *et al.* 1995).

Hybridogenetic organisms like *Poeciliopsis monacha-lucida*, *P. monacha-occidentalis*, and *Rana esculenta* are ultimate examples of nuclear replacement. They substitute a new paternal genome from a sexual population in each generation. Although their hemiclonal genomes may deteriorate, genetic lesions are sheltered by the substitutable paternal genome. Sheltered, non-recombinant, genomes like these should rapidly accumulate nonfunctional genes (Nei 1970; Rice 1994), as found in hybridogenetic *Poeciliopsis* and *Rana* (discussed above). Analysis of mtDNA variation in a monophyletic *P. monacha-occidentalis* lineage suggested its *M* genome has persisted for perhaps 100,000 years (Quattro *et al.* 1992a). Maynard Smith (1992) quipped this is "but an evening gone," but it is enough time for mutational meltdown, according to the simulations of Lynch & Gabriel (1990). Although short on a geological time scale, 100,000 years is mutationally ancient for a clonal lineage. We have no evidence based on allozymes or mtDNA for leakage of paternal genes into these hemiclonal lineages (Avise *et al.* 1992), but tests with other molecular markers are needed.

The permanent association of divergent nuclear genomes in unisexual organisms of hybrid origin creates opportunities to study concerted evolution. Turner (1982) asked "do the selfish sequences of one of the parental species 'take over' the genome?" The answer appears to be yes for nuclear ribosomal RNAs. Several clones of the parthenogenetic lizard *Heteronotia binoei* express only the rRNA pattern of one of the two sexual progenitors, a possible consequence of biased gene conversion (Hillis *et al.* 1991). Various mechanisms of concerted evolution may quickly drive such multi-copy genes to uniformity following the hybrid origins of clones. With the plethora of molecular tools available to biologists, we can now embark on an exciting era of evolutionary research—the detailed molecular dissection of asexual genomes.

5. Summary and conclusions

The NATO Advanced Studies Institute generated many animated discussions about the evolution of sex. I offer a general summary that is based in part on these discussions. It owes its organization to an excellent overview presented and prepared by Africa Gomez and Jean-Christophe Simon. Six main questions were posed.

5.1. Are theories on the maintenance of sex meaningful, testable, and mutually exclusive?

I have presented some of the major theories above. Clearly several theories may have more to do with the origins of sex in prokaryotes and single-celled eukaryotes, and other theories with its maintenance in multicellular eukaryotes. Bacterial sex probably arose as a purely selfish process involving infectious nucleic acids and viruses. Similarly the complex and highly conserved machinery of eukaryotic meiosis may have arisen as a way to facilitate the repair of damaged DNA and maintain the immortality of cell lineages. Once anisogamous gametes and two discrete sexes arose, the cost of sex is primarily contained in the cost of producing males. Perhaps sperm and males arose as ways to parasitize the developmental investment of individuals that produce larger gametes (eggs). Nevertheless, males aren't maintained for that reason, because they are easy enough to eliminate, as is evident in the many forms of uniparental inheritance found in essentially all plant and animal phyla. Sexual mixis may be maintained because it is essential for the repair of damaged DNA and restoration of totipotent development, but it remains to be shown that strictly ameiotic reproduction leads to rapid genomic and developmental deterioration. Substantial theoretical and empirical evidence suggests that mutational meltdown is a problem for strictly asexual lineages. Nevertheless, the rate of meltdown is slow and probably not sufficient to compensate for the twofold demographic cost of males. Both the Red Queen and Tangled Bank models provide some short-term benefits for genotypic diversity that may compensate for the cost of sex, but a clear twofold benefit of sex remains to be demonstrated on time scales relevant to the demographic advantages of uniparental reproduction (Lively & Lloyd 1990). Clearly, in thinking about the evolution of sex, we must separate theories that try to explain its origin from those that attempt to reconcile its maintenance. Many of the models are not mutually exclusive, however. For example, the Tangled Bank and Red Queen models both deal with environmental heterogeneity, but they differ concerning its spatial versus temporal aspects. Both models have underlying frequency- and density-dependent foundations. The key to future research will be to find experimental organisms in which these elements can be disassociated and tested independently. Perhaps protists still retain sufficient diversity in many aspects of mixis to serve as models for such studies.

5.2. How do asexual lineages arise?

Meiotic sex is the ancestral condition for multicellular eukaryotes. Asexuality arises when mictic processes (meiosis and syngamy) are circumvented by somatic reproduction or disrupted during gametogenesis. The variety of cytogenetic mechanisms associated with gametic asexuality are too numerous to cover herein; readers should refer to White (1978), Bell (1982), and Suomalainen et al. (1987). The switch to asexuality in cyclically parthenogenetic organisms occurs regularly in their life cycle and it is reversible under normal circumstances. However, several mechanisms are responsible for the switch to obligate parthenogenesis. Genes that suppress meiosis are found in Daphnia and factors that alter responsiveness to sex-inducing environmental conditions are found in some cyclically parthenogenetic aphids (Hebert 1981; Moran 1992; Hales et al. 1997). For many animals, a small proportion of unfertilized eggs develop spontaneously into zygotes (tychoparthenogenesis), providing opportunities to select for parthenogenesis in the laboratory and wild (Templeton 1982). Infection by symbiotic microorganisms such as Wolbachia suppresses sex in some insects (Stouthamer et al. 1993). Asexuality in the vertebrates and in many insects is associated with hybridization and polyploidy (Schultz 1969; White 1978; Vrijenhoek 1989, 1998). Hybridization can disrupt meiosis and create opportunities for the selection of amictic processes that rescue egg production. Polyploidization may play a similar role, although polyploidy probably arises secondarily in most asexual taxa. An exciting area of research with molecular tools would be to determine whether factors known to stimulate amictic reproduction are encoded by a few genes or genome wide chromosomal interactions.

5.3. Are most clones specialized, or do multipurpose genotypes exist?

Selection in a temporally fluctuating environment should favor the clone with the least variance in fitness, the general-purpose genotype (Lynch 1984). Selection in a spatially heterogeneous (but temporally stable) environment should favor clones that most efficiently use portions of an underexploited niche, i.e. Frozen Niche-Variation. However, the models are not mutually exclusive, as it is possible to envision selection for clones with broad physiological tolerances and yet narrow niches (examples in Vrijenhoek & Pfeiler 1997; Vrijenhoek 1998). If clonal formation from sexual progenitors is frequent, selection for general-purpose clones will be swamped by new diversity. Even if specialized clones have a high probability of extinction, new specialists can be frozen from the sexual progenitors. If clonal origins are rare, however, or if clones have escaped from the range of the progenitors, mutations will be the only source of adaptive variation. Selection may favor general-purpose clones over specialists, in the absence of strong interclonal and interspecific selection. Also, sperm-dependent parthenogens (pseudogamous apomicts, gynogens and hybridogens) are forced to coexist with a suitable sexual host species that provides sperm. The evolution of a superclone is prevented by sperm dependence, because a superclone would outcompete its host and thereby cause its own demise. Similarly, too many specialized clones can eclipse the sexual niche and lead to local extinction of sexual progenitors that rapidly generate new clones. Consequently, selection should favor sexual lineages that are resistant to the production of clonal derivatives (Nunney 1989). Maybe that is why asexual species are so rare.

5.4. Do truly ancient asexual lineages really exist?

This remains an open question, although the burden of proof should be on those who claim the existence of ancient ameiotic clones of multicellular eukaryotes. Most evidence for ancient clones is based on weak inference rather than direct demonstration of genetically diverse, monophyletic asexual clades. However, the bdelloid rotifers remain an interesting enigma. If ancient asexual clades are convincingly demonstrated, we need to ask how they repair DNA damage and escape from Muller's ratchet. Perhaps they escape the ratchet because they do not repair mutations and DNA damage (*e.g.* Lynch & Gabriel 1990), or because their populations are cosmopolitan and effectively infinite, or because they can form dormant cysts that serve as a "seed bank." Nevertheless, the persistence of premeiotic chromosome processing in most asexually reproducing, multicellular eukaryotes (including bdelloids) suggests that covert sexual processes (*e.g.* gene conversion) may be essential for long-term persistence.

5.5. How do asexual taxa persist?

To date, the majority of asexual taxa that have been subjected to molecular analyses are clonally diverse and of recent origin. Perhaps many of these taxa persist in a dynamic equilibrium between clonal formation and extinction. If so, the survival of these taxa requires the persistence of sexual progenitors that can spawn new clones. If clones are too successful, however, the progenitors may be competitively eliminated (Weeks 1993), which also eliminates opportunities for clonal turn-over. Many successful asexual taxa benefit from genotypes that were recently frozen from the sexual gene pool (Vrijenhoek 1979). A little bit of sex may be the best thing for asexual taxa, as is seen in aphids and Daphnia where obligate parthenogens still produce males that exchange genes with the sexual pool (Hebert 1981; Simon *et al.* 1996). Nevertheless, this argument may fail to explain the persistence and diversification of bdelloid rotifers. What mechanisms do they have to help them escape the wrath of DNA damage and Muller's ratchet?

5.6. Can asexual organisms recover sex once it is lost?

Apparently some can. Asexually reproducing plants (*e.g.* allotriploids, AAB) may revert to sex through additional hybridization and balancing of heterologous chromosome sets (*e.g.* allotetraploid, AABB) (Stebbins 1971; Grant 1981). Asexuality in cynipid gall wasps is mediated through the bacterial symbiont *Wolbachia* (Stouthamer *et al.* 1993). Treatment with antibiotics can cure the wasp lineage and result in reversion to biparental sex. Perhaps for different reasons, such cures also happen in nature. Hybridogenetic organisms have a unique way to regenerate mixis. The frog *Rana esculenta* (*RL*) produces hybridogenetic males and females that transmit only the *R* genome to gametes. Mating an *RL* male with an *RL* female produces *RR* progeny that are sexual and resemble the progenitor *R. ridibunda* (Graf & Polls-Pelaz 1989). A similar process is suspected in Iberian cyprinid fish (Alves *et al.* 1998). Although we have no evidence for this process in hybridogenetic *Poeciliopsis*, a different possibility exists. If a *P. monacha-lucida* female mates with a male of *P. monacha*, they produce a *monacha*-like fish with normal meiosis (Vrijenhoek & Schultz 1974; Leslie & Vrijenhoek 1978). A more deviant process apparently gave rise to a new sexual species of *Poeciliopsis* (Vrijenhoek 1989). Hybridogenesis apparently broke down spontaneously in a *P. monacha-occidentalis* lineage and produced a new species with a mosaic genome. Asexuality is probably a dead-end most of the time, but in these rare instances, it also leads to novelty. Schultz (1969) suggested that asexual animals were evolutionary experiments, mostly doomed to failure, but a few novel genotypic combinations might spread and eventually revert to sex. It is instructive, however, that the novelties we see are sexual. Mixis seems to be at the root of evolutionary novelty.

Acknowledgments

I thank the participants in the NATO Advanced Studies Institute, particularly Paul Hebert, Jeff Mitton, and Graham Stone for their energetic discussions. I am indebted to Africa Gomez and Jean-Christophe Simon for their outline of issues regarding the evolution and maintenance of sex, and Curt Lively for helpful suggestions regarding the manuscript. Also, I thank David Welch, William Birky, and Robert Browne for insightful comments regarding putatively ancient asexual organisms.

References

Alves MJ, Coelho MM, Collares-Pereira MJ (1995) The *Rutilus alburnoides* complex (Cyprinidae): evidence for a hybrid origin. *Journal of Zoological Systematic Evolution Research,* **35,** 1-10.

Alves MJ, Coelho MM, Collares-Pereira MJ (1998) Diversity in the reproductive modes of females of the *Rutilus alburnoides* complex (Teleostei, Cyprinidae): a way to avoid the genetic constraints of uniparentalism. *Molecular Biology and Evolution,* in press.

Alves MJ, Coelho MM, Collares-Pereira MJ, Dowling TE (1997) Maternal ancestry of the *Rutilus alburnoides* complex (Teleostei, Cyprinidae) as determined by analysis of cytochrome b sequences. *Evolution,* **51,** 1584-1592.

Angus RA (1980) Geographical dispersal and clonal diversity in unisexual fish populations. *American Naturalist,* **115,** 531-550.

Angus RA, Schultz RJ (1979) Clonal diversity in the unisexual fish *Poeciliopsis monacha-lucida*: a tissue graft analysis. *Evolution,* **33,** 27-40.

Antonovics J (1968) Evolution in closely adjacent plant populations, V. Evolution of self fertility. *Heredity,* **23,** 219-238.

Avise JC, Quattro JM, Vrijenhoek RC (1992) Molecular clones within organismal clones. *Evolutionary Biology,* **26,** 225-246.

Baker HG (1965) Characteristics and modes of origin of weeds. In: *Genetics of Colonizing Species* (eds. Baker HG, Stebbins GL), pp. 147-172. Academic Press, New York.

Bell G (1982) *The Masterpiece of Nature: the Evolution and Genetics of Sexuality.* University of California Press, Berkeley.

Bernstein, H, Byerly, H, Hopf, F, Michod, RE (1985) Genetic damage, mutation and the evolution of sex. *Science,* **229,** 1277-1287.

Bernstein H, Hopf, F, Michod, RE (1988) Is meiotic recombination an adaptation for repairing DNA, producing genetic variation, or both? In: *The Evolution of Sex: an Examination of Current Ideas* (eds. Michod RE, Levin BR), pp. 139-160. Sinauer Associates, Sunderland, Massachusetts.

Beukeboom LW, Vrijenhoek RC (1998) Evolutionary genetics and ecology of sperm-dependent parthenogenesis. *Journal of Evolutionary Biology,* in press.

Bierzychudek P (1985) Patterns in plant parthenogenesis. *Experientia,* **41,** 1255-1264.

Birky CW, Jr. (1996) Heterozygosity, heteromorphy, and phylogenetic trees in asexual eukaryotes. *Genetics,* **144,** 427-437.

Blackman RL (1981) *Species, Sex and Parthenogenesis in the Evolving Biosphere.* Cambridge University Press, Cambridge, U.K..

Bogart JP (1989) A mechanism for interspecific gene exchange via all-female salamander hybrids. In: *Evolution and Ecology of Unisexual Vertebrates* (eds. Dawley RM, Bogart JP), pp. 170-179. Bulletin 466, New York State Museum, Albany, New York.

Bogart JP, Licht LE (1986) Reproduction and the origin of polyploids in hybrid salamanders of the genus *Ambystoma. Canadian Journal of Genetics and Cytogenetics,* **28,** 605-617.

Browne RA (1988) Genetic and ecological divergence of sexual and asexual brine shrimp (*Artemia*) populations in the Mediterranean basin. *National Geographic Research,* **4,** 548-554.

Browne RA (1992) Population genetics and ecology of *Artemia*: insights into parthenogenetic reproduction. *Trends in Ecology and Evolution,* **7,** 232-237.

Browne RA, Bowen S (1990) Population and evolutionary genetics of *Artemia*. In: *Artemia Biology* (eds. Browne RA, Sorgeloos P, Trotman CN), CRC Press, Boca Raton, Florida.

Browne RA, Hoopes CW (1990) Genotypic diversity and selection in asexual brine shrimp (*Artemia*). *Evolution,* **44,** 1035-1051.

Butlin RK, Griffiths HI (1993) Aging without sex? *Nature,* **364,** 680.

Carmona JA, Sanjur OI, Doadrio I, Machurdom A, Vrijenhoek RC (1997) Hybridogenetic reproduction and maternal ancestry of polyploid Iberian fish: the *Tropidophoxinellus alburnoides* complex. *Genetics*, **146**, 983-993.

Case T (1990) Patterns of coexistence in sexual and asexual species of *Cnemidophorus* lizards. *Oecologia*, **83**, 220-227.

Case TJ, Taper ML (1986) On the coexistence and coevolution of asexual and sexual competitors. *Evolution*, **40**, 366-387.

Chao L (1990) Fitness of RNA virus decreased by Muller's ratchet. *Nature*, **348**, 454-455.

Chao L, Tran T, Matthews C (1992) Muller's ratchet and the advantage of sex in the RNA virus f6. *Evolution*, **46**, 289-299.

Charlesworth B, Morgan MT, Charleswort, D (1993) The effect of deleterious mutation on neutral molecular variation. *Genetics*, **134**, 1289-1203.

Christensen B (1980) Constant differential distribution of genetic variants in parthenogenetic forms of *Lumbricillus lineatus* (Enchytraeidae, Oligochaeta) in a heterogeneous environment. *Hereditas*, **92**, 193-198.

Christensen B, Noer H, Theisen BF (1988) Differential response to humidity and soil type among clones of triploid parthenogenetic *Trichoniscus pusillus* (Isopoda, Crustacea). *Hereditas*, **108**, 213-217.

Cimino MC, Schultz RJ (1970) Production of a diploid male offspring by a gynogenetic triploid fish of the genus *Poeciliopsis*. *Copeia*, **1970**, 760-63.

Dybdahl MF, Lively CM (1998) Host-parasite coevolution: evidence for rare advantage and time-lagged selection in natural population. *Evolution* **52**, in press.

Eber, D (1994) Virulence and local adaptation of a horizontally transmitted parasite. *Science*, **265**, 1084-1086.

Elder JF Jr., Schlosser IJ (1995) Extreme clonal uniformity of *Phoxinus eos/neogaeus* gynogens (Pisces: Cyprinidae) among variable habitats in northern Minnesota beaver ponds. *Proceedings of the National Academy of Sciences, USA*, **92**, 5001-5005.

Eshel I, Feldman MW (1970) On the evolutionary effect of recombination. *Theoretical Population Biology*, **1**, 88-110.

Felsenstein J (1981) Skepticism toward Santa Rosalia, or why there are so few kinds of animals. *Evolution*, **35**, 124-138.

Fisher RA (1930) *The Genetical Theory of Natural Selection*. Oxford University Press, Oxford.

Futuyma DJ, Cort RP, van Noordwijk I (1984) Adaptation to host plants in the fall cankerworm (*Alsophila pometaria*) and its bearing on the evolution of host affiliation in phytophagous insects. *American Naturalist*, **123**, 287-296.

Ghiselin MT (1974) *The Economy of Nature and the Evolution of Sex*. University of California Press, Berkeley.

Glesener RR, Tilman D (1978) Sexuality and the components of environmental uncertainty: clues from geographic parthenogenesis in terrestrial animals. *American Naturalist*, **112**, 659-673.

Goddard KA, Dawley RM (1990) Clonal inheritance of a diploid nuclear genome by a hybrid freshwater minnow (*Phoxinus eos-neogaeus*, Pisces: Cyprinidae). *Evolution*, **44**, 1052-1065.

Goddard KA, Schultz RJ (1993) Aclonal reproduction by polyploid members of the clonal species *Phoxinus eos-neogaeus (Cyprinidae)*. *Copeia*, **1993**, 650-660.

Graf JD, Polls-Pelaz M (1989) Evolutionary genetics of the *Rana esculenta* hybrid complex. In: *Evolution and Ecology of Unisexual Vertebrates* (eds. Dawley R, Bogart J), pp. 289-302. Bulletin 466, New York State Museum, Albany, New York.

Grant V (1981) *Plant Speciation*, 2nd edn. Columbia University Press, New York.

Haigh J (1978) The accumulation of deleterious genes in a population—Muller's ratchet. *Theoretical Population Biology*, **14**, 251-257.

Hales DF, Tomiu J, Wöhrmann, K, Sunnucks P (1997) Evolutionary and genetic aspects of aphid biology: a review. *European Journal of Entomology*, **94**, 1-55.

Hamilton WD, Henderson, P, Moran N (1981) Fluctuation of environmental and coevolved antagonist polymorphism as factors in the maintenance of sex. In: *Natural Selection and Social Behavior* (eds. Alexander RD, Tinkle D), pp. 363-381. Chiron Press, New York.

Hanley KA, Fisher RN, Case TJ (1995) Lower mite infestations in an asexual gecko compared with its sexual ancestors. *Evolution*, **49**, 418-426.

Hebert PDN (1974) Ecological differences among genotypes in a natural population of *Daphnia magna*. *Heredity*, **33**, 327-337.

Hebert PDN (1981) Obligate asexuality in *Daphnia*. *American Naturalist*, **117**, 784-789.

Hebert PDN, Crease T (1983) Clonal diversity in populations of *Daphnia pulex* reproducing by obligate parthenogenesis. *Heredity*, **51**, 353-369.

Hedges SB, Bogart JP, Maxson LR (1992) Ancestry of unisexual salamanders. *Nature*, **356**, 708-710.

Hickey DA (1982) Selfish DNA: a sexually-transmitted nuclear parasite. *Genetics*, **101**, 519-531.

Hickey DA, Rose MR (1987) The role of gene transfer in the evolution of eukaryotic sex. In: *The Evolution of Sex: an Examination of Current Ideas* (eds. Michod RE, Levin BR), pp. 161-175. Sinauer Associates, Sunderland, Massachusetts.

Hillis DM, Moritz, C, Porter, CA, Baker, RJ (1991) Evidence for biased gene conversion in converted evolution of ribosomal DNA. *Science,* **251,** 308-310.

Huff DR, Peakall R, Smouse PE (1993) RAPD marker variation within and among natural populations of outcrossing Buffalograss, *Buchloe dactyloides* (Nutt.) Engelm. *Theoretical and Applied Genetics,* **86,** 927-939.

Hurst LD, Hamilton WD, Ladle RJ (1992) Covert sex. *Trends in Ecology and Evolution,* **7,** 144-145.

Innes DJ (1989) Genetics of *Daphnia obtusa*: Genetic load and linkage analysis in a cyclical parthenogen. *Journal of Heredity,* **80,** 6-10.

Jaenike J, Parker ED Jr., Selander RK (1980) Clonal niche structure in the parthenogenetic earthworm *Octolasion tyrtaeum. American Naturalist,* **116,** 196-205.

Jagiello G, Ducayen M, Fang JS, Graffeo J (1976) Cytological observations in mammalian oocytes. *Chromosomes Today,* **5,** 43-64.

Jokela J, Lively CM, Fox JA, Dybdahl MF (1997) Flat reaction norms and 'frozen' phenotypic variation in clonal snails (*Potamopyrgus antipodarum*). *Evolution,* **51,** 1120-1129.

Judson OP, Normark BB (1996) Ancient asexual scandals. *Trends in Ecology and Evolution,* **11,** 41-46.

Kraus F (1989) Constraints on the evolutionary history of the unisexual salamanders of the *Ambystoma laterale-texanum* complex as revealed by mitochondrial DNA analysis. In: *Evolution and Ecology of Unisexual Vertebrates* (eds. Dawley RM, Bogart JP), pp. 218-227. Bulletin 466, New York State Museum, Albany, New York.

Kraus F, Miyamoto MM (1990) Mitochondrial genotype of a unisexual salamander of hybrid origin is unrelated to either of its nuclear haplotypes. *Proceedings of the National Academy of Sciences, USA,* **87,** 2235-2238.

Leslie JF, Vrijenhoek RC (1978) Genetic dissection of clonally inherited genomes of *Poeciliopsis* I. Linkage analysis and preliminary assessment of deleterious gene loads. *Genetics,* **90,** 801-811.

Leslie JF, Vrijenhoek RC (1980) Consideration of Muller's ratchet mechanism through studies of genetic linkage and genomic compatibilities in clonally reproducing *Poeciliopsis. Evolution,* **34,** 1105-1115.

Levin BR (1987) The evolution of sex in bacteria. In: *The Evolution of Sex: an Examination of Current Ideas* (eds. Michod RE, Levin BR). Sinauer Associates, Sunderland, Massachusetts.

Li W-H (1997) *Molecular Evolution.* Sinauer Associates, Sunderland, Massachusetts.

Lim NRW (1998) Genetic analysis of predatory efficiency in natural and laboratory made hybrids of *Poeciliopsis* (Pisces: Poeciliidae). *Behaviour,* **135,** 83-98.

Little TJ, Hebert PDN (1996) Ancient asexuals: scandal or artifact? *Trends in Ecology and Evolution,* **11,** 296.

Lively CM (1987) Evidence from a New Zealand snail for the maintenance of sex by parasitism. *Nature,* **328,** 519-521.

Lively CM, Craddock, C Vrijenhoek RC (1990) The Red Queen hypothesis supported by parasitism in sexual and clonal fish. *Nature,* **344,** 864-866.

Lively CM, Lloyd, DG (1990) The cost of biparental sex under individual selection. *American Naturalist,* **135,** 489-500.

Lloyd DG (1988) Benefits and costs of biparental and uniparental reproduction in plants. In: *The Evolution of Sex: an Examination of Current Ideas* (eds. Michod RE, Levin BR), pp. 233-252. Sinauer Associates, Sunderland, Massachusetts.

Lynch M (1984) Destabilizing hybridization, general-purpose genotypes and geographical parthenogenesis. *The Quarterly Review of Biology,* **59,** 257-290.

Lynch M, Bürger, R, Butcher, D, Gabriel, W (1993) The mutational meltdown in asexual populations. *Journal of Heredity,* **84,** 339-344.

Lynch M, Gabrie W (1990) Mutational load and the survival of small populations. *Evolution,* **44,** 1725-1737.

Martínez-Torres D, Carrió R, Latorre A *et al.* (1997) Assessing the nucleotide diversity of three aphid species. *Journal of Evolutionary Biology,* **10,** 459-477.

Maynard Smith J (1962) Disruptive selection, polymorphism and sympatric speciation. *Nature,* **195,** 60-62.

Maynard Smith J (1971) The origin and maintenance of sex. In: *Group Selection* (ed. Williams GC), Aldine Atherton, Chicago.

Maynard Smith J (1978) *The Evolution of Sex.* Cambridge University Press, Cambridge, U.K..

Maynard Smith J (1986) Contemplating life without sex. *Nature,* **324,** 300-301.

Maynard Smith J (1992) Clonal histories: age and the unisexual lineage. *Nature,* **356,** 661-662.

Michod RE (1995) *Eros and Evolution: a Natural Philosophy of Sex.* Addison-Wesley, Reading, Massachusetts.

Michod RE, Levin, BR (1987) *The Evolution of Sex: an Examination of Current Ideas.* Sinauer Associates, Sunderland, Massachusetts.

Moore WS (1977) A histocompatibility analysis of inheritance in the unisexual fish *Poeciliopsis 2 monacha-lucida. Copeia*, **1977**, 213-223.

Moor WS (1984) Evolutionary ecology of unisexual fishes. In: *Evolutionary Genetics of Fishes* (ed. Turner BJ), pp. 329-398. Plenum Press, New York.

Mora NA (1992) The evolution of aphid life cycles. *Annual Review of Entomology*, **37**, 321-348.

Moritz C (1991) The origin and evolution of parthenogenesis in *Heteronotia binoei* (Gekkonidae): Evidence for recent and localized origins of widespread clones. *Genetics*, **129**, 211-219.

Moritz C, McCallum, H, Donellan, S, Roberts, JD (1991) Parasite loads in parthenogenetic and sexual lizards (*Heteronotia binoei*): support the Red Queen hypothesis. *Proceedings of the Royal Society of London B*, **224**, 145-149.

Muller HJ (1932) Some genetic aspects of sex. *American Naturalist*, **66**, 118-138.

Muller HJ (1964) The relation of mutation to mutational advance. *Mutation Research*, **1**, 2-9.

Nei M (1970) Accumulation of nonfunctional genes in sheltered chromosomes. *American Naturalist*, **104**, 211-222.

Nunney L (1989) The maintenance of sex by group selection. *Evolution*, **43**, 245-257.

Ohta, T (1992) The nearly neutral theory of molecular evolution. *Annual Review of Ecology and Systematics*, **23**, 263-286.

Parker ED, Selander RK, Hudson RO, Lester, LJ (1977) Genetic diversity in colonizing parthenogenetic cockroaches. *Evolution*, **31**, 836-842.

Perez ML Valverde JR, Batuecas B *et al.* (1994) Speciation in the *Artemia* genus: mitochondrial DNA analysis of bisexual and parthenogenetic brine shrimp. *Journal of Molecular Evolution*, **38**, 156-168.

Petren K, Bolger DT, Case TJ (1993) Mechanisms in the competitive success of an invading sexual gecko over and asexual native. *Science*, **259**, 354-358.

Quattro JM, Avise JC, Vrijenhoek RC (1991) Molecular evidence for multiple origins of hybridogenetic fish clones (Poeciliidae: *Poeciliopsis*). *Genetics*, **127**, 391-398.

Quattro JM, Avise JC, Vrijenhoek RC (1992a) An ancient clonal lineage in the fish genus *Poeciliopsis* (Atheriniformes: Poeciliidae). *Proceedings of the National Academy of Sciences, USA*, **89**, 348-352.

Quattro JM, Avise JC, Vrijenhoek RC (1992b) Mode of origin and sources of genotypic diversity in triploid fish clones (*Poeciliopsis*: Poeciliidae). *Genetics*, **130**, 621-628.

Rice WR (1994) Degeneration of a nonrecombining chromosome. *Science*, **263**, 230-232.

Roughgarden J (1972) Evolution of niche width. *American Naturalist*, **106**, 683-718.

Schartl, M Nanda, I Schlupp I *et al.* (1995) Incorporation of subgenomic amounts of DNA as compensation for mutational load in a gynogenetic fish. *Nature*, **373**, 68-71.

Schenck RA, Vrijenhoek RC (1989) Coexistence among sexual and asexual forms of *Poeciliopsis*: foraging behavior and microhabitat selection. In: *Evolution and Ecology of Unisexual Vertebrates* (eds. Dawley R, Bogart J), pp. 39-48. Bulletin 466, New York State Museum, Albany, New York.

Schlosser IJ, Doeringsfeld MR, Elder JF,(1997) Niche relationships of clonal and sexual fish in a heterogeneous landscape. *Ecological Monographs*, **79**, 953-968.

Schultz RJ (1969) Hybridization, unisexuality and polyploidy in the teleost *Poeciliopsis* (Poeciliidae) and other vertebrates. *American Naturalist*, **103**, 605-619.

Schultz RJ, Fielding E (1989) Fixed genotypes in variable environments. In: *Evolution and Ecology of Unisexual Vertebrates* (eds. Dawley R, Bogart J), pp. 32-38. Bulletin 466, New York State Museum, Albany, New York.

Schultz RJ, Kallman KD (1968) Triploid hybrids between the all-female teleost *Poecilia formosa* and *Poecilia sphenops*. *Nature*, **219**, 280-282.

Seger J, Hamilton WD (1988) Parasites and sex. In: *The Evolution of Sex: an Examination of Current Ideas* (eds. Michod RE, Levin BR), pp. 176-211. Sinauer Associates, Sunderland, Massachusetts.

Selander RK, Yang SY, Lewontin RC, Johnson WE (1971) Genetic variations in the horseshoe crab (*Limulus polyphemus*), a phylogenetic "relic". *Evolution*, **24**, 402-414.

Semlitsch RD (1993) Asymmetric competition in mixed populations of tadpoles of the hybridogenetic *Rana esculenta* complex. *Evolution*, **47**, 510-519.

Semlitsch RD, Hotz H, Guex G-D (1997) Competition among tadpoles of coexisting hemiclones of hybridogenetic *Rana esculenta*: support for the Frozen Niche Variation model. *Evolution*, **51**, 1249-1261.

Simmons MJ, Crow JF (1977) Mutations affecting fitness in *Drosophila* populations. *Annual Review of Genetics*, **11**, 49-78.

Simon JC, Martinez D, Latorre AM, Hebert PDN (1996) Molecular characterization of cyclic and obligate parthenogens in the aphid *Rhopalosiphum padi* (L.). *Proceedings of the Royal Society of London B*, **263**, 481-486.

Spinella DG, Vrijenhoek RC (1982) Genetic dissection of clonally inherited genomes of *Poeciliopsis*. II. Investigation of a silent carboxylesterase allele. *Genetics*, **100**, 279-286.

Spolsky CM, Phillips CA, Uzzell T (1992) Antiquity of clonal salamander lineages revealed by mitochondrial DNA. *Nature*, **356**, 706-708.

Stebbins GL (1971) *Chromosomal Evolution in Higher Plants*. Arnold, London.

Stouthammer R, Breeuwer JA, Luck RF, Werren JH (1993) Molecular identification of microorganisms associated with parthenogenesis. *Nature,* **361,** 66-68.

Sunnucks P, Barro PJD, Lushai G, Maclean N, Hales DF (1997) Genetic structure of an aphid studied using microsatellites: cyclic parthenogenesis, differentiated lineages, and host specialization. *Molecular Ecology,* **6,** 1059-1073.

Sunnucks P, England PR, Taylor AC, Hales DF (1996) Microsatellite and chromosome evolution of parthenogenetic *Sitobion* aphids in Australia. *Genetics,* **144,** 747-756.

Suomalainen E, Saura A, Lokki J (1987) *Cytology and Evolution in Parthenogenesis*. CRC Press, Boca Raton, Florida.

Templeton AR (1982) The prophecies of parthenogenesis. In: *Evolution and Genetics of Life Histories* (eds. Dingle H, Hegmann JP), pp. 75-102. Springer-Verlag, Berlin.

Thompson V (1976) Does sex accelerate evolution? *Evolutionary Theory,* **1,** 131-156.

Turner BJ (1982) The evolutionary genetics of a unisexual fish. In: *Mechanisms of Speciation* (ed. Barigozzi C), pp. 265-305. Liss, New York.

Turner BJ, Elder JF, Laughlin TF, Davis WP, Taylor DS (1992) Extreme clonal diversity and divergence in populations of a selfing hermaphroditic fish. *Proceedings of the National Academy of Sciences, USA,* **89,** 10643-10647.

Van Valen L (1973) A new evolutionary law. *Evolutionary Theory,* **1,** 1-30.

Vandel A (1928) La parthénogénèse géographique contribution a l'étude biologique et cytologique de la parthénogénèse naturelle. *Bulletin Biologique de la France et de la Belgique,* **62,** 164-281.

Vinogradov AE, Borkin LJ, Gunther R, Rosanov JM (1990) Genome elimination in diploid and triploid *Rana esculenta* males: cytological evidence from DNA flow cytometry. *Genome,* **33,** 619-627.

Vrijenhoek RC (1978) Coexistence of clones in a heterogeneous environment. *Science,* **199,** 549-552.

Vrijenhoek RC (1979) Factors affecting clonal diversity and coexistence. *American Zoologist,* **19,** 787-797.

Vrijenhoek RC (1984a) Ecological differentiation among clones: the frozen niche variation model. In: *Population Biology and Evolution* (eds. Wöhrmann K, Loeschcke V), pp. 217-231. Springer-Verlag, Heidelberg.

Vrijenhoek RC (1984b) The evolution of clonal diversity in *Poeciliopsis*. In: *Evolutionary Genetics of Fishes* (ed. Turner BJ), pp. 399-429. Plenum Press, New York.

Vrijenhoek RC (1985) Animal population genetics and disturbance: the effects of local extinctions and re-colonizations on heterozygosity and fitness. In: *The Ecology of Natural Disturbance and Patch Dynamics* (eds. Pickett STA, White P), pp. 265-285. Academic Press, New York.

Vrijenhoek RC (1989) Genetic and ecological constraints on the origins and establishment of unisexual vertebrates. In: *Evolution and Ecology of Unisexual Vertebrates* (eds. Dawley R, Bogart J), pp. 24-31. Bulletin 466, New York State Museum, Albany, New York.

Vrijenhoek RC (1998) Animal clones and diversity. *Bioscience,* in press.

Vrijenhoek RC, Angus RA, Schultz RJ (1978) Variation and clonal structure in a unisexual fish. *American Naturalist,* **112,** 41-55.

Vrijenhoek RC, Marteinsdottir G, Schenck, RE (1987) Genotypic and phenotypic aspects of niche diversi-fication in fishes. In: *Community and Evolutionary Ecology of North American Stream Fishes* (eds. Matthews W, Heins D), pp. 245-250. University of Oklahoma Press, Norman.

Vrijenhoek RC, Pfeiler E (1997) Differential survival of sexual and asexual *Poeciliopsis* during environ-mental stress. *Evolution,* **51,** 1593-1600.

Vrijenhoek RC, Schultz RJ (1974) Evolution of a trihybrid unisexual fish (*Poeciliopsis*, Poeciliidae). *Evolution,* **28,** 205-319.

Weeks SC (1993) The effects of recurrent clonal formation on clonal invasion patterns and sexual persis-tence: a Monte Carlo simulation of the frozen niche variation model. *American Naturalist,* **141,** 409-427.

Weeks, SC, Gaggiotti OE, Spindler KP, Schenck RE, Vrijenhoek RC (1992) Feeding behavior in sexual and clonal strains of *Poeciliopsis*. *Behavioral Ecology and Sociobiology,* **30,** 1-6.

Weider LJ (1993) A test of the "general-purpose" genotype hypothesis: differential tolerance to thermal and salinity stress among *Daphnia* clones. *Evolution,* **47,** 965-969.

Weider LJ, Hebert PDN (1987) Ecological and physiological differentiation among low-Arctic clones of *Daphnia pulex*. *Ecology,* **68,** 188-198.

Weissman A (1889) *Essays upon Heredity and Kindred Biological Problems*. Claredon Press, Oxford.

Wetherington JD, Schenck RA, Vrijenhoek RC (1989) Origins and ecological success of unisexual *Poeciliopsis*: the Frozen Niche Variation model. In: *The Ecology and Evolution of Poeciliid Fishes* (eds. Meffe GA, Snelson FF, Jr.), pp. 259-276. Prentice Hall, Englewood Cliffs, N.J..

White MJD (1978) *Modes of Speciation*. Freeman, San Francisco.

Williams GC (1975) *Sex and Evolution*. Princeton University Press, Princeton, N.J..

Williams,GC, Mitton JB (1973) Why Reproduce Sexually? *Journal of Theoretical Biology,* **39,** 545-554.

Williams GS (1971) Introduction. In: *Group Selection* (ed. Williams GS), Aldine Atherton, Chicago.

Wright JW, Lowe CH (1968) Weeds, polyploids, parthenogenesis and the geographical and ecological distribution of all-female species of *Cnemidophorus*. *Copeia*, **1968,** 128-138.

Advances in Molecular Ecology
G.R. Carvalho (Ed.)
IOS Press, 1998

Parentage Analysis in Plants: Mating Systems, Gene Flow, and Relative Fertilities

Andrew Schnabel

*Department of Biological Sciences, Indiana University South Bend,
South Bend, Indiana 46615 USA, e-mail: aschnabe@iusb.edu*

This chapter deals with the reconstruction of mating and dispersal processes in natural and experimental plant populations. Within the past fifteen years, the study of mating and dispersal processes in plants has been greatly expanded due to (i) the development of methods for assessing parentage of individual progeny; and (ii) an increase in the diversity and availability of molecular genetic markers. Most attention has been focused on the use of maternal progeny arrays to estimate short-term rates of pollen gene flow between populations and to examine patterns of pollen dispersal and male fertility variation within populations. The earliest studies relied solely on exclusion methods, but it was almost immediately realized that many gene flow events were not being detected, and that unique parentage could not be determined for a large proportion of the non-immigrant offspring in most natural populations. As a consequence, methods for maximum-likelihood estimation of gene flow and male fertilities have been introduced. Less effort has been devoted to the inference of parentage using dispersed seeds and seedlings, but all of the currently available models can be adapted to this situation as well. I begin this chapter with a short review of single-locus and multilocus methods for estimating the proportions of self-fertilization and outcrossing events for individuals and populations. This provides a motivation for the broader question of parentage analysis, focusing first on the use of multilocus data to estimate levels of pollen gene flow. I then review the methods available for estimating relative fertilities of individual parents within populations, focusing on the strengths and weaknesses of each method. I conclude with some statements about currently unanswered problems with parentage models and some suggestions about novel or insufficiently explored uses to which parentage analysis may be put in the future.

1. Introduction

Many fundamental evolutionary and ecological questions require an understanding of mating processes in natural populations. The behavioural, ecological, and genetic phenomena that affect mating and reproductive success in populations of sexually reproducing organisms ultimately determine how the relative frequencies of alleles and genotypes change from generation to generation. For several reasons, the study of mating processes in plants is especially complex, and therefore, especially interesting. First, plants exhibit a wide variety of breeding systems, such as hermaphroditism, dioecy, monoecy, gynodioecy, and androdioecy. Second, the mating systems of plants can include complete random mating, complete self-fertilization, apomixis, assortative mating, or some combination of these modes of reproduction. Third, plants cannot move about to seek suitable mates or habitats, and therefore they rely on wind, water or complex interactions with animals to effect pollination and dispersal of progeny.

In this chapter, I will describe currently available analytical methods for investigating the breeding structure of plant populations. An initial brief description of traditional methods for estimating selfing and outcrossing rates will serve as a backdrop for a more extensive discussion of genealogy reconstruction methods, which are concerned with the determination of parentage for progeny of one or more cohorts. Parentage analyses can either estimate the most likely pair of parents for each progeny or can determine patterns of parentage at the populational level. In any case, the two most immediate results are estimates of gene flow, or the proportion of progeny that resulted either from pollen or seed immigration into the population, and relative male and female fertilities, which are the proportions of the non-immigrant progeny that can be attributed to each potential parent. Estimates of relative fertility should be correlated with overall reproductive success, and therefore with fitness (Devlin & Ellstrand 1990a; Snow & Lewis 1993).

Given some knowledge of parentage for a set of progeny, numerous questions about the breeding biology and genetic structure of a population can be addressed, such as (i) Is fertility variation greater in males or females? (ii) How variable are male and female fertilities over several generations or breeding seasons? (iii) What is the effect on male, female, and overall reproductive success of characteristics such as plant size and age, spatial location relative to safe germination sites, clonal growth, reproductive effort, inflorescence size, flower size and shape, and nectar production rates? (iv) What are the scales and patterns of effective pollen and seed dispersal? (v) How do various pollinator species differ in their ability to effect seed production or to disperse pollen within and between populations? (vi) How do various seed dispersers differ in their ability to effect dispersal between populations? and (vii) What is the genetically effective size of the population? Moreover, estimates of fertility variation and patterns of gene flow are relevant to the field of conservation biology, which is often concerned with the effects of habitat destruction that leaves populations artificially isolated from one another. In such cases of fragmentation, it is important to know how patterns of gene flow and reproductive success may have been changed through altered interactions with pollinators and seed dispersers, elimination of safe sites for germination, or invasions of weedy competitors or plant pathogens (Bierregaard *et al.* 1992; Levin 1995; Nason & Hamrick 1997; Aldrich & Hamrick 1998). I return to this topic at the end of the chapter.

2. Mating system analysis

One of the first steps in understanding the breeding structure of a plant population is to investigate the relative proportions of progeny produced by self-fertilization (selfing) and cross-fertilization (outcrossing). Qualitative assessments of the mating system can be obtained from the study of floral morphology, results of controlled crosses, and observations of pollinators. These kinds of studies typically indicate whether or not selfing would be expected in a species, but they do not provide quantitative estimates of selfing when it does occur.

Because pollen grains are very small and short-lived, it is essentially impossible to observe individual mating events or to determine directly the genotype of individual male gametophytes. The study of plant mating systems therefore necessarily involves a reconstruction of mating events from genotypic data of maternal individuals and their progeny. As pointed out by many authors (*e.g.* Clegg 1980), one of the great advantages of studying plant breeding structure is the relative ease with which such family units can be sampled. For many species, seeds can be sampled directly from the maternal plant. Because allozymes show codominant inheritance and are sufficiently variable in many plant species, they are particularly well-suited to provide the necessary genotypic data and are

Table 1: Expected distribution of progeny genotypes under the mixed mating model, assuming only two alleles at a locus (after Clegg 1980). In this table, p and q are frequencies of the two alleles, A_1 and A_2, where $p = 1 - q$; s and t are the relative rates of selfing and outcrossing ($s = 1 - t$).

Maternal Genotype	Progeny Genotype		
	A_1A_1	A_1A_2	A_2A_2
A_1A_1	$s + tp$	tq	0
A_1A_2	$s/4 + tp/2$	$1/2$	$2/4 + tq/2$
A_2A_2	0	tp	$s + tq$

still the most popular choice as genetic markers for the estimation of selfing rates in both natural and experimental populations (Karron et al. 1995; Cruzan 1998). Newer molecular markers, however, such as microsatellites, RAPDs (Random Amplified Polymorphic DNA), and AFLPs (Amplified Fragment Length Polymorphisms), are now also widely available (Dow & Ashley 1995; Parker *et al.* 1998).

2.1. Single-locus mating model

To estimate mating system parameters, it is necessary to specify a statistical model of the mating process. For the past 20 years, the most commonly used model in plants has been the mixed mating model (Clegg 1980; Brown *et al.* 1989), which assumes that (i) each zygote results from either self-fertilization or random outcrossing; (ii) pollen allele frequencies are uniform over all maternal individuals; (iii) the probability of outcrossing is independent of maternal genotype; (iv) no selection affecting the genetic markers used occurs between the time of fertilization and the time of the genetic assay. Under these assumptions, the expected progeny frequencies in the sample can be specified explicitly (Table 1). The mating parameters of the model are t, the rate of outcrossing, and p, the pollen allele frequency. These are estimated by means of maximum likelihood based on data from several progeny arrays (Ritland 1986, 1990).

2.2. Multilocus mating model

The most commonly used models for multilocus estimation of outcrossing rates are those of Shaw *et al.* (1981) and Ritland & Jain (1981). Ritland (1983, 1984, 1986), in particular, has published a series of excellent papers dealing with various aspects of plant mating system estimation and has developed a computer software package that is freely available (Ritland 1990). In multilocus models, mating events are divided into two categories: discernible and nondiscernible (ambiguous). For example, comparison of progeny alleles with maternal alleles in Table 2 indicates that progeny 1 and 3 resulted from an outcrossing event, whereas the origin of progeny 2 is ambiguous, because it could have resulted from either outcrossing or selfing. Multilocus estimation of outcrossing therefore takes into account discernible outcrosses as well as the probability of not detecting an outcross when it, in fact, has occurred. Violations of some assumptions of the mixed mating model do not affect multilocus estimates of outcrossing as seriously as they affect single-locus estimates (Ritland & Jain 1981).

Table 2: Hypothetical data set for estimating outcrossing events from multilocus data (after Shaw *et al.* 1981). Asterisks signify loci that discriminate each progeny as an outcross.

	Loci				
Progeny No.	**A**	**B**	**C**	**D**	**E**
			Maternal Genotype		
	11	22	12	13	23
			Progeny Genotypes		
1	11	22	12	13	13*
2	11	22	22	11	33
3	11	12*	12	23*	13*

2.3. Practical considerations in mating system studies

Mating system studies are typically large in scope, requiring the sampling of multiple maternal families and hundreds of progeny (*e.g.* Rieseberg *et al.* 1998). Assuming that time and money are limited, it is important to think about optimising sample sizes and numbers of marker loci assayed. For example, the probability of detecting outcrossing events obviously increases with additional genetic data. Thus, accuracy of the estimates is increased either through increasing number of loci or by choosing loci with more alleles or more even allele frequencies (Shaw *et al.* 1981; Shaw & Brown 1982). Both Shaw & Brown (1982) and Ritland & Jain (1981) show, however, that under most situations, 3-6 codominant loci will be sufficient to obtain accurate multilocus estimates. Moreover, Shaw & Brown (1982) have shown that (i) when selfing levels are high, it is most efficient to sample few loci for the maximum possible number of progeny; and (ii) when selfing levels are very low, it is most efficient to score many loci even if progeny sample sizes suffer.

3. Exclusion analysis and gene flow estimation

Although application of single-locus and multilocus mating system models to family data provides valuable information about the breeding structure of plant populations (*e.g.* Pellmyr *et al.* 1997; Loveless *et al.* 1998), many questions of interest require more detailed knowledge of mating structure and dispersal patterns. In essence, traditional mating system analyses use genetic data to divide a set of progeny into two categories, the relative proportions produced by selfing and by outcrossing. It is useful in many studies, however, to subdivide these progeny further. For example, if one could divide the outcrossed portion of the maternal progeny arrays into those that had been sired by local males and those that had been sired by males from outside the study area, then one would have an estimate of the amount of pollen gene flow entering the population. Similarly, for a set of dispersed progeny, such as a set of tree saplings for which individual ages are known, it might be useful to estimate what proportion of those progeny arose by local mating and seed dispersal, by pollen immigration with local seed dispersal, or by seed immigration. Ultimately, in a full genealogical reconstruction, all gene flow events would be detected, and each possible parent within the population would be assigned a proportion of the non-immigrant progeny. In this way, the analysis of a single set of progeny not only would provide estimates of selfing and outcrossing, but would simultaneously provide direct estimates of several other aspects of the breeding structure, such as reproductive success, the distribution of effective pollen dispersal within the population, and levels of pollen or seed immigration.

Prior to the advent of molecular markers, the extent of gene flow between natural plant populations was inferred from measurements of pollen and seed dispersal distributions within populations (Levin & Kerster 1974; Handel 1983; Hamrick & Schnabel 1985). For example, observations of pollinator movements in many species suggested that most pollen was transferred between near neighbours and long-distance pollen transfer was rare. These types of studies, however, provide little useful information concerning true gene flow, and have been shown repeatedly even to underestimate actual effective dispersal patterns (Hamrick & Schnabel 1985; Fenster 1991a; Campbell 1991; Karron et al. 1995). In this section of the chapter, I will introduce single-parent (paternity) and parent-pair exclusion analysis using molecular markers, and discuss the use of these techniques in the direct estimation of gene flow in natural and experimental plant populations.

3.1. Introduction to exclusion analysis

Exclusion analysis uses multilocus genotypic data to differentiate between genetically compatible and incompatible parents for individual progeny. For plant species, exclusion analysis has been used most widely to estimate rates of pollen gene flow between populations (e.g. Ellstrand & Marshall 1985; Ellstrand et al. 1989; Devlin & Ellstrand 1990a; Kohn & Casper 1992; Godt & Hamrick 1993; Arias & Rieseberg 1994; Broyles et al. 1994; Schnabel & Hamrick 1995; Nason et al. 1996, 1998; Chase et al. 1996b; Stacy et al. 1996; Dow & Ashley 1996, 1998; Goodell et al. 1997). Paternity exclusion analyses compare exactly the same type of multilocus, maternal family data presented in Table 2 against multilocus genotypic data of all possible male parents in a population to identify the specific fathers that contributed to those progeny (cf. Table 2 and Table 3).

The first step in a paternity exclusion analysis is to determine the multilocus haploid genotype of the paternal gamete for each progeny, which is accomplished by comparison of maternal with progeny diploid genotypes and subtraction of maternal alleles (Table 3). Haploid pollen genotypes can then be compared locus by locus against all diploid paternal genotypes within the population, and incompatible males (i.e. those that do not possess the gametic allele at a particular locus) can be eliminated. For example, in Table 3, the only possible father for Progeny 1 is Father 1, because Father 2 is incompatible at Loci A, B, D, and E, and both the maternal plant and Father 3 are impossible fathers based on Locus E. In contrast, both the maternal plant and Father 1 are possible fathers for Progeny 2, thereby representing a possible self-fertilization event (cf. Table 2). In an exclusion analysis, there

Table 3: Hypothetical genotypes for five codominant loci in a population consisting of one maternal family and three possible paternal individuals.

	Locus				
	A	**B**	**C**	**D**	**E**
Maternal plant	11	22	12	13	23
Progeny 1	11	22	12	13	13
Paternal Gamete	1	2	1 or 2	1 or 3	1
Progeny 2	11	22	22	11	33
Paternal Gamete	1	2	2	1	3
Progeny 3	11	12	12	23	13
Paternal Gamete	1	1	1 or 2	2	1
Possible Father 1	12	22	22	13	23
Possible Father 2	22	11	12	22	23
Possible Father 3	11	12	11	13	33

Table 4: Hypothetical genotypes at three loci for a maternal plant and 10 progeny from a singly-sired fruit. For each locus, the diploid genotype of the paternal individual can be determined precisely.

Locus	Maternal Genotype	Progeny Genotypes										Paternal Genotype
		1	2	3	4	5	6	7	8	9	10	
A	11	11	12	12	11	12	12	11	12	12	11	12
B	12	22	12	12	12	11	11	22	12	11	12	12
C	13	23	12	12	12	23	12	23	23	12	12	22

is no way to determine which of two or more possible fathers is the correct father. Finally, Progeny 3 has no possible fathers in this population and therefore must have arisen by pollen gene flow from a plant located outside the population. In general, gene flow events can be inferred when none of the potential pollen donors within a study population could have sired a given seed. In a large sample of progeny, the proportion of the total seed sample for which no fathers were found constitutes a minimum estimate of successful pollen migration into a population.

An especially powerful means of paternity exclusion exists when all seed within a fruit are sired by the same male parent (*i.e.* all seeds are full sibs). In this case, the complete diploid genotype of the male parent can be reconstructed (see example in Table 4), which results in extremely high exclusion probabilities and essentially unambiguous determination of all gene flow events (Broyles *et al.* 1994; Chase *et al.* 1996b; Nason *et al.* 1996, 1998). The use of full-sib paternity analysis is limited, however, by the small number of taxa that have the specialized pollination syndromes that result in the production of full-sib arrays. The best-known examples are (i) those taxa that disperse their pollen in packets sufficiently large to sire all seeds within a single ovary, such as the pollinia of milkweeds and orchids (Broyles & Wyatt 1990, 1991; Broyles *et al.* 1994) or polyads of many mimosoid legumes (Muona *et al.* 1991; Chase *et al.* 1996b); and (ii) tropical figs, which have a tightly coevolved relationship with their wasp pollinators such that a female wasp carries pollen from only a single tree and pollinates all the pistillate flowers of a single syconium (Nason *et al.* 1996, 1998).

3.2. Extensions of exclusion analysis

At present, paternity exclusion is the most powerful method for obtaining direct, short-term estimates of pollen gene flow in natural populations. Both Schnabel & Hamrick (1995) and Dow & Ashley (1996) have suggested, however, that successful pollination by a foreign gamete may not be equivalent to successful establishment of that gamete's genes in the local gene pool, which is a requirement included in most working definitions of gene flow (*e.g.* Endler 1977). For example, gene flow might be significantly less than that estimated through paternity analysis if the resulting progeny were at a selective disadvantage relative to progeny produced by local pollen. The reverse situation might also hold, if seeds resulting from gene flow were less inbred than those produced by local matings (Levin 1981; Fenster 1991b). In particular, highly localized seed dispersal patterns might result in near-neighbour adults being full or half sibs, which might lead to a selective advantage for progeny sired by distant males relative to near-neighbour males.

For many perennial plants (especially trees), it might therefore be useful to estimate patterns of gene movement using dispersed progeny (seeds, seedlings, or saplings). In this case, the basic exclusion procedure can be extended such that potential parents are first excluded individually and then the remaining parent pairs are tested for compatibility with the progeny individual (Meagher & Thompson 1986, 1987). Because neither parent is known in advance, exclusion of a possible parent for a given offspring requires that no alleles be shared between the two diploid individuals at one or more loci (see examples in Table 5). This more general exclusion method is less powerful than traditional paternity exclusion and thus requires more genetic and demographic information about a population. For example, if one has identified a series of seedling cohorts to be used in assessing temporal variation in gene flow rates, then the assumption must be made that the current set of potential parents is the same as the set present when the oldest seedling cohort was produced (e.g. Schnabel & Hamrick 1995). In this kind of analysis, unambiguous seed gene flow events for monoecious or hermaphroditic species can be obtained only when all possible parents are excluded individually. For dioecious species, pollen and seed gene flow events can be identified separately by exclusion of either all potential male parents or all potential female parents. Pollen gene flow is also strongly suggested for self-incompatible species when all but one parent is excluded. On the other hand, the subset of immigration events inferred through the exclusion of parent pairs is always a composite of the two types of gene flow. In their respective studies of two temperate tree species, however, Dow & Ashley (1996, 1997) and Schnabel & Hamrick (1995) argued that most of the immigration uncovered through parent-pair exclusion represents pollen gene flow. These arguments were based on estimates of high pollen flow detected through traditional paternity analyses and on observations of highly localized patterns of primary seed dispersal.

3.3. Estimating cryptic gene flow

Except perhaps for full-sib paternity analyses in very small populations (e.g. Broyles et al. 1994; Nason et al. 1998), the number of immigration events detected through exclusion analysis (i.e. apparent gene flow) will underestimate the actual number of immigration events (i.e. total gene flow), because a certain percentage of immigrant gametic genotypes will mimic local gametic genotypes. This problem is especially acute when attempting to estimate gene flow from dispersed progeny, because the exclusion probabilities are much lower in that case. To compensate for this limitation, Devlin & Ellstrand (1990a) developed a Monte Carlo method for obtaining a maximum-likelihood estimate of total pollen gene flow and thereby estimating the amount of "cryptic" gene flow that goes undetected by exclusion analysis alone. Several studies using allozyme data suggest that estimates of total pollen gene flow can be approximately twice as great as levels of apparent

Table 5: Hypothetical genotypes for five codominant loci to be used in an exclusion analysis assuming that the progeny represent dispersed seeds or seedlings for which neither parent is known in advance. Individual parents can be excluded only when they share no alleles with a given progeny individual at one or more loci. Two compatible parents for Progeny 1 are found within the population, but Progeny 2 and 3 represent gene flow events. Seed gene flow is indicated for Progeny 2, because all parents are excluded individually, whereas lack of a compatible parent pair for Progeny 3 indicates a gene flow event, but cannot differentiate between pollen and seed gene flow.

Progeny and Possible Parents	Locus				
	A	B	C	D	E
Progeny 1	11	22	12	13	13
Progeny 2	11	22	22	11	33
Progeny 3	11	12	12	23	13
Parent 1	11	22	12	33	23
Parent 2	12	22	22	23	13
Parent 3	22	11	12	22	23
Parent 4	11	12	11	13	22

gene flow (Ellstrand *et al.* 1989; Broyles *et al.* 1994; Schnabel & Hamrick 1995). On the other hand, Broyles *et al.* (1994) adapted the method of Devlin & Ellstrand (1990a) to the case of full-sib paternity exclusion in *Asclepias exaltata* (poke milkweed) and concluded that the full-sib analysis detected all gene flow events in their progeny arrays. Interestingly, when Broyles *et al.* (1994) reanalysed their data using a standard paternity exclusion method (*i.e.* assuming that seeds within fruits were half-sibs), the Devlin & Ellstrand (1990a) method underestimated total pollen gene flow compared to results obtained from the full-sib analysis (Table 6). Finally, although no published reports presently exist, it is also possible to modify the method of Devlin & Ellstrand (1990a) to estimate total gene flow from exclusion analysis on dispersed progeny (JD Nason, personal communication).

4. Methods for estimation of relative male and female fertilities

Parentage analyses are capable of a far greater level of resolution than simply determining proportions of immigrant progeny or rates of selfing and outcrossing. Using non-immigrant progeny, parentage analyses can also estimate relative male or female fertilities, which broadly defined, are the proportions of the progeny sampled that can be attributed to each potential parent. Because these estimates should be correlated with reproductive success, they can be used to test hypotheses about the effects of various ecological, morphological, or developmental factors on fitness. One can also use fertility estimates to construct patterns of effective pollen and seed dispersal movement (*e.g.* Meagher & Thompson 1987; Karron *et al.* 1995; Schnabel *et al.* 1998). Several methods for the determination of parentage in plant populations have been proposed and will be discussed in turn below.

4.1. Exclusion analysis

As discussed in greater detail above, exclusion analysis compares multilocus offspring genotypes with those of possible parents and eliminates those parents that are genetically incompatible with the offspring. Exclusion analysis is most powerful when singly-sired

Table 6: Single-season estimates of % immigrant pollen in five populations of *Asclepias exaltata* (poke milkweed) (from Broyles *et al.* 1994). The percentage of immigrant pollen was estimated assuming that progeny within fruits were either full sibs (progeny array analysis) or half sibs (seed-by-seed analysis).

Population name	Isolation distance (km)	No. fruits sampled	No. seeds sampled	Immigrant pollen (%)	
				Seed-by-seed (95% C.I.)	Progeny array
Mile Post 54	0.05	53	636	33.4 (29.6-36.5)	41.5
Lewis Mountain	0.05	22	264	38.3 (32.6-43.2)	50.0
Skyland Lodge	0.20	37	528	17.9 (14.9-20.9)	37.8
Old Rag Overlook	0.40	54	672	25.4 (22.2-27.7)	46.3
South Skyland	0.80	33	396	13.7 (10.4-16.7)	30.3
Fisher's Gap	1.00	24	288	24.2 (19.1-28.1)	29.2
Mean	0.50	37	464	25.5	39.2
Standard Deviation	0.36	14	175	9.2	8.4

fruits are sampled directly from maternal plants, because in that case, the full diploid genotype of the paternal parent can be reconstructed and compared with those in the population (Broyles & Wyatt 1990, 1991). For single-seeded or multiply-sired fruits, however, unique identification of paternal parents is less likely, because often only a partial paternal gametophytic genotype can be reconstructed by subtracting maternal alleles, and often several males within a population are capable of producing the same pollen genotype (Table 3). Exclusion of all but the correct parent or parents for dispersed progeny is even more difficult, because no prior genetic information about either parent is known, and exclusion is possible only when a potential parent shares no alleles with an offspring individual at one or more loci (Schnabel & Hamrick 1995; Dow & Ashley 1996; Schnabel et al. 1998).

Thus, even when exclusion probabilities are high, unique identification of a parent is rare, and more often than not, several genetically compatible parents can be found for a large proportion of the offspring sampled (e.g. Meagher 1986). Because exclusion analysis offers no way to determine which of those several possible parents is the most likely parent, a substantial amount of the data must be discarded. Moreover, simulations conducted by Devlin et al. (1988) suggest that exclusion analysis alone does not allow for accurate estimation of mating patterns or reproductive success even when exclusion probabilities are as high as 97%.

4.2. Most-likely method

In the plant literature, Meagher (1986) and Meagher & Thompson (1986, 1987) were the first to present a set of models for estimating the statistical likelihood of parentage when one or neither of the parents is initially known. Following the notation of Meagher (1986), consider the case of assigning paternal likelihoods for a given set of offspring on a particular mother. Let B be the known maternal individual of offspring C, and let D be a possible father of C, where multilocus genotypes of these individuals are designated by g_B, g_C, g_D. The likelihood that D is the true male parent (MP) of C is calculated based on segregation probabilities as

$$L(MP = D) = \frac{T(g_C \mid g_B, g_D)}{T(g_C \mid g_B)}$$

where $T(g_C \mid g_B, g_D)$ is the Mendelian transition probability of the offspring genotype given the genotypes of the mother and putative father and $T(g_C \mid g_B)$ is the probability of the offspring genotype given that the maternal gamete unites randomly with possible paternal gametes. Likelihood scores are calculated for each possible father, and the individual with the highest likelihood is chosen as the true father, while all other fathers are discarded. A similar approach can be used to identify most likely pairs of parents in the case when neither parent is known in advance (Meagher & Thompson 1986). Thus, this method, like exclusion analysis, identifies particular mother-father-offspring triplets.

The most-likely method has received three major criticisms (Devlin et al. 1988; Brown et al. 1989). First, because for any single locus the transition probability is higher when a non-excluded parent is homozygous than when the parent is heterozygous (e.g. $T(A_1A_1 \mid A_1A_1, A_1A_1) = 1.0$, but $T(A_1A_1 \mid A_1A_1, A_1A_2) = 0.5$), the method overestimates the fertilities of parents that are homozygous at many loci. Second, the parent with the highest likelihood score is typically chosen arbitrarily to be the true parent with little regard to the relative likelihood of other possible parents. Third, there is no way to resolve tie scores. Both of these latter two problems result in potentially valuable data being discarded.

Despite these criticisms, however, the most-likely method does recover considerable useful information about fertility variation in a population (Smouse & Meagher 1994), and as with other parentage models, the accuracy of the results increases with increasing exclusion probabilities (Devlin *et al.* 1988).

4.3. Fractional method

Recognising the problems of the most-likely method, Devlin *et al.* (1988) developed a method of paternity analysis that calculates likelihoods in the same way as the most-likely method, but assigns each male a fraction of the paternity, instead of assigning sole paternity to the most likely male. The fraction assigned to any particular male is determined by its likelihood of paternity relative to the likelihoods of all other possible fathers. For example, if the likelihood scores for three possible males are 0.4, 0.8, and 0.3, then the fractional paternity score for those males would be $0.4/(0.4 + 0.8 + 0.3) = 0.27$, $0.8/(0.4 + 0.8 + 0.3) = 0.53$, and $0.3/(0.4 + 0.8 + 0.3) = 0.2$. Under this model, for any offspring C with known female parent B, the probability that individual D^* is the male parent of C is

$$\text{Prob}(MP = D^* \mid FP = B,\ O = C) = \frac{T(g_C \mid g_B, g_{D^*})P(MP = D^* \mid FP = B)}{\sum T(g_C \mid g_B, g_D)P(MP = D \mid FP = B)}$$

Averaged across the entire sample of offspring (either for individual mothers or for the population as whole), this analysis provides an estimate of relative male fertilities, or the fraction of the total sample sired by each possible father. Compared with simple exclusion and the most-likely method, the fractional method has the advantages of being unbiased with respect to paternal genotype and of using all the available offspring data (Devlin *et al.* 1988; Smouse & Meagher 1994). Based on the results of computer simulations, Devlin *et al.* (1988) also argue that the fractional method is the most reliable method for estimating gene movement and reproductive success over a wide range of exclusion probabilities.

The term $P(MP = D^* \mid FP = B)$ in the equation above is the prior probability of paternity for D^* given all the ecological and genetic parameters of the population that make him more or less likely to be the father of offspring O. These parameters might include differences in fecundity or phenology among males or differences in distances between males and females (Adams *et al.* 1992). Although such differences among males are likely to be of ecological and evolutionary importance, the form of the function that maps these differences to individual probabilities of paternity is unknown. Because the goal of many studies is to use the fertility estimates to investigate the influence of ecological or genetic variables on prior probabilities, a fractional analysis typically assumes that the prior probabilities are constant across all possible male parents (*e.g.* Devlin *et al.* 1988). This assumption introduces a conservative bias in the analysis such that the fertilities of high-fertility males are underestimated and the fertilities of low-fertility males are overestimated (Devlin & Ellstrand 1990b).

To address this problem of assigning prior probabilities, Roeder *et al.* (1989) have developed a maximum-likelihood estimator of relative fertilities based on the fractional method. Their model requires that (i) the number of progeny sampled be greater than the number of fertilities to be estimated; and (ii) each of the possible parents has a unique multilocus genotype. A maximum-likelihood solution is obtained using one of several available iterative algorithms (Roeder *et al.* 1989; Smouse & Meagher 1994), and statistical tests can then be employed to investigate those factors that might cause variation in the fertility estimates (Snow & Lewis 1993; Smouse & Meagher 1994; Conner *et al.* 1996).

The maximum-likelihood model of Roeder *et al.* (1989) has recently been extended by JD Nason (see example in Schnabel *et al.* 1998) to the maximum-likelihood estimation of maternal fertilities from genotypic data on dispersed seeds and seedlings. This approach to inferring maternity is appropriate when a model of random mating can be assumed in the population, and it can be used to identify maternal half-sib family groups, to estimate realized seed dispersal distances and effective population sizes, and to test hypotheses concerning relationships between female fertility and factors such as spatial location, plant size or age, and reproductive effort. In populations where determination of progeny age is possible, maternity analysis can also generate estimates of individual female fertility for progeny cohorts of successive age, thereby allowing near lifetime estimates of female fertility for long-lived plants and tests of variability in female fertility over time (Schnabel *et al.* 1998).

5. Practical considerations in parentage studies

Several factors need to be considered prior to beginning any parentage analysis. First, even more so than with mating system analyses, the accuracy of parentage inference will depend on the amount of available genetic variation in the study populations, which will affect the exclusion probability, or the probability that a randomly chosen adult will be excluded as the parent of an offspring. In general, exclusion probabilities increase with increasing numbers of loci assayed, numbers of alleles per locus, and evenness of allele frequencies at a given locus (Chakraborty *et al.* 1988; Brown *et al.* 1989), and are higher for a set of markers with codominant inheritance, such as allozymes or microsatellites, than for a comparable set of dominant markers (Snow & Lewis 1993), such as RAPDs or AFLPs.

Most published parentage studies to date have used allozyme markers, which at best typically provide 10-20 polymorphic loci with 2-3 alleles/locus and allele frequencies at each locus that are often highly skewed in favour of one common allele (*e.g.* Ellstrand & Marshall 1985; Meagher 1986; Schnabel & Hamrick 1995). Other more recently developed molecular markers, however, offer considerably greater levels of variation. Among these newer markers, microsatellites and AFLPs appear to offer the greatest potential for parentage analyses. Although the development of microsatellites can be very time consuming and often results in only a small number of scorable loci (*e.g.* Dow *et al.* 1995; Chase *et al.* 1996a; Aldrich *et al.* 1998), the small number of studies published to date appears to indicate that each locus may have many alleles within a population, thereby resulting in extremely high exclusion probabilities (Chase *et al.* 1996b; Dow & Ashley 1996, 1997). At nearly the opposite end of the spectrum, AFLPs are very easily developed and often result in more than 100 reliably scorable loci (Vos *et al.* 1995; Lin *et al.* 1996; L. Rieseberg, personal communication). Unfortunately, AFLP markers, like the much less reliable RAPD markers, exhibit dominant/recessive inheritance, which precludes the identification of heterozygotes and greatly lowers the exclusion power of each individual locus (Snow & Lewis 1993). Thus, dominant markers will probably be useful only in paternity studies (Lewis & Snow 1992; Milligan & McMurry 1993), whereas allozymes and microsatellites will be applicable also to parentage analyses on dispersed progeny.

Second, even for species with high genetic variability and high probabilities of exclusion, the ability to detect gene flow events and accurately assess relative fertilities becomes increasingly limited as the number of potential parents increases. The main reason for this is that as the number of parents increases, so too does the probability that two or more parents will be able to produce the same gametic genotype or will actually share the same diploid genotype. Thus, in populations with many hundreds of possible parents, even very strong genetic data that result in exclusion probabilities as high as 99% will rarely be able to assign unique parentage to the majority of progeny or detect the majority of gene flow events. Most parentage analyses, and especially exclusion studies, have therefore typically been confined to fairly small populations of fewer than 100 possible parents (*e.g.* Devlin *et al.* 1992, Kohn & Casper 1992). Studies sites must therefore be carefully chosen to balance the strength of the genetic data with the spatial scale of interest (*e.g.* Adams & Birkes 1991; Campbell 1991). Finally, for any gene flow study, it is important to know the distance of the target population from potential sources of immigrants, and for species that are more or less continuously distributed over space, it is also useful to know the average density of individuals across the landscape. For example, with information on both distances to pollen sources and densities of fig trees within continuous tropical forest, Nason *et al.* (1998) were able to use full-sib paternity exclusion to determine that the size of the effective breeding units for some neotropical fig species can be as much as tens to hundreds of km^2.

6. Future directions in the use of parentage analysis

Ever since it was proposed as a means of studying plant breeding biology (Ellstrand 1984; Ellstrand & Marshall 1985; Hamrick & Schnabel 1985; Meagher 1986), parentage analysis has proven to be the best method for obtaining direct, quantitative estimates of gene flow and relative fertilities in natural and artificial populations. As discussed in previous sections of this chapter, both technical and theoretical advances have now overcome some of the original limitations presented by simple exclusion analysis and by the original likelihood models of Meagher & Thompson (1986, 1987). For example, although allozymes were originally the genetic markers of choice for paternity analysis, and are still widely used (*e.g.* Stacy *et al.* 1996; Emms *et al.* 1997; Goodell *et al.* 1997; Nason *et al.* 1998), newer molecular markers, especially microsatellites and AFLPs, provide the opportunity to conduct parentage studies in species for which allozyme variability is low or for which collection of live tissue is difficult (Parker *et al.* 1998). Among the newer types of genetic markers, microsatellite loci appear to have the greatest potential, because they exhibit codominant inheritance and often have large numbers of alleles within a single population (*e.g.* Dow & Ashley 1996, 1998; Chase *et al.* 1996b; Dayanandan *et al.* 1997; Aldrich *et al.* 1998). The increased use of these powerful molecular markers will certainly allow expanded application of paternity analyses to larger populations than was previously possible and of parent-pair and maternity analyses on dispersed progeny.

Accompanying the discovery of newer, and potentially more informative, molecular markers has been the development of sophisticated likelihood methods for analysing parentage data. Likelihood models are necessary for the proper analysis of parentage data, because unique assignment of parentage for all progeny is never possible in a natural population, even with very high exclusion probabilities, and some degree of uncertainty will therefore always be introduced into the results (*e.g.* Chase *et al.* 1996b; Dow & Ashley 1997). At present, the most widely applicable likelihood models are those of Devlin & Ellstrand (1990) for the estimation of total gene flow (cryptic + apparent) and of Roeder *et al.* (1989) for the estimation of individual fertilities. Unlike simple exclusion analyses, each of these likelihood methods also estimates the variance in the gene flow or fertility values.

Still undeveloped, however, is a method for simultaneous estimation of gene flow and fertilities from the same set of progeny data. All likelihood models for fertility estimation assume complete population isolation (Meagher 1986; Devlin *et al.* 1988; Roeder *et al.* 1989; Smouse & Meagher 1994; Schnabel *et al.* 1998), but some level of gene flow is nearly always seen in natural populations. For example, Schnabel & Hamrick (1995) used the method of Roeder *et al.* (1989) to investigate the relationship between male fertility variation and intermate distances in the temperate tree species, *Gleditsia triacanthos*, but approximately 25% of the seeds analysed had arisen as a result of pollen immigration and had to be excluded from the fertility analyses. More troublesome, however, was the estimation of an approximately equal number of cryptic gene flow events using methods of Devlin & Ellstrand (1990). By including cryptic gene flow progeny in their fertility analysis, Schnabel & Hamrick (1995) implicitly assumed that the gene flow events were spread randomly among the maternal plants from which progeny were sampled and that there was little variation in the ability to discriminate among potential male parents. It is unknown whether either of these assumptions is valid and more generally how the inclusion of these extra progeny affects the final maximum-likelihood fertility estimates. Some progress in solving this problem has recently been made by JD Nason (discussed briefly in Sork *et al.* 1998), who has modified the basic Roeder *et al.* (1989) method such that nearby populations (sources of immigrant pollen and seeds) are effectively treated as additional possible parents. This approach apparently simultaneously recovers both the correct vector of fertility values and the correct level of total gene flow.

In addition to unanswered methodological questions, several classes of empirical questions concerning dispersal and mating have only begun to take advantage of parentage data or are yet to apply these methods. First, parentage analysis has yet to be used extensively in the study of hybrid zones, where estimates of mating systems and reproductive success of parental versus hybrid individuals might be useful in understanding the dynamics of the hybridization process (Rieseberg *et al.* 1998, Rieseberg, this volume). Second, parentage analysis has great potential for assessing the effects of pollinator behaviour on reproduction and dispersal. For example, when a particular species has several different pollinators, experiments could be designed to test the effects of each pollinator on various mating and dispersal parameters (JL Hamrick, personal communication). Similarly, parentage analysis could be used to test for differences in pollen dispersal patterns between two or more species that shared the same pollinator or suite of pollinators. Third, as a recent set of studies has confirmed (*e.g.* Broyles & Wyatt 1995; Karron *et al.* 1995; Conner *et al.* 1996; Emms *et al.* 1997; Goodell *et al.* 1997), parentage analysis is extremely useful in experimental populations where the effects of individual demographic or reproductive traits on fertility and gene flow can be explicitly tested. In many cases, the experimental population can be designed to allow perfect exclusion and exact parentage assignment for all progeny (*e.g.* Karron *et al.* 1995; Emms *et al.* 1997).

Finally, parentage analyses can make substantial contributions to our understanding of the conservation of genetic diversity for species experiencing habitat fragmentation and consequent reductions in population sizes. The rapid fragmentation of once continuous habitats and the destruction of residual migration corridors have raised questions about reduced reproductive success and alterations in dispersal patterns for plant species within the remaining fragments. These questions are important to conservation biologists, because they affect decisions about which fragments might be the most deserving of protection and about how to manage those areas once they are protected.

It is generally unknown whether newly created fragments will become genetically isolated over time, or whether gene flow levels will be sufficiently high to help maintain genetic diversity in the overall metapopulation in the face of reductions in diversity within individual populations due to genetic drift. For example, parentage analysis in *Gleditsia triacanthos* (honey locust) populations (Schnabel *et al.* 1998) revealed that only a small number of female trees were producing most of the progeny in two study sites over periods as long as 20 years. The authors suggested that if such extremely skewed distributions of long-term female reproductive success were common in plant populations, then effective population sizes within small, isolated fragments may be sufficiently reduced to allow relatively rapid losses of genetic variation by genetic drift.

A recent increase in the number of pollen gene flow studies is beginning to address some of these questions in tropical trees (Hamrick & Murawski 1990; Chase *et al.* 1996b; Stacy *et al.* 1996; Nason *et al.* 1996, 1997, 1998; Nason & Hamrick 1997; Aldrich & Hamrick 1998), but many fewer data are available on changes in gene flow patterns for species with other growth forms (*e.g.* vines). Nearly all of the published studies, however, have addressed only one or two years of gene flow, so the question of how fragmentation will affect long-term patterns of gene flow and reproduction within isolated or semi-isolated fragments is still largely unaddressed (Sork *et al.* 1998). At least for long-lived woody species, longer-term patterns might best be addressed in the future by combining ecological studies of seed survival and germination with parentage analyses on naturally established progeny (*e.g.* Dow & Ashley 1996; Schnabel *et al.* 1998, Aldrich & Hamrick 1998). Especially useful might be cases in which age or size cohorts can be identified among seedlings and saplings within a fragment or when fragments of different known ages can be used. As previously discussed, the use highly polymorphic molecular markers will be central to the success of such studies.

Acknowledgements

Discussions with MD Loveless, JD Nason, JL Hamrick, and LH Rieseberg provided several ideas for this chapter. G Carvalho, JL Hamrick and an anonymous reviewer made several useful suggestions for improving an earlier version of the manuscript.

References

Adams WT, Birkes DS (1991) Estimating mating patterns in forest tree populations. In: *Biochemical Markers in the Population Genetics of Forest Trees*, (eds. Fineschi S, Malvolti ME, Cannata F, Hattemer HH), pp. 157-172. SPB Academic Publishing, The Hague.

Adams WT, Griffin AR, Moran GF (1992) Using paternity analysis to measure effective pollen dispersal in plant populations. *American Naturalist*, **140**, 762-780.

Aldrich P, Hamrick JL (1998) Reproductive dominance of pasture trees in a fragmented tropical forest mosaic. *Science*, **281**, 103-105.

Aldrich P, Hamrick JL, Chavarriaga P, Kochert G (1998) Microsatellite analysis of demographic genetic structure in fragmented populations of the tropical tree *Symphonia globulifera*. *Molecular Ecology*, in press.

Arias DM, Rieseberg LH (1994) Gene flow between cultivated and wild sunflowers. *Theoretical and Applied Genetics*, **89**, 655-660.

Bierregaard ROJ, Lovejoy TE, Kapos V, dos Santos AA, Hutchings RW (1992) The biological dynamics of tropical rainforest fragments: a prospective comparison of fragments and continuous forest. *BioScience*, **42**, 859-866.

Brown AHD, Burdon JJ, Jarosz AM (1989) Isozyme analysis of plant mating systems. In: *Isozymes in Plant Biology*, (eds. Soltis DE, Soltis PS), pp. 73-86. Dioscorides Press, Portland, OR.

Broyles SB, Schnabel A, Wyatt R (1994) Evidence for long-distance pollen dispersal in milkweeds (*Asclepias exaltata*). *Evolution*, **48**, 1032-1040.

Broyles SB, Wyatt R (1990) Paternity analysis in a natural population of *Asclepias exaltata*: multiple paternity, functional gender, and the "pollen donation" hypothesis. *Evolution*, **44**, 1454-1468.

Broyles SB, Wyatt R (1991) Effective pollen dispersal in a natural population of *Asclepias exaltata*: the influence of pollinator behavior, genetic similarity, and mating success. *American Naturalist*, **138**, 1239-1249.

Broyles SB, Wyatt R (1995) A reexamination of the pollen-donation hypothesis in an experimental population of *Asclepias exaltata*. *Evolution*, **49**, 89-99.

Campbell DR (1991) Comparing pollen dispersal and gene flow in natural population. *Evolution*, **45**, 1965-1968.

Chakraborty R, Meagher T, Smouse PE (1988) Parentage analysis with genetic markers in natural populations. I. The expected proportion of offspring with unambiguous paternity. *Genetics*, **118**, 527-536.

Chase M, Kesseli R, Bawa K (1996a) Microsatellite markers for population and conservation genetics of tropical trees. *American Journal of Botany*, **83**, 51-57.

Chase M, Moller C, Kesseli R, Bawa K (1996b) Distant gene flow in tropical plants. *Nature*, **383**, 398-399.

Clegg MT (1980) Measuring plant mating systems. *BioScience*, **30**, 814-818.

Conner JK, Rush S, Kercher S, Jennetten P (1996) Measurements of natural selection on floral traits in wild radish (*Raphanus raphanistrum*) II. Selection through lifetime male and total fitness. *Evolution*, **50**, 1137-1146.

Cruzan MB (1998) Genetic markers in plant evolutionary ecology. *Ecology*, **79**, 400-412.

Dayanandan S, Bawa KS, Kesseli R (1997) Conservation of microsatellites among tropical trees (Leguminosae). *American Journal of Botany*, **84**, 1658-1663.

Devlin B, Clegg J, Ellstrand NC (1992) The effect of flower production on male reproductive success in wild radish populations. *Evolution*, **46**, 1030-1042.

Devlin B, Ellstrand NC (1990a) The development and application of a refined method for estimating gene flow from angiosperm paternity analysis. *Evolution*, **44**, 248-259.

Devlin B, Ellstrand NC (1990b) Male and female fertility variation in wild radish, a hermaphordite. *American Naturalist*, **136**, 86-107.

Devlin B, Roeder K, Ellstrand NC (1988) Fractional paternity assignment, theoretical development and comparison to other methods. *Theoretical and Applied Genetics*, **76**, 369-380.

Dow BD, Ashley MV, Howe HF (1995) Characterization of highly variable (GA/CT)n microsatellites in the bur oak, *Quercus macrocarpa. Theoretical and Applied Genetics*, **91**, 137-141.

Dow BD, Ashley MV (1996) Microsatellite analysis of seed dispersal and parentage of saplings in bur oak, *Quercus macrocarpa. Molecular Ecology*, **5**, 615-627.

Dow BD, Ashley MV (1997) Factors influencing male mating success in bur oak, *Quercus macrocarpa. New Forests*, **6**, 1-21.

Dow BD, Ashley MV (1998) High levels of gene flow in bur oak revealed by paternity analysis using microsatellites. *Journal of Heredity*, **89**, 62-70.

Ellstrand NC (1984) Multiple paternity within fruits of the wild radish, *Raphanus sativus. American Naturalist*, **123**, 819-828.

Ellstrand NC, Marshall DL (1985) Interpopulation gene flow by pollen in wild radish, *Raphanus sativus. American Naturalist*, **126**, 606-616.

Ellstrand NC, Devlin B, Marshall DL (1989) Gene flow by pollen into small populations, data from experimental and natural stands of wild radish. *Proceedings of the National Academy of Sciences, USA*, **86**, 9044-9047.

Emms SK, Stratton DA, Snow AA (1997) The effect of inflorescence size on male fitness: experimental tests in the andromonoecious lily, *Zigadenus paniculatus. Evolution*, **5**, 1481-1489.

Endler JA (1977) *Geographic Variation, Speciation, and Clines*. Princeton University Press, Princeton.

Fenster CB (1991a) Gene flow in *Chamaecrista fasciculata* (Leguminosae) I. Gene dispersal. *Evolution*, **45**, 398-409.

Fenster CB (1991b) Gene flow in *Chamaecrista fasciculata* (Leguminosae) II. Gene establishment. *Evolution*, **45**, 410-422.

Godt MJW, Hamrick JL (1993) Patterns and levels of pollen-mediated gene flow in *Lathyrus latifolius. Evolution*, **47**, 98-110.

Goodell K, Elam DR, Nason JD, Ellstrand NC (1997) Gene flow among small populations of a self-incompatible plant: an interaction between demography and genetics. *American Journal of Botany*, **84**, 1362-1371.

Hamrick JL, Murawski D (1990) The breeding structure of tropical tree populations. *Plant Species Biology*, **5**, 157-165.

Hamrick JL, Schnabel A (1985) Understanding the genetic structure of plant populations: some old problems and a new approach. In: *Lecture Notes in Biometrics 60. Population Genetics in Forestry*, (ed. Gregorious HR), pp. 50-70. Springer Verlag, Berlin.

Handel SN (1983) Pollination ecology, plant population structure, and gene flow. In: *Pollination Biology*, (ed. Real L), pp. 163-211. Academic Press, New York.

Karron JD, Thumser NN, Tucker R, Hessenauer AJ (1995) The influence of population density on outcrossing rates in *Mimulus ringens. Heredity*, **75**, 175-180.

Karron JD, Tucker R, Thumser NN, and Reinartz JA (1995) Comparison of pollinator flight movements and gene dispersal patterns in *Mimulus ringens. Heredity*, **75**, 612-617.

Kohn JR, Casper BB (1992) Pollen-mediated gene flow in *Cucurbita foetidissima* (Cucurbitaceae). *American Journal of Botany*, **79**, 57-62.

Levin DA, Kerster HW (1974) Gene flow in seed plants. *Evolutionary Biology*, **7**, 139-220.

Levin DA (1981) Dispersal versus gene flow in plants. *Annals of the Missouri Botanical Garden*, **68**, 233-253.

Levin DA (1995) Plant outliers: an ecogenetic perspective. *American Naturalist*, **145**, 109-118.

Lewis PO, Snow AA (1992) Deterministic paternity exclusion using RAPD markers. *Molecular Ecology*, **1**, 155-160.

Lin JJ, Kuo J, Matthews BF (1996) Identification of molecular markers in soybean comparing RFLP, RAPD, and AFLP DNA mapping techniques. *Plant Molecular Biology Reporter*, **14**, 156-169.

Loveless MD, Hamrick JL, Foster RB (1998) Population structure and mating system of *Tachigali versicolor*, a monocarpic neotropical tree. *Heredity*, in press.

Meagher TR (1986) Analysis of paternity within a natural population of *Chamaelirium luteum*. I. Identification of most-likely male parents. *American Naturalist*, **128**, 199-215.

Meagher TR (1991) Analysis of paternity within a natural population of *Camaelirium luteum*. II. Male reproductive success. *American Naturalist*, **137**, 738-752.

Meagher TR, Thompson E (1986) The relationship between single parent and parent pair genetic likelihoods in genealogy reconstruction. *Theoretical Population Biology*, **29**, 87-106.

Meagher TR, Thompson E (1987) Analysis of parentage for naturally established seedlings of *Chamaelirium luteum* (Liliaceae). *Ecology*, **68**, 803-812.

Milligan BG, McMurry KC (1993) Dominant vs. codominant genetic markers in the estimation of male mating success. *Molecular Ecology*, **2**, 275-283.

Muona O, Moran GF, Bell JC (1991) Hierarchical patterns of correlated matings in *Acacia melanoxylon*. *Genetics*, **127**, 619-626.

Nason JD, Aldrich PR, Hamrick JL (1997) Dispersal and the dynamics of genetic structure in fragmented tropical tree populations. In: *Tropical Forest Remnants: Ecology, Management, and Conservation of Fragmented Communities* (eds. Laurance WF, Bierregaard JRO), in press. The University of Chicago Press, Chicago.

Nason JD, Hamrick JL (1997) Reproductive and genetic consequences of forest fragmentation: two studies of neotropical canopy trees. *The Journal of Heredity*, **88**, 264-276.

Nason JD, Herre EA, Hamrick JL (1996) Paternity analysis of the breeding structure of strangler fig populations: evidence for substantial long-distance wasp dispersal. *Journal of Biogeography*, **23**, 501-512.

Nason JD, Herre EA, Hamrick JL (1998) The breeding structure of a tropical keystone plant resource. *Nature*, **391**, 685-687.

Parker PG, Snow AA, Schug MD, Booton GC, Fuerst PA (1998) What molecules can tell us about populations: choosing and using a molecular marker. *Ecology*, **79**, 361-382.

Pellmyr O, Massey LK, Hamrick JL, Feist MA (1997) Genetic consequences of specialization: yucca moth behavior and self-pollination in yuccas. *Oecologia*, **109**, 273-290.

Rieseberg LH, Baird SJE, Desrochers AM (1998) Patterns of mating in wild sunflower hybrid zones. *Evolution*, **52**, 713-726.

Ritland K (1983) Estimation of mating systems. In: *Isozymes in Plant Breeding and Genetics , Part A*, (eds. S D Tanksley, T J Orton), pp. 289-302. Elsevier, Amsterdam.

Ritland K (1984) The effective proportion of self-fertilization with consanguineous matings in inbred populations. *Genetics*, **106**, 139-152.

Ritland K (1986) Joint maximum likelihood estimation of genetic and mating structure using open-pollinated progenies. *Biometrics*, **42**, 25-53.

Ritland K (1990) A series of FORTRAN computer programs for estimating plant mating systems. *Journal of Heredity*, **81**, 235-237.

Ritland K, Jain SK (1981) A model for the estimation of outcrossing rate and gene frequencies using n independent loci. *Heredity*, **47**, 35-52.

Roeder K, Devlin B, Lindsay BG (1989) Application of maximum likelihood methods to population genetic data for the estimation of individual fertilities. *Biometrics*, **45**, 363-379.

Schnabel A, Hamrick JL (1995) Understanding the population genetic structure of *Gleditsia triacanthos* L.: The scale and pattern of pollen gene flow. *Evolution*, **49**, 921-931.

Schnabel A, Nason JD, Hamrick JL (1998) Understanding the population genetic structure of *Gleditsia triacanthos* L.: seed dispersal and variation in female reproductive success. *Molecular Ecology*, in press.

Shaw DV, Brown AHD (1982) Optimum number of marker loci for estimating outcrossing in plant populations. *Theoretical and Applied Genetics*, **61**, 321-325.

Shaw DV, Kahler AL, Allard RW (1981) A multilocus estimator of mating system parameters in plant populations. *Proceedings of the National Academy of Sciences USA*, **78**, 1298-1302.

Smouse PE, Meagher TR (1994) Genetic analysis of male reproductive contributions in *Chamaelirium luteum* (L.) Gray (Lileaceae). *Genetics*, **136**, 313-322.

Snow AA, Lewis PO (1993) Reproductive traits and male fertility in plants: empirical approaches. *Annual Review of Ecology and Systematics*, **24**, 331-351.

Sork VL, Campbell D, Dyer R, *et al.* (1998) *Proceedings from a Workshop on Gene Flow in Fragmented, Managed, and Continuous Populations. National Center for Ecological Analysis and Synthesis, Santa Barbara, CA. Research Paper No.3.* Available at "http://www.nceas.ucsb.edu/papers/ geneflow/"

Stacy EA, Hamrick JL, Nason JD, Hubbell SP, Foster RB, Condit R (1996) Pollen dispersal in low-density populations of three neotropical tree species. *American Naturalist*, **148**, 275-298.

Vos P, Hogers R, Bleeker M *et al.* (1995) AFLP: a new technique for DNA fingerprinting. *Nucleic Acids Research*, **23**, 4407-4415.

Advances in Molecular Ecology
G.R. Carvalho (Ed.)
IOS Press, 1998

Population Identification in Pelagic Fish: the Limits of Molecular Markers

Lorenz Hauser[1] and Robert D. Ward[2]

[1]*Molecular Ecology and Fisheries Genetics Laboratory, Department of Biological Sciences, University of Hull, Hull HU6 7RX, U.K.*
e-mail: l.hauser@biosci.hull.ac.uk

[2]*CSIRO Marine Research, GPO Box 1538, Hobart, Tasmania 7001, Australia*
e-mail: bob.ward@marine.csiro.au

Pelagic fish dominate the world's fisheries, constituting one of the few major food sources harvested from wild populations. The management of this resource is thus of prime importance, though basic biological information, especially relating to population structure, is often lacking. Molecular markers have been applied extensively to the identification of self-recruiting populations, though few studies have provided the clear-cut information desired by management bodies. Such misunderstanding between managers and molecular biologists arises primarily from their different interests: while managers are primarily concerned with essentially self-recruiting populations as management units, which may have considerable exchange with other such units, molecular biologists can only identify relatively isolated populations with very restricted gene flow. Pertinent ecological features of pelagic fish, such as large population sizes and high migration rates, however, lead to expectations of low genetic differentiation among even relatively isolated populations, and are confirmed here by a compilation of molecular data from large (tunas, billfish) and small (mostly clupeoid) pelagic fish. In contrast, within-population genetic variability is typically far smaller than expected from census population sizes, probably due to high demographic instability and biased reproductive success in many species. A comparison of the suitability of allozymes, mitochondrial DNA (mtDNA) and microsatellites for the identification of pelagic fish populations suggests that allozymes and microsatellites are more powerful than mtDNA RFLP studies. Microsatellite data are currently scarce for pelagic fish; data suggest, however, that they are more likely to reveal significant differentiation among closely related populations than allozymes, even though F_{ST} values may be similar or lower.

1. Introduction

Much has been heard recently of the plight of world fisheries, and of the limits of a resource once believed to be infinite. The widely publicised collapse of well-known stocks, such as Peruvian anchoveta, North Sea herring and Newfoundland cod (Beverton 1990; FAO 1993), are only a few examples illustrating a general trend of depletion in the world's fisheries. It has been estimated that 70% of fish stocks require urgent intervention to prevent over-exploitation and allow the recovery of overfished populations (Garcia & Newton 1997; Garcia & Grainger 1997). Furthermore, landings in the last few decades have shifted significantly from large piscivorous fishes to less valuable smaller planktivorous fishes and invertebrates, possibly reflecting changes in marine food webs (Pauly *et al.* 1998). While optimistic fisheries experts estimate that the world's annual sustainable catch may stabilise at around 100 million metric tons (mt), 10 million mt above the current annual yield, they also stress that to reach this goal more appropriate means of fisheries management and environmental protection have to be achieved (McGoodwin 1990). There is a clear need for improved fisheries management, based on sound advice from a range of different economic, social and scientific disciplines.

Molecular methods can be extremely powerful tools in fisheries management by enabling the identification of relatively isolated populations which will react independently to exploitation and may differ in the parameters used in fishery models (*e.g.* growth, mortality, recruitment). The potential of molecular analysis has resulted in the search for the 'holy grail' of the perfect stock marker by eagerly embracing each new technical development (Ferguson 1994), often without the necessary consideration of the ecology of the species and the pertinent features of its environment. Furthermore, there have often been substantial discrepancies between the questions asked by fishery managers (who primarily want the identification of self-recruiting stocks) and the results delivered by molecular ecologists (who can identify genetically differentiated and more or less reproductively isolated populations) (Carvalho & Hauser 1994). Such misunderstandings often result in dissatisfied fishery managers, who may consequently disregard molecular data and thus be unaware of the valuable insights into the population dynamics of exploited fish resulting from molecular studies.

Pelagic fish dominate the world's fisheries, making up 12 of the top 15 marine fisheries by tonnage (Table 1). Most of these are small clupeoids inhabiting coastal waters, some of which (including the two top species) are harvested mainly for agricultural feed, while the skipjack and yellowfin tunas are oceanic epipelagic species used for human consumption. Considering the importance of pelagic fish, surprisingly little is known about their ecology, in particular regarding the temporal and spatial dynamics of populations, the effects of hydrographic features on their distribution, and indeed their population structure. Nevertheless, there is a plethora of molecular studies, few with the clear-cut information on population structure desired by management bodies, but many with important insights in population dynamics and evolution.

Table 1: Nominal catches for the 15 principal marine fish species in 1995. mt: metric tonnes (FAO 1997).

Rank	Species		Ecotype	mt x 10^6
1	Peruvian anchovy	*Engraulis ringens*	coastal pelagic	8.64
2	Chilean jack mackerel	*Trachurus murphyi*	coastal pelagic	4.96
3	Alaskan pollock	*Theragra chalcogramma*	demersal / semi-pelagic	4.69
4	Atlantic herring	*Clupea harengus*	coastal pelagic	2.33
5	Skipjack tuna	*Katsuwonus pelamis*	epipelagic	1.56
6	Chub mackerel	*Scomber japonicus*	epi-mesopelagic	1.56
7	South American pilchard	*Sardinops sagax*	coastal pelagic	1.50
8	Atlantic cod	*Gadus morhua*	demersal	1.26
9	Largehead hairtail	*Trichiurus lepturus*	demersal	1.24
10	European pilchard	*Sardina pilchardus*	coastal pelagic	1.21
11	Yellowfin tuna	*Thunnus albacares*	epipelagic	1.05
12	Japanese anchovy	*Engraulis japonicus*	coastal pelagic	0.97
13	Atlantic mackerel	*Scomber scombrus*	coastal pelagic	0.79
14	Capelin	*Mallotus villotus*	coastal pelagic	0.75
15	Japanese pilchard	*Sardinops melanostictus*	coastal pelagic	0.73

In this paper, we will address three major points concerning genetics and pelagic fish management:

1. Genetic population structure and the definition of units for fisheries management: Are genetically differentiated populations (the geneticist's unit) and essentially self-recruiting fish stocks (the fishery manager's unit) the same? If not, how do they differ and how does any difference affect the interpretation of molecular data?

2. Ecological factors affecting patterns of genetic diversity in pelagic fish: How do demographic and ecological factors affect the genetic structure of pelagic species?

3. Molecular approaches to the identification of pelagic fish populations: Has the application of molecular markers helped to clarify the population structure of pelagic fish? Are some molecular markers more suitable than others?

2. Genetic population structure and the definition of units for fisheries management

The idea that species should be managed at some subspecific level can be traced back to the turn of the century, when two pioneering fishery biologists, F. Heincke and J. Hjort, established that the preferred unit of study for fisheries management should be the local self-sustaining population rather than the typological species (Sinclair 1988; Carvalho & Hauser 1994). Despite the long-standing notion of subspecific fishery units, there is no universally applicable definition of the term "stock". In fact, there is a wide range of stock definitions, depending on who is defining, and why (Carvalho & Hauser 1994). Often, stocks are defined by managers as a group of fish exploited in a specific area or by a specific method ("fishery stock", Smith *et al.* 1990). Though this definition may facilitate the collection of catch and effort data, and the application of management measures, it does not necessarily represent the true substructuring of fish species. To overcome this problem, various biological stock definitions have been put forward. A good working definition is that of Ihssen *et al.* (1981): "a stock is an intraspecific group of randomly mating individuals with temporal and spatial integrity". This concept covers many of the definitions given by other authors; the aspect which varies is the degree of spatial and temporal integrity.

"Harvest stocks" may be defined as "locally accessible fish resources in which fishing pressure on one resource has no effect on the abundance of fish in another contiguous resource" (Gauldie 1988). In contrast to most stock definitions, this concept does not imply any genetic or phenotypic differences between stocks. It only describes a group of individuals whose abundance depends to a very much larger degree on recruitment and mortality (especially that caused by fishing) than on immigration and emigration. There may be sufficient exchange with other groups to prevent the development of biological differences. For example, two stocks of yellowtail flounder (*Limanda ferruginea*), with an estimated exchange rate of about 10 % and presumably genetically homogeneous for neutral markers, reacted independently to exploitation (Brown *et al.* 1987).

On the other extreme of the continuum of stock integrity is the "genetic stock", defined as "a reproductively isolated unit, which is genetically different from other stocks" (Jamieson 1973; Ovenden 1990). In this definition, the degree of integrity is very high, as often very few migrants are sufficient to prevent the development of detectable genetic differentiation between conspecific stocks (Gyllensten 1985; Waples 1987; Ward *et al.* 1994).

These two interpretations of the definition by Ihssen *et al.* (1981), the harvest and the genetic stock, represent respectively the units that fishery managers are interested in and the populations that molecular geneticists are able to identify. Clearly, the level of exchange among populations differs considerably in these two definitions, highlighting the major limitation of molecular markers, that is their high sensitivity to low levels of gene flow among populations (Carvalho & Hauser 1994). Gene flow rates of a few individuals per generation would mean that populations cannot be distinguished genetically and would appear to be panmictic, yet for fisheries management an exchange of up to 10% between populations may justify treatment as separate stocks. Thus results are only of practical value for the management if differences are detected, and increasingly sophisticated molecular markers are being employed in attempts to detect genetic differentiation. Nevertheless, even with the most sensitive molecular markers, the discrepancy in gene flow levels between a harvest stock and a genetic stock still exists, and molecular markers alone may not suffice to identify populations with small degrees of isolation. The integration of molecular data with results from phenotypic markers such as morphometrics, parasites, otolith microchemistry and population parameters, as well as with information on the ecology of the species, its demography and migrations, and oceanographic features will provide more powerful insights into the population structure of exploited fish species than any one technique alone.

3. Ecological factors affecting patterns of genetic diversity in pelagic fish

In this section we seek to review the major ecological attributes of pelagic fish and indicate how these attributes might be related to levels of genetic variation both within and between populations (Fig. 1). Pelagic fish occupy open coastal and/or oceanic waters, with few discernable physical barriers to gene flow, and are frequently extremely good swimmers that may migrate long distances. In these respects they differ from many demersal or benthic species, which might be restricted to particular depth ranges and are unable, at least as adults, to cross deep water; demersal fish are often less active swimmers, and often have more localised distributions. Pelagic fish also typically have very large population sizes, although these are frequently characterised by pronounced short-term and long-term instabilities. Schooling is another common attribute of pelagic fish which may

Figure 1: Environmental (Env.), ecological (Ecology) and genetic (Genetics) factors affecting the evolution of genetic differentiation in pelagic fish. Arrows denote effects, which can be positive or negative. See text for details.

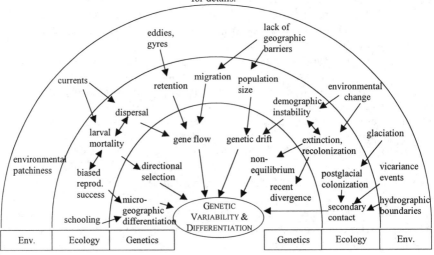

impact on genetic population structure. Finally, most pelagic fish are highly fecund and mortality rates are high, arguably allowing selection to have a greater role in shaping genetic structure than in less fecund k-selected species. Of course some of these attributes also hold for other classes of fish, but generally to a lesser degree.

It seems clear that pelagic fish typically show less genetic differentiation among populations than other classes of fish. For example, the mean F_{ST} for allozymes is 0.026 in small pelagics (17 cases, 10 species, Table 2) and 0.009 in within-ocean comparisons of the large pelagic species (4 cases and species, Table 3), compared to 0.062 in marine fish generally (57 species), 0.108 in anadromous fish (7 species) and 0.222 in freshwater fish (49 species) (Ward et al. 1994). Such low differentiation probably reflects some of the features listed above, and consideration of these factors may help us to understand the evolution of genetic differentiation in pelagic fish. The integration of ecological and molecular information is thus a crucial, though often neglected, element in the interpretation of genetic variation.

3.1. An open environment

The most important feature of the pelagic habitat in population genetics terms is the lack of obvious geographical barriers to gene flow. Generally, the more fragmented nature of freshwater habitats results in a higher degree of population isolation in freshwater and anadromous species than in marine fish where populations are usually less clearly delineated (Ward et al. 1994). Physical barriers to migration among lakes and rivers often prevent migration and gene flow, leading to the evolution of genetically differentiated and locally adapted populations. In contrast, even largely self-recruiting populations of pelagic fish may exchange sufficient migrants to remain genetically homogenous, and thus are often inseparable with molecular methods.

Despite this lack of physical barriers, hydrographic features in the oceans often represent boundaries and contain fish populations within defined areas (Cushing 1982). Most tunas and billfish are found in tropical and warmer temperate waters, and migration patterns are influenced by temperature tolerances, with food and salinity requirements also influencing movement. Such tolerances are generally lower for spawning and larval survival, and so the geographic ranges suitable for spawning and early development are often narrower than the adult distribution. For example, the lower temperature limit to spawning of swordfish (Xiphias gladius) limits their reproduction to the southern Atlantic and the Mediterranean, even though they migrate much further north in the Atlantic (Kotoulas et al. 1995). Southern bluefin tuna (Thunnus maccoyii) spawn only in warm waters between Java and north-west Australia, yet feeding grounds are in southern waters between 30° and 50°S (Caton 1991). Larval survival often depends on sufficient food availability, with very narrow environmental 'windows' for optimal survival and growth (Pitcher & Hart 1982; Cury & Roy 1989). Such environmental windows can limit the successful recruitment of pelagic fish both spatially and temporally, and thus represent effective hydrographic boundaries to distribution, especially in less migratory small pelagic species.

More subtle hydrographic and ecological boundaries may separate more or less reproductively isolated populations of the same species, though the mechanisms of this separation are poorly understood. For example, two stocks of Mediterranean anchovies (Engraulis encrasicolus) have been identified in the Adriatic by allozyme electrophoresis (Bembo et al. 1996b): one population inhabits the shallow and relatively eutrophic coastal areas in the north and the west of the Adriatic, the other is restricted to the deeper, more oligotrophic central part which is influenced by water exchange with the Ionian Sea. Independent circulatory systems in the north and the south of the Adriatic (Zore-Armanda

Table 2: Heterozygosities and F_{ST} values observed in small pelagic species, together with the geographic area surveyed and the number of samples (N_1) and sample sizes (N_2). The marker used, the number of loci examined (allozymes and microsatellites) or the part of the mtDNA molecule examined by RFLP and the numbers of restriction enzymes used (mtDNA) are shown. All mtDNA studies used RFLP analysis. H_1 = % mean heterozygosity per locus or haplotype diversity (mtDNA), H_2 = range of sample heterozygosities. Allozyme heterozygosities are based on all loci (polymorphic and monomorphic).

Sig: significance of F_{ST}: ns: not significant, *: $P<0.05$, **: $P<0.01$, ***: $P<0.001$. n/a: not available.

Species	Geographic Area	Marker	N_1	N_2	H_1	H_2	F_{ST}	sig	Ref.
Atlantic herring *Clupea harengus*	North Sea, Baltic, Celtic, Norway, Barents	allozymes (27)	10	25-50	5.4	4.6-7.7	0.049	***	a
	W & E Atlantic	allozymes (40)	6	40-56	6.5	6.2-6.8	0.004	ns	b
	Norway, Baltic	allozymes (17)	17	30-100	8.6	7.8-9.2	0.001	*	c
	North Sea, Irish Sea, Baltic, Celtic, NE Atlantic	allozymes (27)	27	23-100	4.5	4.2-5.0	0.002	ns	d
	North Sea, Baltic, Celtic, Norway, W Atlantic	allozymes (6)	28	40-255	n/a	n/a	0.163	***	e
	as above, but excluding Norwegian fjords	allozymes (6)	21	40-159	n/a	n/a	0.001	***	e
	North Sea, Baltic, Celtic, Norway	mtDNA (ND3/4: 6)	5	50	89	87-92	0.013	**	a
	North Sea, Baltic, Celtic, Norway	mtDNA (ND5/6: 6)	5	50	89	84-94	0.004	ns	a
	North Sea, Kattegat	mtDNA (whole: 12)	7	16-38	85	76-93	0.009	ns	f
	NW Atlantic	mtDNA (whole: 16)	4	8-26	91.1	85-96	0.003	ns	g
	Norway, Barents	microsatellites (4)	5	50	90	89-92	0.035	***	h
Pacific herring *Clupea pallasi*	North Pacific, Bering Sea	allozymes (40)	18	21-100	8.3	6.7-10	0.007	**	i
	North Pacific Bering Sea	microsatellites (5)	7	50	88.9	84-92	0.036	***	j
European anchovy *Engraulis encrasicolus*	Adriatic, Ionian, Aegean	allozymes (24)	13	40-50	5.8	4.1-8.9	0.034	***	k
	Adriatic, Ionian, Aegean	mtDNA (ND5/6: 6)	7	20	88	79-95	0.016	*	l
Cape anchovy *Engraulis capensis*	South Africa	allozymes (31)	31	n/a	11.5	n/a	0.0015	ns	m
Northern anchovy *Engraulis mordax*	California	allozymes (10)	32	48-120	n/a	n/a	0.006	***	n
Spanish sardine *Sardinella aurita*	W & E Atlantic	allozymes (25)	4	30-99	0.6	0.3-0.9	-0.001	ns	o
	Gulf Mexico, Florida, Brazil	allozymes (41)	6	20-45	2.5	2.5	0.026	***	p
	Gulf Mexico, Florida, Brazil	mtDNA (whole: 10)	2	28-29	77	77	0.059	***	q
Med. sardines *Sardina pilchardus*	W Mediterranean	allozymes (15)	10	35-68	13.0	11-16	0.074	**	r
	NE Mediterranean	allozymes (22)	9	30-50	3.0	2-4	0.022	***	s
	NE Mediterranean	mtDNA (ND3/4: 6)	6	16-19	78.2	70-85	0.000	ns	s
Jack mackerel *Trachurus japonicus*	coasts of Japan	allozymes (18)	15	22-50	3.3	2.2-4.5	0.002	ns	t
King mackerel *Scomberomorus cavalla*	W Atlantic Gulf Mexico	allozymes (1)	12	12-57	41.5	2.1-50	0.189	***	u
	W Atlantic Gulf Mexico	mtDNA (whole: 14)	12	31-59	n/a	n/a	-0.013	ns	u
Kapenta *Limnothrissa miodon*	Lake Tanganyika	allozymes (29)	13	21-50	6.6	5.7-7.6	0.006	***	v
	Lake Tanganyika	mtDNA (ND5/6: 6)	9	19-45	88.8	87-96	0.000	ns	v

References: a, Turan 1997; b, Grant 1984; c, Ryman et al. 1984; d, King et al. 1987; e, Jorstad et al. 1991; f, Dahle & Eriksen 1990; g, Kornfield & Bogdanowicz 1987; h, Shaw et al. 1998a; i, Grant & Utter 1984; j, O'Connell et al. 1998; k, Bembo et al. 1996a; l, Bembo et al. 1996b; m, Grant 1985; n, Hedgecock et al. 1994; o, Chikhi et al. 1998; p, Wilson & Alberdi 1991; q, Tringali & Wilson 1993; r, Ramon & Castro 1997; s, Carvalho et al. 1994; t, Kijima et al. 1985; u, Gold et al. 1997; v, Hauser et al. 1998.

Table 3: Extent of genetic diversity among samples within oceans (F_{ST}) in large pelagic species. See Table 2 for further explanation. All mtDNA studies used RFLP analysis. Ocean abbreviations: P=Pacific Ocean, I=Indian Ocean, A=Atlantic Ocean, M=Mediterranean Sea

Species	Ocean	Marker	N_1	N_2	H_1	H_2	F_{ST}	sig	Ref.
Thunnus albacares	P	mtDNA (whole: 12)	5	19-20	84.7	82-86	-0.015	ns	a
	P	mtDNA (whole: 2)	6	40-176	68.0	63-71	0.012	*	b
	P	allozyme (4)	6	39-175	36.0	34-38	0.027	**	b
	P	microsatellites (6)	5-8	34-285	78.3	77-81	0.001	*	c
	I	mtDNA (whole: 2)	2	21,91	71.1	70,73	0.009	ns	b
Thunnus maccoyii	I	mtDNA (whole: 3)	3	179-189	46.6	40-53	0.003	ns	d
	I	allozymes (6)	3	188-214	40.1	40-40	-0.006	ns	d
Thunnus obesus	P	mtDNA (control: 2)	9	62-101	82.3	79-85	0.001	ns	e
	P	mtDNA (control: 3)	2	17,125	49.2	58,40	0.036	ns	f
	P	microsatellites (4)	9	64-103	63.2	62-65	0.001	ns	e
	A	mtDNA (control: 3)	2	41,43	69.7	63,77	0.048	*	f
Thunnus thynnus thynnus	A	allozymes (1)	2	675, 381	46.1	46, 46	-0.001	ns	g
	A	microsatellites (5)	2	16, 44	49.8	48, 50	0.035	ns	h
	M	microsatellites (5)	2	16, 24	51.0	45, 57	0.188	***	h
Katsuwonus pelamis	P	allozymes (4)	6-23	53-1063	n/a	n/a	0.011	**	i
Thunnus alalunga	P	mtDNA (ATPase: 2)	9	31-56	64.1	60-69	-0.006	ns	j
	A	mtDNA (ATPase: 2)	3	34-75	33.4	22-43	0.002	ns	j
Xiphias gladius	P	mtDNA (whole: 8)	3	42-59	64.8	56-75	0.000	ns	k
	P	mtDNA (control: 4)	6	21-53	93.3	92-96	-0.001	ns	l
	I	mtDNA (control: 4)	2	27,35	94.1	92-96	-0.001	ns	l
	A	mtDNA (control: 4)	3	26-59	85.3	80-92	0.023	*	l
	A	mtDNA (control: 3)	6	17-31	61.1	54-68	0.014	ns	m
Makaira nigricans	A	mtDNA (whole: 11)	2	25,31	93.2	90-97	0.002	ns	n
Istiophorus platypterus	A	mtDNA (whole: 12)	2	13,23	68.2	63-74	0.026	ns	n
Tetrapturus albidus	A	mtDNA (whole: 12)	2	17,18	44.7	31,59	0.030	ns	n
Tetrapturus audax	P	mtDNA (whole: 10)	4	36-47	78.7	69-8	0.053	***	o

References

a, Scoles & Graves 1993; b, Ward et al. 1997; c, Ward & Grewe, *unpublished*; d, Grewe et al. 1997; e, Grewe & Hampton 1998; f, Alvarado Bremer et al. 1998; g, Edmunds & Sammons 1973; h, Broughton & Gold, 1997; i, Richardson 1983; j, Chow & Ushiama 1995; k, Grijalva-Chon et al. 1994; l, Chow et al. 1997; m, Alvarado Bremer et al. 1996; n, Graves & McDowell 1995; o, Graves & McDowell 1994.

1969) reinforce such discontinuities, as evidenced by the presence of several endemic fish in northern waters (Tortonese 1983). Similar genetic heterogeneity in relation to hydrographic boundaries was found by mtDNA analysis in both the Adriatic and the Aegean Sea (Magoulas *et al.* 1996). Another hydrographic discontinuity separates genetically differentiated populations of sardine (*Sardina pilchardus*) along the Almerian-Oran front in the Eastern Mediterranean (Ramon & Castro 1997), again supported by independent zoogeographic evidence (Quesada *et al.* 1995; Saavedra *et al.* 1993). The important point of such studies is that it is often insufficient to collect samples from fishing ports without consideration of exact sampling locations and the ecological and hydrographic features of the area. In the above anchovy study, for example, landings from different ports showed no genetic differentiation, as the range of fishing vessels exceeded the distribution of the local stock (DG Bembo, *pers. comm.*), and the existence of the two populations would have remained undetected without a regular, scheduled sampling programme including all major zoogeographic areas of the Adriatic.

3.2. High dispersal abilities

In adaptation to the uniform and vast habitat of the open oceans, most pelagic fish are extremely good swimmers and may migrate long distances. For example, the exchange rate of eastern and western Atlantic bluefin tuna is estimated at about 2-3% per year (Suzuki 1991; National Research Council 1994) and there are instances of trans-Atlantic recoveries of yellowfin tuna tags (ICCAT 1992). Bigeye tuna in the Pacific Ocean have been recorded as moving more than 7000 km in two years, although most movements are within the 2000 km range (Grewe & Hampton 1998). Such extensive migrations, coupled with lifespans of up to 40 years (southern bluefin tuna, J Gunn, *pers. comm.*) indicate extensive geographic ranges of populations, and genetic differentiation may therefore be very limited even on a large geographic scale. Nevertheless, in some species, genetic differentiation may be maintained, presumably by homing to natal areas, despite extensive mixing of feeding populations: swordfish, for example, are known to migrate through the Straits of Gibraltar, but Atlantic and Mediterranean populations still show significantly different mtDNA haplotype frequencies (Kotoulas *et al.* 1995).

Relatively little is known about the migration abilities of small pelagic fish: North Sea herring may swim 900 to 1200 miles on their annual migrations (Cushing 1975), while sprat (*Sprattus sprattus*) only move between deeper offshore water and estuaries in the English Wash (Johnson 1970). Nevertheless, it is the number of migrants among spawning groups which will determine their genetic differentiation. Return rates to spawning grounds in Atlantic herring estimated from tagging studies appear to be high (75-95%, Wheeler & Winters 1984), though tagging of adult fish can only prove repeated use of the same spawning ground rather than homing to natal sites. Indeed, there is increasing evidence for social transmission of migration and homing patterns from adult herring to recruiting juveniles, with varying proportions of migrants between populations (McQuinn 1997). Considering the relatively high straying rates from previous spawning sites estimated from tagging studies (5-25%, Wheeler & Winters 1984), the gene flow caused by such migrants is likely to minimise genetic differentiation at neutral molecular markers. The weak genetic differentiation among populations of small pelagic fish (Table 2) suggests that similar processes determine the population structure of other pelagic fish, with significant gene flow even among populations that may be largely self-recruiting. Thus it may sometimes be impossible to detect genetic differentiation among spawning groups which are demographically independent and should be managed separately, highlighting the need for consideration of ecological data before formulating guidelines for fishery managers.

In addition to such active dispersal by adult fish, pelagic larvae may be transported over great distances, and so provide an efficient means of gene flow among populations. Indeed, inverse relationships between genetic inter-population heterogeneity and dispersal capabilities inferred from larval duration was found in several species of eastern Pacific shorefishes (Waples 1987) as well as in Great Barrier Reef species (Doherty *et al.* 1995). However, such high dispersal potential does not always translate into high gene flow over large areas, as illustrated in a wide range of marine invertebrates with pelagic larvae and significant genetic differentiation among populations (Avise 1994). Oceanographic features such as currents or eddies play an important role in dispersal and retention of pelagic larvae, and may also strongly affect larval mortality. In walleye pollock (*Theragra chalcogramma*), a semi-pelagic gadoid fish, larvae tend to be concentrated in eddies which may contain higher phyto- and zooplankton concentrations and thus better conditions for larval survival (Bailey *et al.* 1997). Such eddies also retain larvae in the coastal areas near the Alaska penninsula, and protect them from drift into the fast westward Alaskan Stream. In contrast, in stormy years larvae are rapidly swept out into the current, where they experience high mortality. Therefore, gene flow between the Gulf of Alaska and the eastern Bering Sea are impeded by geographical barriers (Alaskan peninsula), retention in eddies and high mortality of vagrants, and, indeed, recent mtDNA RFLP and microsatellite studies provided evidence for genetically differentiated stocks in these two areas (Bailey *et al.* 1997). Similar retention within relatively small areas has been reported in Pacific herring (*Clupea pallasi*), with few larvae collected in offshore areas between nursery regions (Hay & McCarter 1997). In some demersal fish on subantarctic islands, retention mechanisms appear to be efficient enough to allow an extended pelagic larval phase despite low fecundity and potential losses of larvae into the rapid West Wind Drift (White 1998). These examples show that dispersal capacity and thus gene flow not only depend on larval duration, but also on local oceanographic conditions and the fate of vagrants.

3.3. Population sizes and demography

The very feature which renders pelagic fish particularly suitable to commercial exploitation, their typically large population sizes, also has important consequences for the distribution of genetic variance within and between populations. Population genetics theory predicts that large populations should maintain high levels of genetic variability at neutral loci, because the loss of genetic diversity due to drift is lower, and so mutations can accumulate over time (Kimura 1983). Furthermore, very large populations are expected to harbour many very rare alleles which would remain undetected in the sample sizes typically employed in molecular studies (Ryman 1993; Ryman *et al.* 1995). In populations in mutation-drift equilibrium, the number of alleles at a selectively neutral locus with a given mutation rate increases disproportionally with population size (Crow & Kimura 1970). For example, populations of 10^2, 10^4, 10^6 and 10^8 are expected to have 1.00, 1.02, 4 and 323 alleles per locus, respectively, assuming a mutation rate of 10^{-7} and an effective population size of half the census number of individuals (Ryman *et al.* 1995). Population crashes to 1% of the original size would then have very different genetic effects, depending on the initial size of the population: while a reduction from 10^4 to 10^2 individuals would result in a loss of only 2 % of alleles, a larger population (10^8 individuals) would lose 99 % of its alleles. For natural populations, the estimates of expected numbers of alleles are probably overestimates because of violations of assumptions such as mutation-drift equilibrium and absence of selection (Nei *et al.* 1975; Nei 1987). The general conclusion still holds, however, that very large populations harbour, and may lose, disproportionally more alleles than small ones. Although the above expectations were formulated for selectively neutral loci, the exposure to a new environment may rapidly increase the adaptive significance of previously neutral alleles. These considerations indicate that population crashes of pelagic fish may have considerable effects on their genetic composition, even though these effects may remain undetected in molecular studies employing conventional sample sizes of 50-100 individuals (Ryman et al. 1995).

In agreement with theoretical expectations based on their large population sizes, many small pelagic fish have relatively high mtDNA haplotype diversities (mean of five species 84.2% (Table 2), compared to 66.8% in nine large pelagics (Table 3), and 49.5% in six salmonid species (Hauser 1996)). At allozyme loci, however, heterozygosity levels are similar to marine fish generally (small pelagic fish: 5.9% (Table 4), compared to 5.3% in large pelagic species (Table 4) and 5.9% in 57 species of marine fish (Ward et al. 1994)). Under neutral expectations, small pelagic species with populations sizes in the billions should have mean heterozygosities of around 99% (Chikhi et al. 1998). One explanation for

Table 4: Heterozygosity estimates for allozyme loci in marine pelagic species. Average species heterozygosity estimates are estimated by averaging values of multiple populations or studies, where available. The average figures for groups are means ± standard error. A table of most of the clupeids is given in Chikhi et al. 1998.

Group	Species	Loci	Heterozygosity	Ref.
Small pelagics	Sardina pilchardus	15-22	0.130-0.030	a, b
	Sardinella longiceps	19	0.008	c
	Sardinella aurita	25-41	0.003-0.060	d, e, f
	Sardinella maderensis	18	0.105	g
	Sardinops sagax caerulea	27	0.010	h
	Sardinops melanosticta	22	0.064	i
	Ethmalosa fimbriata	24	0.015	j
	Clupea harengus	25-44	0.040-0.073	k, l, m
	Clupea pallasi	40	0.087	n
	Opisthonema bulleri	29	0.053	o
	Opisthonema libertate	29	0.064	o
	Opisthonema medirastre	29	0.092	o
	Engraulis encrasicolus	24	0.065	p
	Engraulis capensis	31	0.115	q
	Engraulis mordax	38	0.075	h
	Trachurus japonicus	18	0.034	r
	Average of 16 species	26.66±1.70	0.059±0.008	
Large pelagics	Auxis thazard	38	0.038	s
	Euthynnus affinis	38	0.048	s
	Katsuwonus pelamis	38	0.054	s
	Thunnusa thynnus thynnus	38	0.049	s
	Thunnus alalunga	38	0.068	s
	Thunnus maccoyii	38	0.065	s
	Thunnus albacares	38	0.063	s
	Thunnus obesus	38	0.068	s
	Xiphias gladius	26	0.018	t
	Makaira nigricans	35	0.061	u
	Average of 10 species	36.50±1.20	0.053±0.005	
All pelagics	Average of 26 species	30.37±1.49	0.057±0.005	

References
a, Ramon & Castro 1997; b, Carvalho et al. 1994; c, Menezes 1994; d, Chikhi et al. 1998; e, Wilson & Alberdi 1991; Kinsey et al. 1994; g, Chikhi et al. unpublished; h, Hedgecock et al. 1989; i, Fujio & Kato 1979; j, Gourene et al. 1993; k, Kornfield et al. 1982; l, Grant 1986; m, Andersson et al. 1981; n, Grant & Utter 1984; o, Hedgecock et al. 1988; p, Bembo et al. 1996a; q, Grant 1985; r, Kijima et al. 1985; s, Elliott & Ward 1995; t, Grijalva-Chon et al. 1996; u, Shaklee et al. 1983.

this discrepancy is that populations are unlikely to have reached mutation-drift equilibrium since the last major climatic change (Nei & Grauer 1984; Bowen & Grant 1997). The time required to reach equilibrium is approximately the reciprocal of the mutation rate (Nei *et al.* 1975), and for slowly mutating allozyme loci it may take millions of years to attain equilibrium diversity values (Chikhi *et al.* 1998). New alleles increase in frequency by genetic drift, and so the increase in heterozygosity after a bottleneck is slower in large populations than in small ones (Maruyama & Fuerst 1984). Expanding populations are expected to show an excess of rare alleles (Maruyama & Fuerst 1984) and 'star phylogenies' of mtDNA sequences, with clusters of very closely related haplotypes and large divergences among clusters (Rogers & Harpending 1992; Rogers 1995). Excess of rare allozyme alleles and 'star phylogenies' have been empirically demonstrated in several pelagic species (Magoulas *et al.* 1996; Grant & Leslie 1996; Bowen & Grant 1997; see Grant & Bowen 1998 for a review), supporting the notion that indeed many pelagic populations may not yet have reached equilibrium heterozygosities for allozyme loci. In contrast, the higher mutation rate and smaller effective population size (Birky *et al.* 1989) of mtDNA would reduce the time required to attain equilibrium haplotype diversities considerably, even though mtDNA is expected to lose more variability in population bottlenecks than nuclear markers. It seems unlikely, however, that allozyme heterozygosities so much lower than expected from population sizes reflect only population fluctuations on a geological time scale, as population bottlenecks would have had to be very small or very long (Chikhi *et al.* 1998).

Superimposed on geological time-scale fluctuations is the high short-term demographic instability of many small pelagic fish. Often these fluctuations are attributed exclusively to fishing pressure (Blaxter & Hunter 1982), but there is increasing evidence that the instability of coastal pelagic fish populations is a natural phenomenon (Cury 1993), perhaps an adaptation to spatially and temporally fluctuating hydrographic conditions and productivity (Lowe-McConnell 1987). Scale counts in anaerobic sediments (Baumgartner *et al.* 1992; deVries & Pearcy 1982; Shackelton 1986) have revealed large fluctuations in population size in many small pelagic fish with no apparent regularity (Cury 1993). Such population fluctuations would reduce the long-term effective population size considerably and thus reduce the genetic variability maintained in populations, even if each population 'crash' has relatively little effect (Hedgecock *et al.* 1989).

In addition to fluctuations on geological and ecological time-scales, decreased genetic diversity may be partly due to the high variance in reproductive success of many marine animals (Hedgecock 1994), especially highly fecund species like pelagic fish. Biotic, hydrological and meteorological conditions may affect some cohorts more than others, and minor differences in the timing of spawning may result in large differences in reproductive success among spawners (see also match-mismatch hypothesis, Cushing 1972). After hatching, larvae need to find food within an extremely short period to prevent starvation, and larval survival often depends on the chance encounter of a suitable plankton patch. The generally weak relationship between adult stock and recruitment in many pelagic fish is likely to be one of the ecological consequences of this unpredictable and density-independent reproductive success of spawners (Hedgecock 1994). Genetically, biased reproductive success reduces effective population size and thus genetic variability (Nelson & Soulé 1987), especially in highly fecund pelagic species where relatively few parents could contribute large numbers of offspring to the next generation if their larvae find suitable conditions.

Other explanations for levels of allozyme diversity lower than expected include selection, and artefacts like biased choice of loci and scoring errors (Chikhi *et al.* 1998). While these factors may be important in specific studies, they are unlikely to be a general explanation. It is more likely that the large and unstable populations of pelagic fish are not in mutation-drift equilibrium and therefore that equilibrium models are inappropriate for such species.

More important for the identification and discrimination of essentially self-recruiting populations is the effect of large population size on the evolution of genetic differentiation among isolated groups. Even in the absence of gene flow, large populations will diverge by genetic drift relatively slowly at selectively neutral loci. Furthermore, in semi-isolated populations, it may take millions of generations to reach an equilibrium between genetic drift and gene flow (Palumbi 1996), and only then will genetic differentiation fully reflect the reproductive isolation among extant populations. However, major climatic changes in the Pleistocene have affected marine environments globally, and have significantly altered species distributions (Briggs 1995) and oceanic circulation patterns (Duplessy 1982). The 10,000 years since the last major glaciation may thus have been insufficient for some species to have accumulated detectable genetic differentiation at neutral molecular markers, even if populations were completely isolated after the colonization of their current habitats (Ferguson 1994). The very limited genetic inter-population heterogeneity usually found in pelagic fish may be as much the result of recent population isolation and expansion as high levels of extant gene flow. Such considerations are particularly important where the conservation of genetic diversity is a defined management aim: species which appear genetically homogeneous and thus panmictic may consist of locally adapted populations, as genes under selection would diverge much more rapidly than neutral molecular markers (Ryman *et al.* 1995). Another consequence of the likely non-equilibrium conditions is that estimates of the numbers of migrants (N_em) derived from F_{ST} statistics (where $F_{ST} = 1/(1+4N_e m)$ for nuclear genes, Wright 1943) will be erroneous, as such derivations assume equilibrium between genetic drift and migration.

3.4. Schooling

Notwithstanding the low levels of genetic differentiation observed on a large geographic scale (Section 4), several studies on pelagic fish have detected small but statistically significant genetic differences among samples collected from proximate localities within a short time interval (*e.g.* skipjack tuna, *Katsuwonus pelamis*, Sharp 1978; blueback herring, *Alosa aestivalis*, Smith & Tolliver 1987; blue grenadier, *Macruronus novaezelandiae*, Milton & Shaklee 1987; South African anchovy, *Engraulis capensis*, Grant 1985; jackass morwong, *Cheilodactylus macropterus,* Richardson 1982; northern anchovy, *Engraulis mordax*, Hedgecock *et al.* 1994, Spanish sardine, *Sardinella aurita*, Wilson & Alberdi 1991, Kinsey *et al.* 1994; Lake Tanganyika sardine, *Limnothrissa miodon*, Hauser *et al.* 1998). These differences were variously explained by sampling errors, insufficient sample sizes, selection, the immigration of individuals from unknown and genetically differentiated populations, and microgeographic genetic structure caused by biased reproductive success and schooling behaviour (Hedgecock 1994; Hedgecock *et al.* 1994). Recently, the evidence for genuine microgeographic genetic differentiation is increasing, as studies on fish and marine invertebrates indicate that aggregations of pelagic larvae may be genetically heterogeneous on a very small geographic scale (Campton *et al.* 1992; Ruzzante *et al.* 1997). For this differentiation among larval assemblages to be detectable in schools of adult fish, the exchange among schools would have to be negligible, and schools would have to represent long-term stable groups rather than opportunistic aggregations for the short-term benefit of individual fish (Pitcher & Parrish 1993).

The temporal stability of schools of pelagic fish, however, is uncertain, and there is evidence of extensive mixing of individuals over short time intervals. In skipjack tuna

(*Katsuwonus pelamis*) tagging experiments suggest that complete mixing of schools may take place within months (Bayliff 1988) or even weeks (Hilborn 1991), though schools may consist of smaller, more stable subunits (Hilborn 1991). Similarly, life history studies of minnows (*Phoxinus phoxinus*) have shown that individuals may join several different schools during a lifetime (Mills 1987). In Atlantic herring (*Clupea harengus*), acoustic surveys showed frequent splitting and joining of schools, suggesting continuous adjustment of school size to environmental conditions and low school stability (Pitcher *et al.* 1996). On the other hand, highly significant morphometric differences among proximate samples of the Lake Tanganyika sardine (*Limnothrissa miodon*) suggest that schools are not random assemblages of fish, and that there is relatively little mixing among schools (Hauser *et al.* 1998).

A mechanism which may maintain school integrity even after temporary mixing is assortative grouping (Hedgecock *et al.* 1994), or 'phenotype matching' (Crozier 1987), that is when fish actively join similar individuals. The size-selective schooling behaviour of many species (Pitcher & Parrish 1993) may suggest a preference for similar individuals, which may extend to individuals similar in shape. Fish of similar size and shape are probably the same age and may have grown up in the same nursery area, and thus may descend from the same spawning group. Alternatively, fish may prefer to school with familiar conspecifics, as shown in guppies (*Poecilia reticulata,* Magurran *et al.* 1994), and such familiar fish may well originate from the same nursery area. However, the level of school integrity in pelagic fish and its mechanisms remain uncertain and require further clarification.

High variation in reproductive success, combined with a high temporal stability of schools, and consequent microgeographic differentiation may have important consequences both for the evolution and the management of pelagic fish. The responses to selective pressures and thus processes of adaptive divergence may be far more complex and indeterminate than under simple population models (Hedgecock 1994). Furthermore, high variation in reproductive success reduces the effective population size, probably explaining the often high discrepancies between census and genetically effective population sizes in many marine organisms (Hedgecock *et al.* 1992) and may provide a means for speciation by shifting-balance evolutionary processes (Barton & Charlesworth 1984; Barton 1989).

In fishery terms, schooling fish are particularly vulnerable to overexploitation, because modern fish-finding devices (*e.g.* spotter planes, sonar) are able to detect schools at a large distance, and thus catch per unit effort is largely independent of fish abundance. As a consequence, catchability (proportion of the stock caught per unit effort, Hilborn & Walters 1992) increases as abundance declines (Mackinson *et al.* 1997), and the stock may collapse even if effort is reduced (Pitcher & Parrish 1993). Such an effect would be particularly apparent in species showing random schooling, because depleted schools would join to form fewer, but equally large, schools (Carvalho *et al.* 1994). In contrast, species with high school fidelity would show a decrease in average school size as progressively more schools are depleted, a development which could be detected as a reduction in catch per unit effort. In addition, such species may recover faster from a stock collapse, as each of the partially depleted schools would represent a separate refuge. Because of such effects on the resilience to exploitation and the speed of population recovery, an understanding of genetic relationships among schools and larger assemblages presents a major challenge for fishery geneticists.

3.5. High larval mortality

Most pelagic fish are highly fecund, and consequently mortality rates are high. Most of the mortality occurs during the egg and larval stages (Pitcher & Hart 1982): mortality of the adults varies between 5 and 10% per year, compared to 2-10% per day in eggs and larvae. This high egg/larval mortality clearly offers ample opportunities for selection to operate, as small differences in adaptation among genotypes may have significant effects on survival and thus affect genotype frequencies. In practical terms, this offers the possibility of 'nursery stocks' (Smith *et al.* 1990) where different selection pressures at different locations of a panmictic population could produce the impression of several isolated subpopulations (Ward & Grewe 1994). Clearly, coding loci such as allozyme loci are more likely to be prone to such effects than non-coding loci, and indeed, several fish species show evidence for selection on allozyme loci (*e.g.* cod, *Gadus morhua,* Mork & Sundnes 1985; sand flounder, *Rhombosolea plebeia,* Smith 1987; killifish, *Fundulus heteroclitus*, Powers *et al.* 1991; desert pupfish, *Poeciliopsis monacha,* Vrijenhoek *et al.* 1992). Selection is usually only detectable at a few loci (Lewontin & Krakauer 1973; Slatkin 1987), whereas differentiation due to reproductive isolation and random genetic drift should affect most loci. In species with low genetic variability, however, where genetic differentiation relies on very few loci, it may be difficult to decide whether the observed patterns reflect genuine population structure or selection. In theory, it is possible to detect such selective effects by taking samples regularly as the cohort ages, though sampling of the very early stages (eggs, early larvae) may be difficult in many pelagic species.

In long-lived fish like tuna and billfish, the existence of genetic differentiation in adults, even if due to differential selection, may provide valuable insights into migration patterns (PJ Smith, *pers. comm.*). As most of the mortality occurs during the egg and larval phase, differences in allele frequencies among adult samples caused by selection are likely to reflect differential mortality of early life-history stages in different nursery areas, and thus may indicate that there is only little exchange of adult fish among areas. Such results are somewhat similar to morphometric data, as environmental effects on morphological characters are likely to be most pronounced during the early stages of ontogeny (Buckmann 1950; Cushing 1955), and so any morphometric differences are likely to reflect the origin of fish from different nursery areas (Junquera & Perez-Gandaras 1993) rather than the short-term history in environmental conditions of a specific sample of fish. Even though neither loci under selection nor morphometrics can prove reproductive isolation, they can provide information on migration patterns and thus on short-term effects of local exploitation in long-lived fish.

3.6. Conclusions

In summary, some of the ecological, demographic and historical features of pelagic fish are expected to limit genetic differentiation between populations. This is not to say that molecular genetics cannot usefully contribute to the identification of populations of pelagic fish, but indicates that the ecology of pelagic fish and pertinent features of their habitat pose specific problems not encountered elsewhere. While logistic constraints often limit the samples that can be obtained, consideration of hydrographic features, known migration routes and population assessment from biological data is vital for molecular data to be applied successfully to population identification in pelagic fish. In addition, it will often be necessary to include information on past distribution and demography in the interpretation of molecular data, as extant patterns of population structure may reflect historical extinctions, dispersals and vicariances rather than contemporary gene flow, and thus estimates of migrant numbers from molecular data could be misleading. The interactive collection of genetic, ecological and oceanographic data is thus a vital prerequisite for the study of population structure in pelagic fish.

4. Molecular approaches to the identification of pelagic fish populations

It is apparent from the above discussion that using genetics to delimit populations of pelagic fish is not an easy task, and increasingly sophisticated molecular genetic techniques are being applied (Park & Moran 1994; Ward & Grewe 1994; Carvalho & Hauser 1994; O'Connell & Wright 1997). Here we will consider the three most common approaches: allozymes, mitochondrial DNA (mtDNA) and microsatellites, with two main aims: (1) a review of spatial patterns of genetic differentiation detected in empirical studies on large and small pelagic species, and (2) an assessment of the relative effectiveness of allozyme, mtDNA and microsatellite approaches. Two recent reviews of the genetics of tunas (Ward 1995) and tunas and billfish (Graves 1995) did not consider microsatellite data, which form a significant part of this review.

We restricted ourselves to comparing and contrasting the population structure of large (tunas and billfish) and small (mainly clupeids) pelagic species - space limitation does not permit inclusion of, for example, sharks, although many of these are pelagic.

Where F_{ST} values were not published, we estimated levels of population differentiation using conventional F-statistics (Wright 1969; Weir & Cockerham 1984) based on gene-frequency data from allozymes, mtDNA and microsatellites. We have not included allele size data in our microsatellite analyses and therefore have not calculated R_{ST} (Slatkin 1995); it has been recommended that the conservative approach of using F-statistics be used by fishery geneticists until models of microsatellite mutation are better understood (O'Connell & Wright 1997). For those allozymes and microsatellites where multiple loci were examined in a single study, an average F_{ST} was calculated and its significance level derived by combining significance values for individual loci (Sokal & Rohlf 1995). In addition, a hierarchical analysis of variation between and within oceans was carried out where the data allowed. All analyses were performed using the software package AMOVA (Excoffier *et al.* 1992)

4.1. Large pelagics

Genetic population data were examined for six species of tuna: skipjack (*Katsuwonus pelamis*), albacore (*Thunnus alalunga*), yellowfin (*T. albacares*), bigeye (*T. obesus*), Atlantic northern bluefin (*T. thynnus thynnus*), Pacific northern bluefin (*T. t. orientalis*), and southern bluefin (*T. maccoyii*). Four of these (skipjack, albacore, yellowfin and bigeye) are globally distributed throughout the tropical and subtropical waters of the three major oceans. The Atlantic northern bluefin and the Pacific northern bluefin are restricted to the Atlantic and Pacific oceans respectively (genetic data indicate that these two subspecies are as different from one another as most *Thunnus* species (Sharp & Pirages 1978; Grewe, in Ward 1995; Chow & Kishino 1995; Alvarado Bremer *et al.* 1997) and probably warrant species status). The southern bluefin tuna is essentially an Indian Ocean species, although its feeding range extends to the southern Atlantic and south-west Pacific.

The taxonomic status of some billfish species is still unclear. The blue marlin is considered by some as a single circumtropical species marlin (*Makaira nigricans*, Briggs 1960; Robins & de Sylva 1960; Rivas 1975) but by others (Nakamura 1985) as having distinct Atlantic (*Makaira nigricans*) and Indo-Pacific (*M. mazara*) species. Similarly, the sailfish is recognised by some as a single circumtropical species (*Istiophorus platypterus*,

Morrow & Harbo 1969) but by others as having distinct Atlantic (*I. albicans*) and Indo-Pacific (*I. platypterus*) species (Nakamura 1985). Genetic data favour the single global species view (Graves & McDowell 1995), but we follow the interpretation of Nakamura (1985) here. Genetic population data are available for six billfish species: the globally distributed swordfish (*Xiphias gladius*), the Indo-Pacific sailfish, the Atlantic sailfish, the Atlantic blue marlin, the Atlantic white marlin (*Tetrapturus albidus*) and the Pacific striped marlin (*T. audax*).

Table 5 summarises the results of those data sets, the majority based on mtDNA analysis, that permit an assessment of between-ocean differentiation. Most of these also permit analyses of within-ocean differentiation, making hierarchical analyses possible. Data from six species were available; all showed significant differentiation among samples (F_{ST}). The first yellowfin tuna mtDNA study (Scoles & Graves 1993) gave an F_{ST} of zero, but a subsequent larger study (Ward *et al.* 1997) revealed significant, if very limited (F_{ST} = 0.010), differentiation. One or two early studies, based on very few fish (typically less than 10 per sample), have not been included. Extensive studies (*e.g.* SPC 1981; Fujino *et al.* 1981) of an esterase locus (*EST*) in skipjack tuna, indicated the likelihood of at least four distinct stocks (Atlantic, Indian, Western Pacific, Central-eastern Pacific), but the raw data were not available for our analysis.

The extent of between-sample variation varies from about 1% in yellowfin tuna to nearly 50% in the sailfish (although this estimate is based on only two samples), with a mean taken

Table 5: Results of hierarchical analyses of genetic variation among samples (F_{ST}), among samples within oceans (F_{SO}) and among oceans(F_{OT}). See Tables 2 and 3 for further explanations.

Species	Oceans	Marker	H_1 H_2	N_1 N_2	F_{ST} sig	F_{SO} sig	F_{OT} sig	Ref.
Thunnus albacares	P, A	mtDNA (whole: 12)	84.9 82-86	6 19-20	-0.021 ns	-0.015 ns	-0.006 ns	a
	P, I, A	mtDNA (whole: 2)	68.2 63-73	9 21-176	0.010 **	0.012 *	-0.002 ns	b
	P, I, A	allozyme (4)	36.2 34-39	8 21-175	0.025 **	0.027 **	-0.002 ns	b
Thunnus alalunga	P, A	mtDNA (ATPase: 2)	56.4 21-69	12 31-75	0.092 ***	-0.004 ns	0.096 **	c
Thunnus obesus	P, I, A	mtDNA (control: 3)	55.7 40-77	5 17-125	0.260 ***	0.042 *	0.218 ***	d
Thunnus thynnus thynnus	A, M	microsatellite (5)	50.4 45-56	4 16-44	0.069 ***	0.112 ***	-0.043 ns	e
Xiphias gladius	P, I, A, M	mtDNA (control: 4)	89.6 70-96	13 11-59	0.036 ***	0.005 ns	0.031 **	f
	P, A, M	mtDNA (control: 3)	55.7 15-68	8 16-76	0.191 ***	0.014 ns	0.177 ***	g
Istiophorus platypterus	P, I	mtDNA (whole: 12)	49.9 10,90	2 20,13	0.473 ***	-	0.473 ***	h

References

a, Scoles & Graves 1993; b,Ward *et al.* 1997; c, Chow & Ushiama 1995; d, Avarado Bremer *et al.* 1998; e Broughton & Gold 1997; f, Chow *et al.* 1997; g, Alvarado Bremer *et al.* 1996; h, Graves & McDowell 1995.

across studies of 0.126±0.053. Five species allowed an assessment of the relative contributions of within and between ocean divergence to overall differentiation: in three of these species (albacore tuna, bigeye tuna, swordfish) the differentiation was almost entirely due to inter-ocean differences, in two species (yellowfin, Atlantic bluefin) the within-ocean differentiation exceeded the between-ocean differentiation.

Two studies on global mtDNA variation in swordfish gave disparate absolute values for the F-statistics (i.e. $F_{ST} = 0.036$, Chow *et al.* 1997; $F_{ST} = 0.191$, Alvarado Bremer *et al.* 1996), although both agreed that virtually all the between-sample differentiation was attributable to between-ocean variation. The disparity might be largely related to the pooling of haplotypes into three clades by Alavarado Bremer (1996), while Chow *et al.* (1997) kept their 52 separate haplotypes distinct. In addition the former study focused largely on the Atlantic, the latter on the Indo-Pacific.

Table 3 summarises the within-ocean studies. Eight of the 26 studies and six of the 12 species showed statistically significant instances of within-ocean differentiation. These significant F_{ST} values ranged from 0.001 to 0.053, with an outlier at 0.188. The outlier is from five microsatellite loci in two collections of Atlantic bluefin tuna from the Mediterranean Sea (Broughton & Gold 1997); one of the loci showed no allele overlap in the two samples (Broughton, *pers. comm.*). Given the very low levels of within-ocean divergence between other tuna samples, including those typed for microsatellites, this result needs to be viewed cautiously at present. Overall levels of genetic differentiation were 0.019±0.008, or 0.012±0.004 if the Mediterranean northern bluefin result is omitted.

In the skipjack tuna, the bulk of the observed differentiation was due to clinal or stepped variation for the allozyme locus *EST* ($F_{ST} = 0.041$, $P < 0.001$), with a second locus showing much reduced but still significant differentiation (*GDA*, $F_{ST} = 0.005$, $P < 0.001$) and the other two loci (*ADA, PGI*) no differentiation. These data have led to the rejection of a single panmictic Pacific population, but whether the data are better explained by an isolation-by-distance model or by multiple discrete subpopulations remains uncertain (SPC 1981; Fujino *et al.* 1981). It would be very valuable to examine these interpretations using mtDNA and microsatellite loci.

In the yellowfin tuna, the significant within-ocean differentiation for allozymes reflects differentiation at only one of the four polymorphic allozyme loci. For this locus, *GPI-A*, the F_{ST} value within the Pacific Ocean is about 10%, whereas it is not significantly greater than zero for the other three loci (Ward *et al.* 1994; Ward *et al.* 1997). Furthermore, F_{ST} for mtDNA in the Pacific Ocean is only 0.012 and for microsatellites is only 0.001 (Table 3). Had the *GPI-A* differentiation reflected genetic drift in isolated populations, then we might have expected to see more differentiation in other polymorphic allozymes and microsatellite loci. The GPI-A differentiation may therefore reflect selective forces specific to this locus, while the smaller (yet still significant) F_{ST} values shown by mtDNA and microsatellites may be due to genetic drift in isolated populations.

For both skipjack and yellowfin tuna, the Pacific Ocean differentiation observed is largely in an east-west direction, that is. longitudinal rather than latitudinal, whereas the Pacific populations of striped marlin appeared to have a more patchy distribution of genotypes. Atlantic swordfish populations appear to be differentiated on a north-south but not east-west basis (Alvarado Bremer *et al.* 1996; Chow *et al.* 1997).

The remaining species showed little evidence of genetic population structuring within oceans, despite ocean-wide sampling in most cases. In the southern bluefin tuna, where only a single spawning location is known, this homogeneity is not unexpected; in the other species, with several or numerous spawning grounds, the homogeneity can be ascribed to gene flow among sites.

The mean F_{ST} value for inter-ocean differentiation, 0.105 ± 0.055 (six species, nine cases, Table 5) was about five times that of the mean F_{ST} value for within-ocean differentiation, 0.019 ± 0.008 (11 species, 26 cases, Table 3). The conclusions to be drawn from this survey are (1) most large pelagic fish show between-ocean genetic differentiation and (2) most large pelagic fish show minimal or undetectable within-ocean differentiation, at least with the sample sizes and techniques currently employed.

4.2. Small pelagics

In contrast to the general pattern of genetic subdivision in large pelagic species, that is, between-ocean genetic heterogeneity and within-ocean homogeneity, the genetic population structure of small pelagic species appears to be more varied and more dependent on population history, geography, hydrography and migratory ability of species (Table 2). The high demographic instability together with the limited distribution of many small pelagic species often makes it difficult to disentangle the effects of contemporary gene flow with those of historic population extinctions and recolonizations (Grant & Bowen 1998). For example, Atlantic herring (*Clupea harengus*) show genetic homogeneity across the Atlantic, possibly suggesting significant gene flow between East and West Atlantic coasts, though the lack of genetic differentiation is more likely due to colonization of the NW Atlantic after the last ice-age (Grant 1984). On the other hand, secondary contact of previously isolated populations may increase the observed genetic differentiation: for example, frequency heterogeneity of two deep mtDNA lineages of anchovies (*Engraulis encrasicolus*) within the Mediterranean indicate immigration from the Black Sea after the last glacial period, and subsequent maintenance of genetic differentiation by hydrographic barriers to gene flow in parts of the Aegean and Adriatic (Magoulas *et al.* 1996). Thus historic factors may both enhance and reduce the resolution of molecular markers for the identification of pelagic fish populations, and should be considered in the interpretation of results.

In addition to population history, geographic and hydrographic factors affect the population structure of many small pelagic species. In some species, there is genetic differentiation defined by major geographic ocean basins: for example, the Baltic and Barents Sea sustain genetically differentiated herring populations (Turan 1997). As another example, there are separate subpopulations of both anchovies (Bembo *et al.* 1995, 1996a) and sardines (Carvalho *et al.* 1994) in the Adriatic and Ionian Seas. On an even smaller scale, hydrographic differences may help to sustain the isolation of Atlantic herring in some Norwegian fjords, which can harbour genetically very differentiated populations, though reproductive isolation due to different spawning behaviour may be the main factor separating fjord populations from Atlanto-Scandian herring (Jorstad *et al.* 1991; McQuinn 1997). Hydrographic boundaries may delineate populations within seas, for example the Almeria-Oran front in the Mediterranean Sea for sardines (Ramon & Castro 1997) and the boundary between coastal eutrophic and central oligotrophic waters in the Adriatic for anchovies (Bembo *et al.* 1996b). On the smallest geographic scale, genetic differentiation can be found among very proximate samples (Grant 1985; Wilson & Alberdi 1991; Hedgecock *et al.* 1994; Chikhi *et al.* 1998; Hauser *et al.* 1998), probably reflecting biased reproductive success (Hedgecock *et al.* 1994), containment of larvae in gyres and eddies (Ruzzante *et al.* 1997) or long-term stability of schools (Hauser *et al.* 1998). This range in the extent of differentiation on different geographic scales may at least in part be caused by differences in migratory abilities among small pelagic species (Smith *et al.* 1990), though patterns of historical dispersal may also play an important role (Bowen & Grant 1997).

Most of the small pelagic species in Table 2 are marine, with the exception of kapenta (Lake Tanganyika sardine, *Limnothrissa miodon*). Nevertheless, kapenta shares many of the ecological features of marine pelagics, such as schooling behaviour, high fecundity and short life-span (Coulter 1991a). Furthermore, the expanse of Lake Tanganyika (650 km long, 50 km wide, 570m mean depth) creates a large pelagic realm comparable in size to many coastal marine habitats. Indeed, kapenta shares patterns of genetic variability with many small marine pelagics: relatively low allozyme diversity, high mtDNA haplotype diversity, low overall differentiation at allozymes but homogeneity at mtDNA (Table 2) and significant microgeographic genetic differences (Hauser *et al.* 1998). These characteristics of small pelagic species are therefore likely to be more due to their pelagic life-history, than the marine habitat *per se*.

One of the most intensively investigated marine fish species is the Atlantic herring, which is one of the few pelagic species where microsatellites have already been applied. Indeed, herring is often cited as an example where molecular tools did little to help resolve the stock structure of an exploited species (Carvalho & Hauser 1994). Several stocks are recognised in herring (Parrish & Saville 1965), supported by tag returns (Cushing & Burd 1957; Wheeler & Winters 1984), differences in spawning times (Haegele & Schweigert 1985), morphometrics (Postuma 1974; Rosenberg & Palmen 1982) and rates of growth, recruitment and mortality (Burd 1985). Some of these stocks are even considered as sibling species (Ojaveer 1989). While initial electrophoretic studies, based on few loci and small samples, tended to support this complex stock structure (Lush 1969; Ridgway *et al.* 1970; Lewis & Ridgway 1972), more extensive investigations provided little support for genetic differentiation in North Atlantic herring (Andersson *et al.* 1981; Grant 1984; Ryman *et al.* 1984; King *et al.* 1987). Only one study detected small, but significant differentiation among North Atlantic stocks (Jorstad *et al.* 1991). Some fjord populations in Norway were genetically highly differentiated, although the taxonomic status of herring in these fjords is uncertain and allozyme data suggest that these populations are genetically more similar to Pacific than to Atlantic herring (Jorstad *et al.* 1994). Similarly, herring in the Barents Sea show different allele frequencies at both allozymes and microsatellites, and are thus most likely a separate population from herring in the North Atlantic (Shaw *et al.* 1998a). Interestingly, similar patterns of genetic heterogeneity were found in blue whiting (*Micromesistius poutassou*), where samples from the Barents Sea and a Norwegian fjord were significantly differentiated from North Atlantic and Mediterranean samples at two allozyme loci (Giæver & Stien 1998). Findings of genetic differences between spring and autumn spawners of herring in the western Atlantic (Kornfield *et al.* 1982) were questioned (Smith & Jamieson 1986), and studies using mtDNA analysis revealed no major genetic differentiation between putative stocks (Kornfield & Bogdanowicz 1987). Some evidence for genetic differentiation has, however, been found for Georges Bank herring (Stephenson & Kornfield 1990). Recent allozyme and mtDNA studies show differentiation among Barents Sea, Baltic Sea and North Sea (Turan 1997), confirming the previous distinction of subspecies based on morphological and meristic characters (Ryman *et al.* 1984). Despite, or perhaps because of, the general disappointment about the scarcity of detectable differentiation in Atlantic herring, the results of this intense research effort have led to critical reviews of the typological population concept (Smith & Jamieson 1986) and to more appropriate models of population structure in herring (McQuinn 1997), which may be applicable to other pelagic species.

4.3. Large and small pelagics– comparison of within-ocean differentiation

There is some indication that large pelagic species show less within-ocean differentiation than small pelagics. For example, only 8 of the 26 large pelagic studies (30%) showed significant within-ocean differentiation (Table 3), compared with 17 of 28 small pelagics (61%) (Table 2). Furthermore, the average F_{ST} value of the large pelagic fish, 0.019 ± 0.008 (0.012 ± 0.004 if the Mediterranean bluefin tuna data are omitted) is less than that of the small pelagic fish, 0.027 ± 0.009 (or 0.029 ± 0.009 if the freshwater kapenta is omitted). These differences are not statistically significant owing to high variances, and the results are biased towards those species with multiple studies. Nonetheless, these data do suggest that samples of large pelagic fish might show less population differentiation than samples of small pelagic fish, despite generally coming from more widely separated areas. If true, this is likely to be due to the higher migratory powers of the large pelagic species.

This conclusion is certainly preliminary and needs to be tested with additional studies. The possible confounding effects of different marker classes need to be examined in a larger dataset, as more studies of large than small pelagic species were based on mtDNA analysis. While theory suggests that this should, if anything, have increased levels of differentiation among populations, these assumed differences in efficacy of mtDNA and nuclear DNA for defining populations do not seem to be fully borne out in practise.

4.4. Comparison of the techniques

While advantages and disadvantages of particular molecular markers have been discussed elsewhere (Park & Moran 1994; Ward & Grewe 1994; O'Connell & Wright 1997), further considerations in relation to the specific ecological and demographic features of pelagic fish are warranted.

Descriptions of population structure derived from genetic data generally assume selective neutrality of the markers, with differences in gene frequencies held to reflect genetic drift, migration, and mutation only. However, for any genes under directional selection, the high juvenile mortality of pelagic fish offers ample opportunity for selection to cause significant genetic differentiation even in the presence of considerable gene flow. In some instances, levels of differentiation at one allozyme locus can considerably exceed those of other markers (including other allozyme loci), and then caution has to be exercised in using these loci to deduce population structure: such differences may reflect directional selection at specific loci rather than population isolation (*e.g.* GPI-A in yellowfin tuna, Ward *et al.* 1997, PEP-A in king mackerel, Gold *et al.* 1997). In species with low allozyme variability, selective effects are particularly problematic, as little comparison among loci is possible. The neutrality of variation observed in coding regions of mtDNA is also debatable (MacRae & Anderson 1988; Nigro & Prout 1990), and even non-coding DNA like the control region/D-loop may be under selective constraints relating to physical conformation of the DNA molecule and function in gene expression or DNA replication (Park & Moran 1994). Clonal inheritance of mtDNA ensures that all genes are linked, and markers are therefore affected by selection anywhere on the molecule. For population studies, however, and especially for stock structure analyses, small selection differentials may not be statistically detectable (Ferguson 1994), and to our knowledge, genetic differentiation due to selective effects on mtDNA has not been shown in fish. Microsatellites reflect variation in non-coding sequences and are thus more likely to fit the neutral paradigm than mtDNA and, especially, allozyme variation. From this viewpoint, microsatellite and mtDNA analyses may be preferred to allozymes as markers in population studies, though tests for selective effects, such as correlations with environmental gradients and comparison of differentiation detected by different loci / marker systems, may be advisable for all molecular markers.

Notwithstanding the possibility of selective effects, allozymes appear to be powerful genetic markers, which often reveal more genetic differentiation than mtDNA (number of statistically significant tests in Tables 2 and 3: allozymes: 14 out of 21 tests, mtDNA: 7 out of 27 tests). This may seem surprising, as population genetics theory predicts higher levels of differentiation in mtDNA than in allozymes (Birky *et al.* 1989): mtDNA haploidy and maternal inheritance reduce the effective population size to about a quarter, and its higher mutation rate should allow the faster accumulation of genetic variability and a more rapid approach to mutation-drift equilibrium. However, this theoretical potential does not seem to have been realised in the empirical analyses here, which may partly be due to the fact that mtDNA is inherited as a single unit and therefore has to be treated as one locus, a distinct disadvantage compared to multilocus allozyme or nuclear DNA assays. Furthermore, in pelagic species, the extremely high levels of haplotype diversity (Tables 2 & 3), where a high proportion of haplotypes are present only once or twice in the whole data set, considerably reduce the power of conventional population genetic statistics based on contingency tables (Bowen & Grant 1997).

Although mtDNA provided fewer significant test results overall (Tables 2 & 3), it may be the more powerful marker under specific circumstances. For example, although F_{ST} values in *Sardinella aurita* from the Gulf of Mexico, Florida and Brazil were significant for both marker systems (Table 2; Wilson & Alberdi 1991; Tringali & Wilson 1993), only the mtDNA analysis detected differentiation between the Gulf of Mexico and the Brazilian samples. The total differentiation was due to differences among the US samples (Gulf of Mexico, Florida) in the allozymes ($F_{within US}$=0.024***, $F_{between US and Brazil}$=0.004, n.s.), but entirely due to differentiation between the Gulf / Florida populations and the Brazilian samples in mtDNA ($F_{within US}$=0.005, n.s., $F_{between US and Brazil}$=0.098***). The significant genetic differentiation within the Gulf of Mexico and large scale homogeneity detected by allozymes was confirmed by later independent studies (Kinsey *et al.* 1994; Chikhi *et al.* 1998), and may reflect the greater sensitivity of multilocus allozyme data to small scale differentiation caused by non-random association of genotypes, while low allozyme heterozygosity may have prevented the detection of large scale population differences (Chikhi *et al.* 1998). The *Sardinella* data therefore indicate that molecular markers which appear to be generally less powerful may still be better suited to reveal population differentiation under certain conditions. This may particularly be true for markers with different modes of inheritance (*e.g.* nuclear *vs.* mitochondrial markers), mutation or selection (*e.g.* allozymes *vs.* microsatellites). In pelagic species, whose ecology and population dynamics are expected to allow only low-level genetic differentiation, such small differences among marker systems may decide whether population substructuring is detected or not.

The wide range of evolutionary rates between different regions of the mtDNA molecule allows its application to genetic investigations at different taxonomic levels, from intra-specific population studies (*e.g.* Carr & Marshall 1991; Cronin *et al.* 1993) to inter-specific (*e.g.* Billington *et al.* 1991; McVeigh & Davidson 1991; Bernatchez *et al.* 1991) or even inter-family phylogenies (*e.g.* Meyer & Dolven 1992; Milinkovitch *et al.* 1993). It may therefore be possible to increase the power of the analysis by a more detailed assay of the right region rather than coarser analysis of the whole mtDNA genome. Indeed, in Atlantic herring, significant differentiation between the Baltic and Celtic Sea was found at the ND3/4 gene, but not in the ND5/6 region, probably because the larger number of relatively common haplotypes at the ND3/4 gene increased the statistical power of these tests (Turan 1997). It may therefore be advisable in mtDNA studies to investigate several different regions, a task greatly facilitated by the availability of universal PCR primers (Kocher et al. 1989).

Although the majority of fisheries genetics studies to date, and all examples listed in Table 2, 3 and 5, used RFLP analysis, sequencing has with the development of automated sequencers become a feasible alternative even for sample sizes required in population analyses (e.g. Bowen & Grant 1997; Koutoulas et al. 1995). In particular in species with high mtDNA haplotype diversity, detailed sequence information may be useful in weighting nucleotide substitutions for the accurate reconstruction of genetic relationships among haplotypes (Grant et al. 1998). Sequence data allow the distinction between more frequent, and thus more homoplaseous, transitions from rarer transversions, or between synonymous and non-synonymous substitutions, and thus may be more useful to estimate genetic distances among haplotypes than RFLPs where all substitutions have to be weighted equally. However, there is a trade-off between such very detailed information from a short sequence and the less detailed information from a larger fragment (RFLP) or indeed from several loci (allozymes, microsatellites, Hillis et al. 1996).

Microsatellites have so far been applied only in three large and two small pelagic species. Any general conclusions are therefore preliminary, and have to be tested with further studies. However, these five studies allow some interesting comparisons. For example, in yellowfin tuna, the F_{ST} estimated from microsatellites is in fact smaller (0.001) than that of allozymes (0.027) and mtDNA RFLPs (0.012). This difference may partly be due to selection at the GPI-A locus raising the allozyme F_{ST}, but other studies of pelagic species also report higher allozyme than microsatellite F_{ST} values, though differences are much smaller than in yellowfin tuna (e.g. Atlantic herring: 0.049 vs. 0.035, Table 2, Shaw et al. 1998a; veined squid, Loligo forbesi, 0.536 vs. 0.245, Shaw et al. 1998b). Indeed, closer examination of some of the herring results (Shaw et al. 1998a), where allozyme and microsatellite data were collected from the same samples, reveals interesting patterns of differentiation at the two marker systems (Table 6). Within the Atlantic (IC, NS), only the microsatellites detect differentiation, but with increasing isolation, F_{ST} values of allozymes become larger than those of microsatellites: allozyme and microsatellite values are similar between Trondheims Fjord (TF) and the rest, but allozyme F_{ST} values are 2-3 times higher than those of microsatellites in the comparisons between Barents Sea herring (BS) and the other Atlantic herring. This discrepancy becomes even more obvious in the interspecific comparison between Atlantic (IC, NS, TF, BS) and Pacific herring (PC), where the allozymes indicate about 20 times more differentiation than microsatellites, and the microsatellite F_{ST} values are even smaller than in some of the intraspecific comparisons. In

Table 6: F_{ST} estimates from microsatellite and allozyme analysis of Atlantic herring samples (Shaw et al. 1998a). Samples are from Iceland (IC), Norway (NS), Barents Sea (BS) and Trondheinsfjord (TF); PC: Pacific herring for comparison. Probabilities of $F_{ST} > 0$, determined by permutation tests, are indicated: *** p < 0.001.

| | Sample | F_{ST} **Microsatellites** | | | | |
		IC	NS	BS	TF	PC
	IC	-	0.0086***	0.0553***	0.0237***	0.0267***
F_{ST}	NS	0.0006	-	0.1376***	0.0124***	0.0319***
Allozymes	BS	0.1589***	0.0537***	-	0.0521***	0.0520***
	TF	0.0298***	0.0373***	0.1577***	-	0.0301***
	PC	0.7414***	0.7411***	0.7811***	0.6848***	-

contrast, F_{ST} estimates from allozymes and microsatellites are comparable over a wide range of divergences in brown trout (*Salmo trutta*, Estoup *et al.* 1998). The higher resolving power of microsatellites compared to allozymes in closely related populations is most likely due to the higher variability in the former which increase the power of statistical tests, even when F_{ST} values are similar (Estoup *et al.* 1998; Shaw *et al.* 1998a). The discrepancy between herring and brown trout in the relationship of allozyme and microsatellite F_{ST} values among more distantly related populations may be due to the much larger population sizes in herring, which not only reduce genetic drift, but also cause higher microsatellite heterozygosity (0.90 in herring, 0.42 in brown trout) and allelic diversity (mean number of alleles per locus per population: 24.2 in herring, 3.6 in brown trout). The larger number of alleles may increase the incidence of homoplasy, that is mutations to an already existing allele (Shaw *et al.* 1998a), and thus genetic distances among more distantly related populations would be underestimated. In contrast, the probability of homoplasy would be lower in relatively small brown trout populations, which possess only a few alleles due to genetic drift, and so both allozyme and microsatellite F_{ST} values increase with genetic distance at similar rates (Estoup *et al.* 1998). These empirical comparisons confirm theoretical arguments that F_{ST} values from microsatellites only inadequately estimate genetic differentiation among divergent populations in species with large population sizes and high genetic variability (Nauta & Weissing 1996).

The data from pelagic species show that microsatellites and mtDNA often have high and comparable levels of diversity (Tables 2 & 3). Nevertheless, the few studies available suggest that mtDNA is less powerful than microsatellite analysis for population comparisons: 4 out of 6 microsatellite comparisons demonstrated significant differentiation within oceans, while only 7 out of 27 tests showed significant F_{ST} values for mtDNA. Furthermore, in Atlantic herring, where microsatellites and mtDNA RFLPs of the ND5/6 region were examined in the same samples, only the microsatellites demonstrated highly significant differentiation, despite similar levels of diversity (Shaw *et al.* 1998a). Several explanations are possible: first, as discussed above, mtDNA studies are analysing effectively only one locus, while microsatellite analyses typically involve several loci and so are more likely to detect differentiation due to random drift. For example, only two out of six microsatellite loci indicated significant differentiation of yellowfin tuna in the Pacific, but the overall result is still significant (Ward & Grewe, *unpublished*). Second, many mtDNA RFLP studies demonstrated an extremely skewed distribution of allele frequencies, with very few common haplotypes and many haplotypes occurring only once in the dataset (*e.g.* 71 unique haplotypes in 196 Atlantic herring, with only two haplotypes in more than 10 fish, Turan *et al.* 1998). The more even distribution of microsatellite allele frequencies may increase the power of statistical tests (PW Shaw, *pers. comm.*), though this possibility has yet to be tested. Finally, mtDNA analyses are often compromised by ancestral polymorphisms which are much older than the taxa under question (Kornfield & Parker 1997). In contrast, the problem of such ancestral lineages is reduced in microsatellites by recombination and rapid mutation leading to homoplasy. Microsatellites may therefore reflect the more recent demographic history without 'noise' from old diversity patterns (Nauta & Weissing 1996).

One of the problems with the application of microsatellites to fish stock identification is the uncertainty over the appropriate mutation model, and consequently on the appropriate measure of differentiation. Currently, there are two main measures of microsatellite differentiation (O'Connell & Wright 1997): F_{ST} which is derived from the infinite allele model (IAM), and R_{ST} which is related to the stepwise mutation model (SMM). R_{ST} takes the allele sizes into account, thus making R_{ST}, at least in theory, more informative (Slatkin 1995). However the large range in allele sizes in many abundant fish species, both pelagic (e.g. Shaw et al. 1998a) and demersal (e.g. Bentzen et al. 1996), may increase the variance of R_{ST} estimates and thus make them statistically less meaningful (O'Connell & Wright 1997). Furthermore, R_{ST} may be more sensitive to unequal sample sizes (Ruzzante 1998), and give different results than F_{ST} depending on number of samples, nature of genetic differentiation (Bentzen et al. 1996) and locus-specific variation (O'Connell & Wright 1997). In pelagic species, with generally low levels of genetic differentiation, this difference in performance may cause different statistical results between F_{ST} and R_{ST} (e.g. Shaw et al. 1998a,b; O'Connell et al. 1998), and thus introduces ambiguity in the conclusions. Research into mutation processes and the statistical analysis of microsatellite data is therefore urgently needed.

The limited levels of genetic differentiation detected with most markers, even when statistically significant, point to the need to examine large samples to obtain reasonable estimates of differentiation. For example, an early study of mtDNA variation in 10-12 albacore tuna drawn from each of the Atlantic and Pacific Oceans failed to detect differentiation (Graves & Dizon 1989), but as techniques advanced to permit the analysis of larger sample sizes (Chow & Ushiama 1995), a significant F_{ST} value of nearly 10% was found (Table 5). For microsatellites, sample sizes of 50-100 individuals have been shown to provide sufficiently accurate and precise estimates of genetic differentiation, though sample size requirements will depend on the level of genetic variability detected (Ruzzante 1998). In general, sample sizes much below 50 run an unacceptable risk of failing to detect true stock separation, while samples much larger than 100 individuals represent a small increase in statistical power achieved by a substantial increase in work-load and expense.

5. Summary and concluding remarks

The application of molecular genetic analysis has an important role to play in improving the scientific basis for fisheries management, and in ensuring the conservation and sustainable exploitation of marine resources. Pelagic fish form a substantial component of the wild fishery catch and their sustainable harvesting requires, inter alia, improved understanding of population structures. This review shows that because of their ecology and demography, genetic population differentiation in pelagic is fish is both expected and observed to be more limited than in other groups of fish, thereby highlighting the need for an interdisciplinary approach to stock structure analysis.

Fisheries managers generally want genetic analysis to help them identify harvest stocks (i.e. primarily self-recruiting stocks), but because of the extent of gene low in pelagic fish and their propensity to periodic population extinctions and expansions, the genetic stock may in fact contain several harvest stocks. While molecular tools often cannot fully answer the questions posed by managers, they have played an important role in identifying practical problems and misconceptions with the stock concept and in testing current views of the ecology of pelagic fish. For example, the concept that many small pelagic fish have a metapopulation structure with relatively short-lived subpopulations, whose demographic instability is a natural phenomenon exacerbated by fishing pressure, has been supported by molecular data (e.g. Bowen & Grant 1997). Such information cannot provide knowledge of the geographic boundaries between self-recruiting fish stocks sought by fisheries managers, but does provide valuable insights into natural fluctuations in abundance which can then be incorporated into fisheries models (Hilborn & Walters 1992). Furthermore, research on phylogeographic relationships among such populations may allow the reconstruction of colonization routes and the identification of potential sources for recolonization after population extinctions. Close collaboration among scientists from different disciplines, such as oceanography, ecology, fisheries science, palaeontology and molecular genetics, as well as an appreciation of both the limits and the potential of molecular markers will be required to address questions of population structure in pelagic fish.

Many pelagic species are unlikely to be at demographic equilibrium with respect to the effects of gene flow and genetic drift, and present-day levels of differentiation may well reflect past population size and range fluctuations rather than extant gene flow. Nevertheless, genetic differentiation among populations, assuming selective neutrality of markers, still indicates non-panmixia and the need for separate management plans for each genetic stock. The finding of genetic homogeneity among regions, on the other hand, is relatively uninformative for managers - such homogeneity in principle might reflect sufficient levels of gene flow to generate panmixia, or might reflect comparatively recent population separation without extant gene flow. Thus genetic data are extremely useful when they indicate population differences, but much less useful when they do not. In the latter instance, the decision on how many harvest stocks are present has to be based on other, non-genetic methods such as tagging, morphometrics and ecological data.

Another major opportunity for molecular genetic analysis in pelagic fish is the investigation of social structuring within populations, its causes, mechanisms and consequences. As pointed out above, stable social structuring would have important implications for standard fishery models. In addition, the evolution of pelagic fish may be significantly affected by their social structure, and research into the selective effects of schooling may provide valuable insights into speciation in many marine fish and invertebrates (Hedgecock 1994). More sensitive markers, such as microsatellites, have already been used for the investigation of these questions (Ruzzante *et al.* 1997) and will allow further research into the fine-scale structure of pelagic populations in relation to hydrographic features.

While our survey indicated that some molecular markers appear to be more powerful in detecting genetic population structure than others, it also provided examples where supposedly less effective approaches were successful in identifying population differentiation (*e.g.* Wilson & Alberdi 1991; Tringali & Wilson 1993). It is thus important to consider a range of molecular tools, and, if possible, to apply several techniques to the same samples of fish. Such an approach would not only increase the power of the analysis, but also provide information on the mechanisms responsible for population differentiation, such as selection, sex-biased gene flow or genetic drift. Simultaneous employment of several molecular techniques will be crucial where microsatellites are applied to species which are difficult to identify and which are collected by inexperienced field workers. Inclusion of even a small number of mis-identified specimen could easily result in erroneous conclusions about population structure - we therefore strongly recommend that in such circumstances an independent means of species identification (such as mtDNA diagnosis) be routinely included.

Finally, the points discussed here show that an integration of molecular data with ecological information may be even more important in pelagic fish than elsewhere. While such information is sometimes considered in the interpretation of results, its inclusion into the planning and execution of sampling programmes is often neglected, not least because of the logistical problems of obtaining samples from geographically very distant locations. However, the value of the results obtained will be determined largely by the appropriateness of the sampling design (Carvalho & Hauser 1998), and great emphasis should be placed in securing adequate collections from locations determined not only by logistical ease but by hydrological and ecological knowledge. For example, as populations may disperse and mix outside the spawning season, it will often be necessary to collect samples of spawning fish in order to identify self-recruiting populations. In many cases, a time series of samples may be required to investigate the temporal stability of the patterns observed, especially in relation to annual and seasonal variation in hydrographic features affecting distribution.

Acknowledgements

We wish to thank John Gold, Linda Richardson and Richard Broughton for unpublished data, and two anonymous referees and Nick Elliott for useful comments which greatly improved the manuscript. We also thank Paul Shaw for many fruitful discussions, and Miranda Trojanowska for proof-reading and help with the extensive reference list.

References

Alvarado Bremer JR, Mejuto J, Greig TW, Ely B (1996) Global population structure of the swordfish (*Xiphias gladius* L.) as revealed by analysis of the mitochondrial DNA control region. *Journal of Experimental Marine Biology and Ecology*, **197**, 295-310.

Alvarado Bremer JR, Naseri I, Ely B (1997) Orthodox and unorthodox phylogenetic relationships among tunas revealed by the nucleotide sequence analysis of the mitochondrial DNA control region. *Journal of Fish Biology*, **50**, 540-554.

Alvarado Bremer JR, Stequert B, Robertson NW, Ely B (1998) Genetic evidence for inter-oceanic subdivision of bigeye tuna (*Thunnus obesus* Lowe) populations. *Marine Biology*, in press.

Andersson L, Ryman N, Rosenberg R, Stahl G (1981) Genetic variability in Atlantic herring (*Clupea harengus harengus*): description of protein loci and population data. *Hereditas*, **95**, 69-78.

Avise JC (1994) *Molecular Markers, Natural History and Evolution.* Chapman & Hall, London.

Barton NH, Charlesworth B (1984) Genetic revolutions, founder effects, and speciation. *Annual Reviews in Ecology and Systematics*, **15**, 133-164.

Barton NH (1989) Founder effect speciaton. In: *Speciation and Its Consequences* (eds. Otte D, Endler JA), pp. 229-256. Sinauer Associates, Sunderland, Massachusetts, USA.

Baumgartner TR, Souter A, Ferreira-Bartrina V (1992) Reconstruction of the history of Pacific sardine and the northern anchovy populations over the last two millenia from sediments off the Santa Barbara Basin, California. *California Cooperative Oceanic Fisheries Investigations Reports*, **33**, 24-40.

Bailey KM, Stabeno PJ, Powers DA (1997) The role of larval retention and transport features in mortality and potential gene flow of walleye pollock. *Journal of Fish Biology*, **51** (Suppl. A), 135-154.

Bayliff WH (1988) Integrity of schools of skipjack tuna, *Katsuwonus pelamis*, from the eastern Pacific Ocean as determined from tagging data. *Fishery Bulletin*, **86**, 315-323.

Bembo DG, Carvalho GR, Snow M, Cingolani N, Pitcher TJ (1995) Stock discrimination among European anchovies, *Engraulis encrasicolus*, by means of PCR-amplified mitochondrial DNA analysis. *Fisheries Bulletin*, **94**, 31-40.

Bembo DG, Carvalho GR, Cingolani N, Pitcher TJ (1996a) Electrophoretic analysis of stock structure in Northern Mediterranean anchovies. *ICES Journal of Marine Science*, **53**, 115-128.

Bembo DG, Carvalho GR, Cingolani N, Arneri E, Giannetti G, Pitcher TJ (1996b) Allozymic and morphometric evidence for two stocks of the European anchovy *Engraulis encrasicolus* in Adriatic waters. *Marine Biology*, **126**, 529-538.

Bentzen P, Taggart CT, Ruzzante DE, Cook D (1996) Microsatellite polymorphism and the population structure of Atlantic cod (*Gadus morhua*) in the northwest Atlantic. *Canadian Journal of Fisheries and Aquatic Sciences*, **53**, 2706-2721.

Bernatchez L, Colombani F & Dodson JJ (1991) Phylogenetic relationships among the subfamily Coregoninae as revealed by mitochondrial DNA analysis. *Journal of Fish Biology* **39**, 283-290.

Beverton RJH (1990) Small marine pelagic fish and the threat of fishing: are they endangered? *Journal of Fish Biology*, **37** (suppl. A), 5-16.

Billington N, Danzmann TG, Hebert PDN, Ward RD (1991) Phylogenetic relationships among four members of *Stizostedion* (Percidae) determined by mitochondrial DNA and allozyme analyses. *Journal of Fish Biology*, **39**, 251-258.

Birky CW, Fuerst P, Maruyama T (1989) Organelle gene diversity under migration, mutation, and drift: equilibrium expectations, approach to equilibrium, effects of heteroplasmic cells, and comparison to nuclear genes. *Genetics*, **121**, 613-627.

Blaxter JHS, Hunter JR (1982) The biology of clupeoid fishes. *Advances in Marine Biology*, **20**, 1-194.

Bowen BW, Grant WS (1997) Phylogeography of the sardines (*Sardinops* spp.): assessing biogeographic models and population histories in temperate upwelling zones. *Evolution*, **51**, 1601-1610.

Briggs JC (1960) Fishes of worldwide (circumtropical) distribution. *Copeia 1960*, 171-180.

Briggs JC (1995) *Global Biogeography*. Elsevier, New York.

Broughton RE, Gold JR (1997) Microsatellite development and survey of variation in northern bluefin tuna (*Thunnus thynnus*). *Molecular Marine Biology and Biotechnology*, **6**, 308-314.

Brown BE, Darcy GH, Overholtz W (1987) Stock assessment/stock identification: an interactive process. In: *Proceedings of the Stock Identification Workshop* (eds. Kumpf HE, Vaught RN, Grimes CB), pp. 1-24. NOAA-TM-NMFS-SEFC-199 Washington, DC: Department of Commerce.

Buckmann A (1950) Research of the Biological Institute on the ecology of herring fry in the southern part of the North Sea. *Helgolander Wissenschaftliche Meeresuntersuchungen*, **3**, 171-205.

Burd AC (1985) Recent changes in the central and southern North Sea herring stocks. *Canadian Journal of Fisheries and Aquatic Sciences*, **42** (Suppl. 1), 192-206.

Campton DE, Berg CJ, Robison LM, Glazer RA (1992) Genetic patchiness among populations of queen conch *Strombus gigas* in the Florida keys and Bimini. *Fishery Bulletin*, **90**, 250-259.

Carr SM, Marshall HD (1991) Detection of intraspecific DNA sequence variation in the mitochondrial cytochrome b gene of Atlantic cod (*Gadus morhua*) by the polymerase chain reaction. *Canadian Journal of Fisheries and Aquatic Sciences*, **48**, 48-52.

Carr SM, Snellen AJ, Howse KA, Wroblewsi JS (1995) Mitochondrial DNA sequence variation and genetic stock structure of Atlantic cod (*Gadus morhua*) from bay and offshore locations on the Newfoundland continental shelf. *Molecular Ecology*, **4**, 79-88.

Carvalho GR, (1993) Evolutionary aspects of fish distribution: genetic variability and distribution. *Journal of Fish Biology*, **43**, (Suppl. A) 53-73.

Carvalho GR, Hauser L (1994) Molecular genetics and the stock concept in fisheries. *Reviews in Fish Biology and Fisheries*, **4**, 326-350.

Carvalho GR, Hauser L (1998) Advances in the molecular analysis of fish population structure. *Italian Journal of Zoology*, **65**, (Supplement 1), in press.

Carvalho GR, Bembo DG, Carone A *et al.* (1994) Stock discrimination in relation to the assessment of Adriatic anchovy and sardine fisheries. *Final Project Report to the Commission of the European Community, EC XIV-1/MED/91001/A.*

Caton AE (1991) Review of aspects of southern bluefin tuna biology, population and fisheries. In: *World Meeting on Stock Assessments of Bluefin Tunas: Strengths and Weaknesses. Special Report No. 7* (eds. Desiro RB, Bayliff WH), pp. 181-350. Inter-American Tropical Tuna Commission, La Jolla, California.

Chikhi L, Bonhomme F, Agnese J-F (1998) Low genetic variability in a widely distributed and abundant clupeid species, *Sardinella aurita*. New empirical results and interpretations. *Journal of Fish Biology*, **52**, 861-878.

Chow S, Kishino H (1995) Phylogenetic relationships between tuna species of the genus *Thunnus* (Scombridae: Teleostei): inconsistent implications from morphology, nuclear and mitochondrial genomes. *Journal of Molecular Evolution*, **127**, 359-367.

Chow S, Ushiama H (1995) Global population structure of albacore (*Thunnus alalunga*) inferred by RFLP analysis of the mitochondrial ATPase gene. *Marine Biology*, **123**, 39-45.

Chow S, Okamoto H, Uozomi Y, Takeuchi Y, Takeyama H (1997) Genetic stock structure of the swordfish (*Xiphias gladius*) inferred by PCR-RFLP analysis of the mitochondrial DNA control region. *Marine Biology*, **127**, 359-367.

Coulter GW (1991a) Pelagic fish. In: *Lake Tanganyika and its Life* (ed. Coulter GW), pp. 111-138. Oxford University Press. London, Oxford & New York.

Coulter GW (1991b) Fisheries. In: *Lake Tanganyika and its Life* (ed. Coulter GW), pp. 139-150. Oxford University Press. London, Oxford & New York.

Cronin MA, Spearman WJ, Wilmot RL, Patto JC, Bickham JW (1993) Mitochondrial DNA variation in chinook (*Oncorhynchus tsawytscha*) and chum salmon (*O. keta*) detected by restriction enzyme analysis of polymerase chain reaction (PCR) products. *Canadian Journal of Fisheries and Aquatic Sciences*, **50**, 708-715.

Crow JF, Kimura M (1970) *An Introduction to Population Genetics Theory*. Harper and Row, New York.

Crozier RH (1987) Genetic aspects of kin recognition: concept, models and synthesis. In: *Kin Recognition in Animals* (eds. Fletcher DJ, Mitchener CD), pp. 287-331. John Wiley & Sons, New York.

Cury P, Roy C (1989) Optimal environmental window and pelagic fish recruitment success in upwelling areas. *Canadian Journal of Fisheries and Aquatic Sciences*, **46**, 670-680.

Cury P (1993) Catastrophe-type regulation of pelagic fish stocks: adaptive management for evolving resources. In: *The Exploitation of Evolving Resources* (eds. Stokes TK, McGlade JM, Law R), pp. 204-220. Springer-Verlag, Berlin.

Cushing DH (1955) On the autumn spawning herring races of the North Sea. *Journal du Conseil International d'Exploration du Mer,* **21,** 44-60.

Cushing DH, Burd AC (1957) On the herring of the southern North Sea. III. *Fisheries Investigations Series II,* Vol. 10.

Cushing DH (1972) The production cycle and the number of marine fish. *Symposia of the Zoological Society, London,* **29,** 213-232.

Cushing DH (1975) *Marine Ecology and Fisheries.* Cambridge University Press, Cambridge.

Cushing DH (1982) *Climate and Fisheries.* Academic Press, London.

Dahle G, Eriksen AG (1990) Spring and autumn spawners of herring (*Clupea harengus*) in the North Sea Skagerrak and Kattegat; population genetic analysis. *Fishery Research,* **9,** 131-141.

deVries TJ, Pearcy WG (1982) Fish debris in sediments of the upwelling zone off central Peru: a late Quaternary record. *Deep Sea Research,* **29,** 87-109.

Doherty PJ, Planes S, Mather P (1995) Gene flow and larval duration in seven species of fish from the Great Barrier Reef. *Ecology,* **76,** 2373-2391.

Duplessy JC (1982) Glacial to interglacial contrasts in the northern Indian Ocean. *Nature,* **295,** 494-498.

Edmunds PH, Sammons JI (1973) Similarity of genetic polymorphism of tetrazolium oxidase in bluefin tuna (*Thunnus thynnus*) from the Atlantic coast of France and the Western North Atlantic. *Journal of the Fisheries Research Board of Canada,* **30,** 1031-1032.

Elliott NG, Ward RD (1995) Genetic relationships of eight species of Pacific tunas (*Teleostei, Scombridae*) inferred from allozyme analysis. *Marine and Freshwater Research,* **46,** 1021-1032.

Estoup A, Rousset F, Michalakis Y, Cornuet JM, Adriamanga M, Guyomard R (1998) Comparative analysis of microsatellite and allozyme markers: a case study investigating microgeographic differentiation in brown trout (*Salmo trutta*). *Molecular Ecology,* **7,** 339-353.

Excoffier L, Smouse PE, Quattro JM (1992) Analysis of molecular variance inferred from metric distances among DNA haplotypes: application to human mitochondrial restriction data. *Genetics,* **131,** 479-491.

FAO (1993) Review of the state of world marine fishery resources. *FAO Fisheries Technical Paper,* **335.** Food and agriculture Organization of the United Nations, Rome.

FAO (1997) FAO Yearbook 1995. *Fishery Statistics: Catches and Landings,* **80.** Food and agriculture Organization of the United Nations, Rome.

Ferguson A (1994) Molecular genetics in fisheries: current and future perspectives. *Reviews in Fish Biology and Fisheries,* **4,** 379-383.

Fujio, Y and Kato, Y (1979) Genetic variation in fish populations. *Bulletin of the Japanese Society for Scientific Fisheries,* **45,** 1169-1178.

Fujino K, Sasaki K, Okumura S (1981) Genetic diversity of skipjack tuna in the Atlantic, Indian, and Pacific Oceans. *Bulletin of the Japanese Society of Scientific Fisheries,* **47,** 215-222.

Galvin P, Sadusky T, McGregor D, Cross T (1995) Population genetics of Atlantic cod using amplified single locus minisatellite VNTR analysis. *Journal of Fish Biology,* **47** (Suppl. A), 200-208.

Garcia S, Grainger R (1997) Fisheries management and sustainability: a new perspective of an old problem. In: *Developing and Sustaining World Fisheries Resources: The State of Science and Management. 2nd World Fisheries Congress Proceedings* (eds. Hancock DA, Smith DC, Grant A, Beumer JP), pp. 631-654. CSIRO Publishing, Collingwood, Australia.

Garcia S, Newton C (1997) Current situation, trends, and prospects in world capture fisheries. In: *Global Trends: Fisheries Management* (eds. Pikitch EL, Huppert DD, Sissenwine MP), pp. 3-27. American Fisheries Society Symposium 20, Bethesda, Maryland, USA.

Gauldie RW (1988) Tagging and genetically isolated stocks of fish: a test of one stock hypothesis and the development of another. *Journal of Applied Icthyology,* **4,** 168-173.

Giæver M, Stien J (1998) Population genetic substructure in blue whiting based on allozyme data. *Journal of Fish Biology,* **52,** 782-795.

Gold JR, Kristmundsdottir AY, Richardson LR (1997) Mitochondrial DNA variation in king mackerel (*Scomberomorus cavalla*) from the western Atlantic Ocean and Gulf of Mexico. *Marine Biology,* **129,** 221-232.

Gourene AB, Pouyard L,Agnese J.-F. 1993. Importance de certaines characteristiques biologiques dans la structuration génétique des espèces de populations: le cas de *Ethmalosa fimbriata* et *Sarotherodon melanotheron. Journal Ivoirien d'Océanologie et Limnologie d'Abidjan,* **2,** 55-69.

Grant WS (1984) Biochemical population genetics of Atlantic herring, *Clupea harengus. Copeia 1984,* 357-364.

Grant WS, Utter FM (1984) Biochemical population genetics of Pacific herring (*Clupea pallasi*). *Canadian Journal of Fisheries and Aquatic Sciences,* **41,** 856-864.

Grant WS (1985) Biochemical genetic stock structure of the southern African anchovy, *Engraulis capensis* Gilchrist. *Journal of Fish Biology,* **27,** 23-29.

Grant WS, Bowen BW (1998) Shallow population histories in deep evolutionary lineages of marine fishes: insights from sardines and anchovies and lessons for conservation. *Journal of Heredity*, in press.

Grant WS, Clark A-M, Bowen BW (1998) Why RFLP analysis of mitochondrial DNA failed to resolve sardine (*Sardinops*) biogeography: insights from mitochondrial DNA cytochrome b sequences. *Canadian Journal of Fisheries and Aquatic Sciences*, in press.

Grant WS, Leslie RW (1996) Late Pleistocene dispersal of Indian-Pacific sardine populations in an ancient lineage of the genus *Sardinops*. *Marine Biology*, **126**, 133-142.

Graves JE, Dizon AE (1989) Mitochondrial DNA sequence similarity of Atlantic and Pacific albacore tuna (*Thunnus alalunga*). *Canadian Journal of Fisheries and Aquatic Science*, **46**, 870-873.

Graves JE, McDowell JR (1994) Genetic analysis of striped marlin (*Tetrapturus audax*) population structure in the Pacific Ocean. *Canadian Journal of Fisheries and Aquatic Sciences*, **51**, 1762-1768.

Graves JE (1995) Conservation genetics of fishes in the pelagic marine realm. In: *Conservation Genetics: Case Histories from Nature* (eds. Avise JC, Hamrick JL), pp. 335-366. Chapman and Hall, New York.

Graves JE, McDowell JR (1995) Inter-ocean genetic divergence of istiophorid billfishes. *Marine Biology*, **122**, 193-203.

Grewe PM, Elliott NG, Innes BH, Ward RD (1997) Genetic population structure of southern bluefin tuna (*Thunnus maccoyii*). *Marine Biology*, **127**, 555-561.

Grewe PM, Hampton J (1998) An assessment of bigeye (*Thunnus obesus*) population structure in the Pacific Ocean, based on mitochondrial DNA and DNA microsatellite analysis. *CSIRO Marine Research*, Hobart, Australia.

Grijalva-Chon JM, Numachi K, Sosa-Nishizaki O, de la Rosa-Velez J (1994) Mitochondrial DNA analysis of North Pacific swordfish *Xiphias gladius* population structure. *Marine Ecology Progress Series*, **115**, 15-19.

Grijalva-Chon JM, de la Rosa-Velez J, Sosa-Nishizaki O (1996) Allozyme variability in two samples of swordfish, *Xiphias gladius* L., in the North Pacific Ocean. *Fishery Bulletin*, **94**, 589-594.

Gyllensten U (1985) The genetic structure of fish: differences in the intraspecific distribution of biochemical genetic variation between marine, anadromous, and freshwater species. *Journal of Fish Biology*, **26**, 691-699.

Haegele CW, Schweigert JF (1985) Distribution and characteristics of herring spawning grounds and description of spawning behaviour. *Canadian Journal of Fisheries and Aquatic Sciences*, **42**, Suppl. 1, 39-55.

Hauser L (1996) *Genetic and Morphological Differentiation of Native and Introduced Populations of the Lake Tanganyika Sardine, Limnothrissa miodon*. PhD thesis, University of Wales, Swansea.

Hauser L, Carvalho GR, Pitcher TJ (1998) Genetic population structure of the Lake Tanganyika sardine, *Limnothrissa miodon*. *Journal of Fish Biology*, in press.

Hay DE, McCarter PB (1997) Larval distribution, abundance, and stock structure of British Columbia herring. *Journal of Fish Biology*, **51** (Suppl. A), 155-175.

Hedgecock D, Nelson K, Lopez-Lemus LG (1988) Biochemical genetic and morphological divergence among three species of thread herring (*Opisthonema*) in Northwest Mexico. *California Cooperative Oceanic Fisheries Investigations Reports*, **29**, 110-121.

Hedgecock D, Hutchinson ES, Li G, Sly FL, Neslon K (1989) Genetic and morphometric variation in the Pacific sardine, *Sardinops sagax caerulea*: comparisons and contrasts with historical data and with variability in the northern anchovy, *Engraulis mordax*. *Fishery Bulletin*, **87**, 653-671.

Hedgecock D, Chow V, Waples RS (1992) Effective population number of shellfish broodstocks estimated from temporal variances in allele frequencies. *Aquaculture*, **108**, 215-232.

Hedgecock D (1994) Does variance in reproductive success limit effective population size of marine organisms? In: *Genetic and Evolution of Aquatic Organisms* (ed. Beaumont AR), pp. 122-134. Chapman & Hall.

Hedgecock D, Hutchinson ES, Li G, Sly FL, Neslon K (1994) The central stock of northern anchovy is not a randomly mating population. *California Cooperative Oceanic Fisheries Investigation Reports*, **35**, 121-136.

Hilborn R (1991) Modeling the stability of fish schools: exchange of individual fish between schools of skipjack tuna (*Katsuwonus pelamis*). *Canadian Journal of Fisheries and Aquatic Sciences*, **48**, 1081-1091.

Hilborn R, Walters CJ (1992) *Quantitative Fisheries Stock Assessment: Choice, Dynamics and Uncertainty*. Chapman & Hall, New York and London.

Hillis DM, Mable BK, Larson A, Davis SK, Zimmer EA (1996) Nucleic Acids IV: sequencing and cloning. In: *Molecular Systematics* (eds. Hillis DM, Moritz C, Mable BK), pp 321-381. Sinauer Associates, Sunderland, MAS.

ICCAT (1992) Comments on the stock structure of Atlantic yellowfin tuna. *International Commission for the Conservation of Atlantic Tunas. Report for 1990-91, Part II*, pp. 217-220.

Ihssen PE, Booke HE, Casselman JM, McGlade JM, Payne NR, Utter FM (1981) Stock identification: materials and methods. *Canadian Journal of Fisheries and Aquatic Sciences*, **38**, 1838-1855.

Jamieson A (1973) Genetic "tags" for marine fish stocks. In: *Sea Fisheries Research* (eds. Hardin JFR), pp. 91-99. Elek Science, London.

Johnson PO (1970) The Wash sprat fishery. *Fisheries Investigations London*, Series 2, **26** (4).

Jørstad KE, King DPF, Nævdal G (1991) Population structure of Atlantic herring, *Clupea harengus* L. *Journal of Fish Biology*, **39** (Suppl. A), 43-52.

Jørstad KE, Dahle G, Paulsen OI (1994) Genetic comparison between Pacific herring (*Clupea pallasi*) and a Norwegian fjord stock of Atlantic herring *(Clupea harengus)*. *Canadian Journal of Fisheries and Aquatic Sciences*, **51** (Suppl. 1), 233-239.

Junquera S, Perez-Gandaras G (1993) Population diversity in Bay of Biscay anchovy (*Engraulis encrasicolus* L. 1758) as revealed by multivariate analysis of morphometric and meristic characters. *ICES Journal of Marine Science*, **50**, 383-391.

Kijima A, Taniguchi N, Makino H, Ochai A (1985) Degree of genetic divergence and breeding structure of jack mackerel, *Trachurus japonicus*. *Report of the Marine Biology Institue of Kochi University*.

Kimura M (1983) *The Neutral Theory of Molecular Evolution*. Cambridge University Press, Cambrigde.

King DPF, Ferguson A, Moffett IJJ (1987) Aspects of population genetics of herring, *Clupea harengus*, around the British Isles and in the Baltic Sea. *Fisheries Research*, **6**, 35-52.

Kinsey ST, Orsoy T, Bert TM, Mahmoudi B (1994) Population structure of the Spanish sardine *Sardinella aurita*: natural morphological variation in a genetically homogenous population. *Marine Biology*, **118**, 309-317.

Kocher TD, Thomas WK, Meyer A *et al.* (1989) Dynamics of mitochondrial DNA evolution in animals: amplification and sequencing with conserved primers. *Proceedings of the National Academy of Sciences, USA*, **86**, 6196-6200.

Kornfield I, Sidell BD, Gagnon PS (1982) Stock definition in Atlantic herring (*Clupea harengus harengus*): genetic evidence for discrete fall and spring spawning populations. *Canadian Journal of Fisheries and Aquatic Sciences*, **39**, 1610-1621.

Kornfield I, Bogdanowicz SM (1987) Differentiation of mitochondrial DNA in Atlantic herring, *Clupea harengus*. *Fishery Bulletin*, **85**, 561-568.

Kornfield I, Parker A (1997) Molecular systematics of a rapidly evolving species flock: the mbuna of Lake Malawi and the search for phylogenetic signal. In: *Molecular Systematics of Fishes* (eds. Kocher TD, Stepien CA). Academic Press, London.

Kotoulas G, Magoulas A, Tsimenides N, Zouros E (1995) Marked mitochondrial DNA differences between Mediterranean and Atlantic populations of the swordfish, *Xiphias gladius*. *Molecular Ecology*, **4**, 473-481.

Lewis RD, Ridgway GJ (1972) Biochemical studies on the stock structure of herring in the Gulf of Maine, Georges Bank and adjacent areas. *International Committee of Northwest Atlantic Fisheries Research Documents*, **72** (20), 1-15.

Lewontin RC, Krakauer J (1973) Distribution of gene frequency as a test of the theory of the selective neutrality of polymorphisms. *Genetics*, **74**, 175-195.

Lowe-McConnell RH (1987) *Ecological Studies in Tropical Fish Communities*. Cambridge University Press, Cambridge.

Lush IE (1969) Polymorphism of a phosphoglucomutase isoenzyme in the herring (*Clupea harengus*). *Comparative Biochemistry and Physiology*, **30**, 391-395.

Mackinson S, Sumaila UR, Pitcher TJ (1997). Bioeconomics and catchabilty: fish and fishers behaviour during stock collapse. *Fisheries Research*, **31**, 11-17.

MacRae AF, Anderson WW (1988) Evidence for non-neutrality of mitochondrial DNA haplotypes in *Drosophila pseudoobscura*. *Genetics*, **120**, 485-494.

Magoulas A, Tsimenides N, Zouros E (1996) Mitochondrial DNA phylogeny and the reconstruction of the population history of a species: the case of the European anchovy (*Engraulis encrasicolus*). *Molecular Biology and Evolution*, **13**, 178-190.

Magurran AE, Seghers BH, Shaw PW, Carvalho GR (1994) Schooling preferences for familiar fish in the guppy, *Poecilia reticulata*. *Journal of Fish Biology*, **45**, 401-406.

Maruyama T, Fuerst PA (1984) Population bottlenecks and nonequilibrium models in population genetics. I. Allele numbers when populations evolve from zero variability. *Genetics*, **108**, 745-763.

McGoodwin JR (1990) *Crisis in the World's Fisheries. People, Problems and Policies*. Stanford University Press, California.

McQuinn IH (1997) Metapopulations and the Atlantic herring. *Reviews in Fish Biolgy and Fisheries*, **7**, 297-329.

McVeigh HP, Davidson WS (1991) A salmonid phylogeny inferred from mitochondrial DNA restriction analsyis. *Journal of Fish Biology*, **39**, 277-282.

Menezes MR (1994) Little genetic variation in the oil sardine, *Sardinella longiceps* Val., from the western coast of India. *Australian Journal of Marine and Freshwater Research*, **45**, 257-264.

Meyer A, Dolven SI (1992) Molecules, fossils and the origin of tetrapods. *Journal of Molecular Evolution*, **35**, 102-113.

Milinkovitch MC, Orti G, Meyer A (1993) Revised phylogeny of whales suggested by mitochondrial ribosomal DNA sequences. *Nature*, **361**, 346-348.

Mills CA (1987) The life history of the minnow *Phoxinus phoxinus* (L.) in a productive stream. *Freshwater Biology*, **17**, 53-67.

Milton DA, Shaklee JB (1987) Biochemical genetics and population structure of blue grenadier, *Macruronus novaezelandiae* (Hector) (*Pisces : Merlucciidae*), from Australian waters. *Australian Journal of Marine and Freshwater Research*, **38**, 727-742.

Mork J, Sundnes,G (1985) O-group cod (*Gadus morhua*) in captivity: differential survival of certain genotypes. *Helgoländer Meeresuntersuchungen*, **39**, 63-70.

Morrow JE, Harbo SJ (1969) A revision of the sailfish genus *Istiophorus*. *Copeia 1969*, 34-44.

Nakamura I (1985) FAO Species Catalogue. Billfishes of the World. An annotated and illustrated catalogue of marlins, sailfishes, spearfishes and swordfishes known to date. *FAO Fish. Synop. 125*, **5**. FAO, Rome.

National Research Council (1994) *An Assessment of Atlantic Bluefin Tuna*. Washington D.C: National Academy Press.

Nauta MJ, Weissing FJ (1996) Constraints on allele size at microsatellite loci: implications for genetic differentiation. *Genetics*, **143**, 1021-1032.

Nei M, Maruyama T, Chakraborty R (1975) The bottleneck effect and genetic variability in populations. *Evolution*, **29**, 1-10.

Nei M, Grauer D (1984) Extent of protein polymorphism and the neutral mutation theory. *Evolutionary Biology*, **17**, 73-118.

Nei M (1987) *Molecular Evolutionary Genetics*. Columbia University Press, New York.

Nelson K, Soulé M (1987) Genetical Conservation of Exploited Fishes. In: *Population Genetics and Fisheries Management* (eds. Ryman N, Utter F), pp. 345-368. University of Washington Press, Seattle and London.

Nigro L, Prout T (1990) Is there selection on RFLP differences in mitochondrial DNA? *Genetics*, **123**, 551-555.

O'Connell M, Wright JM (1997) Microsatellite DNA in fishes. *Reviews in Fish Biology and Fisheries*, **7**, 331-363.

O'Connell M, Dillon MC, Wright JM, Bentzen P, Merkouris S, Seeb J (1998) Genetic structuring among Alaskan Pacific herring (*Clupea pallasi*) population identified using microsatellite variability. *Journal of Fish Biology*, in press.

Ojaveer E (1989) Population structure of pelagic fishes in the Baltic. *Raports P.V. Reun. Conseil International d'Exploration du Mer*, **190**, 17-21.

Ovenden JR (1990) Mitochondrial DNA and marine stock assessment: a review. *Australian Journal of Marine and Freshwater Research*, **41**, 835-853.

Palumbi SR (1996) Nucleic Acids II: the polymerase chain reaction. In: *Molecular Systematics*, 2nd edn. (eds. Hillis DM, Moritz C, Mable BK), pp. 205-248. Sinauer Associates, Massachusetts, USA.

Park LK, Moran P (1994) Developments in molecular genetic techniques in fisheries. *Reviews in Fish Biology and Fisheries*, **4**, 272-299.

Parrish BB, Saville A (1965) The biology of the north-east Atlantic herring populations. *Oceanographic Marine Biology Annual Review*, **3**, 323-373.

Pauly D, Christensen V, Dalsgaard J, Froese R, Torres F Jr (1998) Fishing down marine food webs. *Science*, **279**, 860-863.

Pitcher TJ, Hart P (1982) *Fisheries Ecology*. Croom-Helm, London.

Pitcher TJ, Parrish JK (1993) Functions of shoaling behaviour in teleosts In: *Behaviour of Teleost Fishes*, 2nd edn. (ed. Pitcher TJ). Chapman & Hall, London.

Pitcher TJ, Misund OA, Ferno A, Totland B, Melle V (1996). Adaptive behaviour of herring schools in the Norwegian Sea as revealed by high-resolution sonar. *ICES Journal of Marine Science*, **53**, 449-452.

Pogson GH, Mesa KA, Boutilier RG (1995) Genetic population structure and gene flow in the Atlantic cod *Gadus morhua*: a comparison of allozyme and nuclear RFLP loci. *Genetics*, **139**, 375-385.

Postuma KH (1974) The nucleus of the herring otolith as a racial character. *Journal du Conseil International d'Exploration du Mer*, **35**, 121-129.

Powers DA, Lauerman T, Crawford D, Smith M, Gonzalez-Villasenor I, DiMichelle L (1991) The evolutionary significance of genetic variation at enzyme synthesizing loci in the teleost *Fundulus heteroclitus*. *Journal of Fish Biology*, **39** (Suppl. A), 169-184.

Quesada H, Beynon CM, Skibinski DOF (1995) A mitochondrial DNA discontinuity in the mussel *Mytilus galloprovincialis* Lmk: Pleistocene vicariance biogeography and secondary intergradation. *Molecular Biology and Evolution*, **12**, 521-524.

Ramon MM, Castro JA (1997) Genetic variation in natural stocks of *Sardinia pilchardus* (sardines) from the western Mediterranean Sea. *Heredity*, **78**, 520-528.

Richardson BJ (1982) Geographical districution of electrophoretically detected protein variation in Australian commercial fishes. II. Jackass morwong *Cheilodactylus macropterus* Bloch and Schneider. *Australian Journal of Marine and Freshwater Research*, **33**, 917-926.

Richardson BJ (1983) Distribution of protein variation in skipjack tuna (*Katsuwonus pelamis*) from the central and south-western Pacific. *Australian Journal of Marine and Freshwater Research*, **34**, 231-251.

Ridgway GJ, Sherburne SW, Lewis RD (1970) Polymorphism in the esterases of Atlantic herring. *Transactions of the American Fisheries Society*, **99**, 147-151.

Rivas LR (1975) Synopsis of biological data on blue marlin, *Makaira nigricans* Lacepede, 1802. In: *Proceedings of the International Billfish Symposium* (eds. Shomura RS, Williams F), pp. 1-16. Kailua-Kona, Hawaii, part 3. US Dept. Commerc., NOAA Tech. Rep. NMFS SSRF-675.

Robins CR, de Sylva DP (1960) Description and relationships of the longbill spearfish, *Tetrapturus belone*, based on western North Atlantic specimens. *Bulletin of Marine Science*, **10**, 383-413.

Rogers AR, Harpending H (1992) Population growth makes waves in the distribution of pairwise genetic differences. *Molecular Biology and Evolution*, **9**, 552-569.

Rogers AR (1995) Genetic evidence for a Pleistocene population explosion. *Evolution*, **49**, 608-615.

Rosenberg R, Palmen LE (1982) Composition of herring stocks in the Skagerrak-Kattegat and the relation of these stocks with those of the North Sea and adjacent waters. *Fisheries Research*, **1**, 83-104.

Ruzzante DE (1998) A comparison of several measures of genetic distance and population structure with microsatellite data: bias and sampling variance. *Canadian Journal of Fisheries and Aquatic Sciences*, **55**, 1-14.

Ruzzante DE, Taggart CT, Cook D (1997) Spatial and temporal variation in the genetic composition of a larval cod (*Gadus morhua*) aggregation: cohort contribution and genetic stability. *Canadian Journal of Fisheries and Aquatic Sciences*, **53**, 2695-2705.

Ryman N (1993) Genetic effects of harvesting and enhancing natural populations. In: *Proceedings of the Norway/UNEP Expert Conference on Biodiversity, 24-28 May 1993.* Directorate for Nature Management (DN) and Norwegian Institute for Nature Research (NINA). Trondheim, Norway.

Ryman N, Lagercrantz U, Anderson L, Chakraborty R, Rosenberg R (1984) Lack of correspondence between genetic and morphologic variability patterns in Atlantic herring (*Clupea harengus*). *Heredity*, **53**, 687-704.

Ryman N, Utter F, Laikre L (1995) Protection of intraspecific biodiversity in exploited fishes. *Reviews in Fish Biology and Fisheries*, **5**, 417-446.

Saavedra C, Zapata C, Guerra A, Alvarez G (1993) Allozyme variation in European populations of the oyster *Ostrea edulis*. *Marine Biology*, **115**, 85-95.

Scoles DR, Graves JE (1993) Genetic analysis of the population structure of yellowfin tuna, *Thunnus albacares*, from the Pacific Ocean. *Fishery Bulletin of the US*, **91**, 690-698.

Shackelton LY (1986) Fossil pilchard and anchovy scales - indicators of past fish populations off Namibia. In: *International Symposium on Long Term Changes in Marine Fish Populations* (eds. Wyatt T, Larraneta MG), pp. 55-68.

Shaklee JB, Brill RW, Acerra R (1983) Biochemical genetics of Pacific blue marlin, *Makaira nigricans*, from Hawaiian waters. *Fishery Bulletin*, **81**, 85-90.

Sharp GD (1978) Behavioural and physiological properties of tunas and their effect on vulnerability to fishing gear. In: *The Physiological Ecology of Tunas* (eds. Sharp GD, Dizo AE), pp. 397-449. New York, Academic Press.

Sharp GD, Pirages SW (1978) The distribution of red and white swimming muscles, their biochemistry, and the biochemical phylogeny of selected scombrid fishes. In: *The Physiological Ecology of Tunas* (eds. Sharp GD, Dizon AE), pp. 41-78. New York, Academic Press.

Shaw PW, Turan C, Wright JM, O'Connell M, Carvalho GR (1998a) Microsatellite DNA analysis of population structure in Atlantic herring (*Clupea harengus*), with direct comparison to allozyme and mtDNA data. *Canadian Journal of Fisheries and Aquatic Sciences*, in press.

Shaw PW, Pierce GJ, Boyle PR (1998b) Subtle population structuring within a highly vagile marine invertebrate, the Veined Squid *Loligo forbesi*, demonstrated with microsatellite DNA markers. *Molecular Ecology*, in press.

Sinclair M (1988) *Marine Populations: an Essay on Population Regulation and Speciation.* University of Washington Press, Seattle & London.

Slatkin M (1987) Gene flow and the geographic structure of natural populations. *Science*, **236**, 787-792.

Slatkin M (1995) A measure of population subdivision based on microstallite allele frequencies. *Genetics,* **139**, 157-162.

Smith MH, Tolliver D (1987) Blueback herring and the stock concept. In: *Proceedings of the stock identification workshop* (eds. Kumpf HE, Vaught RN, Grimes CB, Johnson AG, Nakamura EL). *NOAA Technical Memorandum* NMFS-SEFC-199, Panama City Beach, Florida.

Smith PJ, Jamieson A (1986) Stock discreteness in herrings: a conceptual revolution. *Fisheries Research,* **4**, 223-234.

Smith PJ, Jamieson A, Birley AJ (1990) Electrophoretic studies and stock concept in marine teleosts. *Journal du Conseil International d'Exploration du Mer,* **47**, 231-245.

Smith PJ, Francis RICC, McVeagh M (1991) Loss of genetic diversity due to fishing pressure. *Fisheries Research,* **10**, 309-316.

Smith PJ, Benson PG (1997) Genetic diversity in orange roughy from the east of New Zealand. *Fisheries Research,* **31**, 197-213.

Sokal RR, Rohlf FJ (1995) *Biometry - The Principles and Practice of Statistics in Biological Research,* 2nd edn. W.H. Freeman & Co., New York.

SPC (1981) Report of the Second Skipjack Survey and Assessment Programme Workshop to Review Results from Genetic Analysis of Skipjack Blood Samples. *Skipjack Survey and Assessment Programme. Technical Report No. 6.* Noumea, New Caledonia: South Pacific Commission.

Stephenson RL, Kornfield I (1990) Reappearance of spawning Atlantic herring (*Clupea harengus harengus*) on Georges Bank: population resurgence not recolonisation. *Canadian Journal of Fisheries and Aquatic Sciences,* **47**, 1060-1064.

Suzuki Z (1991) Migration, western Atlantic. In: *World Meeting on Stock Assessment of Bluefin Tunas: Strengths and Weaknesses* (eds. Deriso RB, Bayliff WH), pp. 129-130. La Jolla, California. Inter-American Tropical Tuna Commission.

Tortonese E (1983) Distribution and ecology of endemic elements in the Mediterranean fauna (fishes and echinoderms*). NATO Conf. (Ser I: Medité. OR Ecosystems),* **1**, 57-83.

Tringali MD, Wilson RR (1993) Differences in haplotype frequencies of mtDNA of the Spanish sardine *Sardinella aurita* between specimens from the eastern Gulf of Mexico and southern Brazil. *Fishery Bulletin,* **91**, 362-370.

Turan C (1997) *Population structure of Atlantic herring, Clupea harengus L., in the northeast Atlantic using phenotypic and molecular approaches.* PhD thesis, University of Wales, Swansea.

Turan C, Carvalho GR, Mork J (1998) Molecular genetic analyis of Atlanto-Scandian herring (*Clupea harengus*) populations using allozymes and mitochondrial DNA markers. *Journal of the Marine Biological Association, U.K,* **78**, 1-15.

Utter F, Ryman N (1993) Genetic markers and mixed stock fisheries. *Fisheries,* **18** (8), 11-21.

Vrijenhoek RC, Pfeiler E, Wetherington J (1992) Balancing selection in a desert stream dwelling fish, *Poeciliopsis monacha. Evolution,* **46**, 1642-1657.

Waples RS (1987) A multispecies approach to the analysis of gene flow in marine shore fishes. *Evolution,* **41**, 385-400.

Ward RD, Grewe PM (1994) Appraisal of molecular genetic techniques in fisheries. *Reviews in Fish Biology and Fisheries,* **4**, 300-325.

Ward RD, Woodwark M, Skibinski DOF (1994) A comparison of genetic diversity levels in marine, freshwater and anadromous fish. *Journal of Fish Biology,* **44**, 213-232.

Ward RD (1995) Population genetics of tunas. *Journal of Fish Biology,* **47** (suppl.A), 259-280.

Ward RD, Elliott NG, Innes BH, Smolenski AJ, Grewe PM (1997) Global population structure of yellowfin tuna (*Thunnus albacares*) inferred from allozyme and mitochondrial DNA variation. *Fishery Bulletin US,* **95**, 566-575.

Weir BS, Cockerham CC (1984) Estimating *F*-statistics for the analysis of population structure. *Evolution,* **38**, 1358-1370.

Wheeler JP, Winters GH (1984) Homing of Atlantic herring (*Clupea harengus harengus*) in Newfoundland waters as indicated by tagging data. *Canadian Journal of Fisheries and Aquatic Sciences,* **41**, 108-117.

White BA, Shaklee JB (1991) Need for replicated electrophoretic analyses in multiagency genetic stock identification (GSI) programs: examples from a pink salmon (*Oncorhynchus gorbuscha*) GSI fisheries study. *Canadian Journal of Fisheries and Aquatic Sciences,* **48**, 1396-1407.

White M (1998) Development, dispersal and recruitment: a paradox for survival among Antarctic fish. In: *Fishes of Antarctica: A Biological Overview* (eds. di Prisco G, Pisano E, Clarke A,). Springer Verlag, in press.

Wilson RR, Alberdi PD (1991) An electrophoretic study of Spanish sardine suggests a single predominant species in the eastern Gulf of Mexico. *Canadian Journal of Fisheries and Aquatic Sciences,* **48**, 792-798.

Wright S (1969) *Evolution and the Genetics of Populations (Vol. 2). The Theory of Gene Frequencies.* University of Chicago Press, Chicago.

Zore-Armanda, M (1969) Water exchange between the Adriatic Sea and eastern Mediterranean. *Deep Sea Research,* **16**, 171-178.

Advances in Molecular Ecology
G.R. Carvalho (Ed.)
IOS Press, 1998

Molecular Markers and Natural Selection

Jeffry B. Mitton
Department of Environmental, Population and Organismic Biology
University of Colorado
Boulder, Colorado, USA 80309
e-mail: mitton@colorado.edu

Natural selection is defined as the differential reproduction of genotypes. Advances in molecular methodology now enable genotypes to be identified with allozyme polymorphisms, cleaved polymorphic amplified fragments, anonymous nuclear DNA polymorphisms, and mitochondrial DNA and chloroplast DNA haplotypes. Most molecular markers are expected to be neutral, but intense selection has been detected in some allozyme loci. It is always difficult to determine whether documented examples involve *selection for* allozyme genotypes, or *selection detected by* allozyme genotypes. Similarly, some studies have reported components of fitness to increase with allozyme heterozygosity, but the interpretation of these correlations is controversial.

Comprehensive studies of allozyme polymorphisms have revealed that the alternate genotypes at a locus often differ kinetically, and may have substantial impacts on physiological variation, growth rate, viability, fecundity, and male mating success. Two recent research programs are featured here. The alcohol dehydrogenase (*ADH*) polymorphism in the tiger salamander interacts with levels of oxygen in ponds to produce variability in growth and survival. In pinyon pine, the glycerate dehydrogenase polymorphism (*GLY*) is associated with microgeographic variation in soil moisture, and both growth rates and viabilities on dry sites.

Demographic and genetic studies in red deer and harbour seals have reported that birth weight and neonatal survival increase with variation at microsatellite loci. The high mutation rates of microsatellites may detect differences in levels of inbreeding among individuals.

Loci sharing the same mode of inheritance but revealing strikingly different patterns of geographic variation must be subject to different evolutionary pressures. Studies that compare the geographic variation of allozymes and DNA markers often show discordant patterns of variation. When estimates of gene flow are estimated from values of F_{ST}, allozyme markers usually return higher estimates of gene flow than do DNA markers.

Molecular markers have provided new insights into sexual selection, and provided evidence in support of female choice of "good genes". Studies of sexual selection in butterflies, brine shrimp, and marine snails have revealed male mating success to increase with allozyme heterozygosity.

1. Introduction

The mechanism of natural selection was first described by Darwin and Wallace in the 19th century (Darwin 1859; Eiseley 1958), and has been studied extensively since (Dobzhansky 1970; Ford 1975; Wallace 1975; Endler 1986; Mitton 1997). Natural selection can most succinctly be defined as the differential reproduction of genotypes. It may result in evolution, or it may retain a population at an equilibrium. If we define evolution as a substantial and sustained change in the genetic constitution of a population, we can see that directional selection, such as unrelenting selection for larger body size in Pleistocene mammals, would cause a population to evolve. However, if selection acts primarily against unusual phenotypes, or favours intermediate phenotypes, then it will act to prevent evolution, stabilising phenotypes at an equilibrium (Dobzhansky 1970).

1.1. Identifying targets of selection

Natural selection discriminates among different forms at many levels (Gould 1982), including genotypes at single loci (Williams 1985; Mitton 1997), physiological, morphological and behavioural phenotypes, individuals, family groups (Hamilton 1964; Michod 1982), demes (Wade 1978; Wilson 1997), and species. The identification of the targets of selection is a much debated and important issue (Sober & Lewontin 1982; Brandon & Burian 1984). Many studies have reported evidence of natural selection (Endler 1986; Mitton 1997), but for only a tiny proportion of these is the true target of selection identified unambiguously. For example, geneticists have been studying inbreeding depression (Darwin 1868; Wright 1977) and heterosis (Shull 1948) for more than a century, but the relative contributions of deleterious recessive alleles versus the superior performance of heterozygotes remains a matter of controversy (Frankel 1983; Mitton 1993a, b; Lamkey & Staub 1998). The difficulty of identifying targets of selection is exemplified by the distinction of *selection for* a particular gene or locus versus *selection detected by* that locus. For example, Powers and colleagues have been studying the physiological and developmental consequences of the lactate dehydrogenase (*LDH*) polymorphism in the killifish, *Fundulus heteroclitus*, for more than 25 years, and have produced more than 50 publications (Powers & Schulte 1996). The full amino acid and DNA sequences of the *LDH* alleles are known. Differences in the enzyme kinetics (Place & Powers 1979) of the three genotypes are consistent with predicted genotypic differences in development (Paynter *et al.* 1991), hatching times (DiMichele & Powers 1982a), sustained swimming speeds (DiMichele & Powers 1982b), and geographic variation associated with latitude and temperature (Powers & Place 1978). Yet, after accumulating an immense amount of data implicating *LDH*, the authors are still hesitant to conclude that the *LDH* variation is the *direct* cause of the physiological variation.

Although it is very difficult to demonstrate unequivocally that natural selection discriminates among the alternate genotypes at a locus, the following evidence will demonstrate the direct influence of a gene on physiological, morphological, or behavioural phenotypes and on fitness:

1) functional differences among the gene products of the genotypes at a locus;
2) physiological, morphological, or behavioural differences (phenotypic variation) among the genotypes produced by the gene products;
3) variation in some component of fitness produced by the phenotypic variation.

Without the critical data listed above, biologists are hesitant to ascribe phenotypic consequences to a specific locus because it is difficult to rule out the possibility that the real source of the phenotypic variation is a locus linked to, and in linkage disequilibrium with, the marker locus. In the killifish example, the differences caused by *LDH* variation, or is the *LDH* locus fortuitously in linkage disequilibrium with genes directly regulating development, hatching time, and swimming speed?

The most thorough research programmes on allozymes have identified enzyme kinetic, physiological, and fitness differentials among loci for the leucine aminopeptidase polymorphism in blue mussels, *Mytilus edulis* (Hilbish & Koehn 1985a, b; Koehn & Hilbish 1987), the lactate dehydrogenase polymorphism in the common killifish, *Fundulus heteroclitus* (Powers *et al.* 1994; Powers & Schulte 1996), and the phosphoglucose isomerase polymorphism in sulfur butterflies, *Colias eurytheme* and *C. philodice eriphyle* (Watt *et al.* 1983, 1986; Watt 1992). These research programs meet the stringent requirements listed above and identify the specific targets of natural selection (Mitton 1997).

1.2. Correlations between individual heterozygosity and components of fitness

A large number of empirical studies have reported components of fitness, including developmental stability, growth rate, mating success, and fecundity to increase with heterozygosity at a small number, typically one to twelve, allozyme loci (Zouros & Foltz 1987; Britten 1996; Mitton 1997). Why is it that we can detect increases in fitness with heterozygosity when we categorize individuals with so few loci? There are four possible hypotheses (Mitton 1997): 1) the enzyme loci estimate heterozygosity of the entire genome; 2) polymorphic markers identify individuals with different levels of inbreeding; 3) closely linked genes directly affect the measure of fitness; and 4) the enzyme loci, through control of metabolic reactions, influence components of fitness. Each of these hypotheses is discussed below.

A small number of loci, such as the 1 to 12 polymorphic loci typically employed to measure individual heterozygosity, cannot reliably rank individuals in a population for levels of heterozygosity at hundreds or thousands of polymorphic loci (Mitton & Pierce 1980; Chakraborty 1981). Computer simulations demonstrated that a small number of loci (say 20) might reasonably estimate the heterozygosity of a larger set (perhaps 100) of loci (Mitton & Pierce 1980), but as the proportion of loci sampled decreases, so does the predictive value of heterozygosity estimates.

If individuals vary in their degree of inbreeding, individual heterozygosity will be negatively correlated with the degree of inbreeding. That is, individuals with the lowest level of heterozygosity will be the most inbred, and inbreeding depression will result in a positive correlation between heterozygosity and fitness.

The relationships between heterozygosity and components of fitness might be attributed to genes very tightly linked to the enzyme markers. However, linkage alone will not suffice for this explanation - the allozymes must be in strong linkage disequilibrium with the targets of selection to see a correlated effect through neutral allozyme loci. Linkage disequilibrium will be common in inbred species, and rare in outcrossed species living in large populations. But regardless of the mating system, it is laborious and difficult to gather the data needed to reject this hypothesis.

Because enzymes catalyse metabolic reactions, they control flux in metabolic pathways. Differential fluxes have been measured as a consequence of different genotypes at an enzyme locus (Zamer & Hoffmann 1989; Paynter *et al.* 1991). Furthermore, individual protein polymorphisms can influence whole animal physiology (Frelinger 1972; Koehn *et al.* 1980; DiMichele & Powers 1982b; Watt 1992). If the associations between allozyme heterozygosity and components of fitness are caused by linkage disequilibrium between the allozyme loci and loci directly influencing components of fitness, then any set of marker loci should reveal these correlations. But in the most comprehensive study of the association between allozyme heterozygosity and growth rate, Koehn *et al.* (1988) concluded that associations were strong for some enzymes, particularly those involved with protein cycling, and virtually nil for others. An empirical study of genetic variation and growth in scallops, *Placopecten magellanicus*, demonstrated that protein heterozygosity was correlated with growth rate, but that the heterozygosity of DNA markers was not

(Zouros & Pogson 1993; Pogson & Zouros 1994). These results suggest a direct role for some, but not all, enzymes in the variability of growth rate among individuals.

1.3. Molecular markers are expected to be neutral

Many biologists acknowledge natural selection to have a primary role in the evolution of morphological and physiological traits, but do not expect selection to have a major impact on molecular evolution. There are some good and some bad reasons for this expectation. First of all, mutations in the spacers between genes, in introns, in pseudogenes and the synonymous point mutations in sequences coding for proteins are unlikely to influence any aspect of the phenotype of an organism, and should not be influenced by natural selection. Furthermore, mutations influencing the amino acid sequences of proteins in relatively unimportant portions of the molecule are expected to be neutral. Many patterns in the genetic data are consistent with predictions from neutral theory (Nei 1975; Kimura 1983; Gillespie 1991; Kreitman & Akashi 1995).

Among biologists working with enzyme polymorphisms, the notion of neutrality finds uncritical support in the fit of observed genotypic frequencies to those expected under the Hardy-Weinberg Equilibrium (HWE). The HWE allows us to interconvert allelic frequencies and genotypic frequencies when certain conditions are met, such as random mating and no selection (Hartl & Clark 1997). Although the HWE relies on the assumption of no selection, a satisfactory fit between genotypic proportions observed in natural populations and those expected from the HWE cannot be taken as evidence of no selection; the chi-square (x^2) test is simply not sensitive to violations of this assumption (Wallace 1958). For example, if a population begins in HWE equilibrium, and selection is imposed so that the relative fitnesses are 1, 1-s, and $(1-s)^2$ for homozygote, the heterozygote, and the other homozygote, respectively, the allelic frequencies will change, but the new genotypic distribution will again be in HWE (Table 1). In this example, the selection coefficient is 0.5, so this is an example of intense selection, in which nearly half of the population disappears in the selective calamity. Nevertheless, the genotype frequencies of the survivors fit the HWE expectations perfectly, with a x^2 value of 0. Many population biologists examine population samples for a fit to HWE, and if observed frequencies are in accord, they typically conclude that their genetic markers were selectively neutral. This, however, is a rather incautious interpretation because a single population sample can reveal much about the mating system but it is not likely to reveal anything about natural selection.

Table 1: Demonstration that strong selection may produce a genotypic distribution in Hardy-Weinberg equilibrium.

		Genotypes					
		AA	Aa	aa	f(A)	f(a)	x^2
Initial population		1000	2000	1000	.500	.500	0.0
	Fitnesses	1	(1-s)	$(1-s)^2$			
	s = 0.5	1	0.5	0.25			
Survivors		1000	1000	250	.667	.333	0.0

1.4. The intensity of natural selection

Most molecular markers are likely to be selectively neutral for much of the time. However, the intensities of natural selection that are sometimes detected with enzyme polymorphisms will come as a surprise to theoretical population geneticists, who traditionally use selection coefficients of 0.001 to 0.01 in their models. Selection coefficients estimated with enzyme polymorphisms are occasionally in the range of 0.2 to 0.5 (Mitton 1997), just as they are in morphological studies (Endler 1986). Unfortunately, we do not have sufficient data, at this time, to describe the shape of the distribution of selection coefficients for molecular markers (Kreitman & Akashi 1995).

1.5. Selection varies with the environment

It is important to appreciate that natural selection is a process that is contingent on the environment in which the genotypes are compared. We know that environments vary in both space and time, and consequently we can expect natural selection to vary in a similar way. Most environments are not perfectly stable; they fluctuate daily and seasonally, with changes in weather, oscillation of the tides, and with changes in the population sizes of predators, competitors, prey, and parasites. In the most benign environments, virtually all genotypes fare well. In the very harshest of environments, virtually all genotypes suffer. These environmental conditions may not allow genotypic differences to be expressed, rendering genetic variation neutral in these environments. Conditions imposing moderate degrees of stress are the most likely to elicit differential performance among genotypes, resulting in natural selection. Naturalists appreciate the bewildering diversity of stresses that challenge natural populations, and evolutionary biologists have documented that different

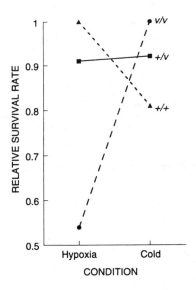

Figure 1: Relative survival rates of Ldh-C genotypes in *Poeciliopsis monacha* during hypoxic and cold stress. Relative survival is determined as the absolute survival rate for that genotype divided by the maximal survival rate under a particular type of stress. From Vrijenhoek (1996).

forms of stress favour alternate genotypes. Through time and space, natural selection varies from weak or absent to intense, favouring one genotype and then another.

The following two examples illustrate the variation in natural selection with environmental fluctuations. The first describes the survival rates for a lactate dehydrogenase polymorphism of desert fish, *Poeciliopsis monacha* (Vrijenhoek 1996). This fish lives in small intermittent streams of western Mexico, and it experiences dramatic shifts in environmental conditions with the seasons. This polymorphism detects intense selection that favours one homozygote during hypoxic stress, and the other homozygote during cold stress (Figure 1). The second example is taken from a long-term study of the colour polymorphism of the African butterfly *Danaus chrysippus*. Male mating success was estimated by the relative proportions of males caught alone versus those copulating (Smith 1975, 1980, 1981). The male mating success of the heterozygote was always the highest (Table 2), but relative performances of the homozygous genotypes switched with the seasons, favouring the dark phenotype during the cool season, and the light phenotype during the hot season.

1.6. Rationale for the following examples

Numerous methods are used to detect natural selection (Endler 1986). For example, selection of DNA sequences can be inferred from comparisons of the ratio of the number of point mutations causing amino acid replacements to the number of synonymous changes (Kreitman & Akashi 1995). The ratio of replacement to synonymous changes was too high in *Drosophila melanogaster*, *D. simulans*, and *D. yakuba*, suggesting that a significant fraction of the amino acid replacements among species was driven by natural selection (McDonald & Kreitman 1991). Strong evidence for balancing selection on the *ADH* polymorphism of *D. melanogaster* was revealed by comparing polymorphic nucleotide sites along an *ADH* cline in the eastern United States (Berry & Kreitman 1993). Selective constraints on coding regions can be measured by comparing the evolutionary rates of coding and non-coding sequences. These methods are indirect, inferring the action of natural selection by comparing observed and expected patterns of mutation or sequence divergence.

Table 2: Male mating success for three colour and pattern phenotypes of the African Butterfly, *Danaus chrysippus*, at Dar es Salaam, Tanzania. Dorippus and aegyptius are homozygous genotypes, and transiens is heterozygous. In all study periods, male mating success is heterogeneous among the phenotypes, and always favors the heterozygote. Extracted and modified from Smith (1981).

| Period | Condition | Phenotypes | | | N |
		dorippus	transiens	aegyptius	
April-August 1975	mated	36	52	23	111
	unmated	269	187	155	611
	mating success	0.54	1.0	0.59	
September 1974-	mated	88	47	2	137
March 1975	unmated	292	113	47	452
	mating success	0.79	1.0	0.14	
April-August 1975	mated	26	40	26	92
	unmated	194	117	45	456
	mating success	0.48	1.0	0.60	

Natural selection on allozyme loci has been demonstrated directly by gathering the data outlined in section 1.1. The most direct way to identify functional differences among allozyme genotypes is to examine the kinetic properties of the enzymes (Hall & Koehn 1983). Measurable differences in enzyme kinetic variables, such as Michaelis constants, k_{cat} s, maximum velocities, and thermal stabilities have the potential to influence the physiology of whole organisms. The majority of kinetic studies of protein polymorphisms have revealed functional differences among genotypes (Koehn *et al.* 1983; Zera *et al.* 1983), although the functional equivalency of electrophoretically differentiable proteins has also been reported (Dykhuizen *et al.* 1984).

Since this volume is intended for molecular ecologists, I have chosen two direct studies of natural selection that have significant components of field studies. The first is a study of the interaction between *ADH* and dissolved oxygen consumption in tiger salamanders. The second is a study of the interaction between glycerate dehydrogenase and soil moisture in pinyon pine. An example of discordant patterns of geographic variation in oysters was included to illustrate how these observations can reveal natural selection. Finally, three studies of sexual selection were chosen to illustrate selection differentials for male mating success, and to further demonstrate intense selection detected by molecular markers.

2. Recent examples of selection detected by molecular markers

2.1. ADH in tiger salamanders

In the ephemeral ponds of western Colorado, tiger salamanders, *Ambystoma tigrinum*, must hatch from eggs, grow as gilled larvae, and metamorphose into terrestrial adults before ponds evaporate in summer. Before a salamander can successfully metamorphose, it must grow beyond a minimal size threshold, absorb its tail fin and external gills, and modify its skin. Salamanders engage in this deadly race in extremely heterogeneous environments; the level of oxygen dissolved in the ponds around Gothic, Colorado, varies from hypoxic (20% saturation) to supersaturated (140% saturation).

The *ADH* polymorphism of the tiger salamander is associated with oxygen consumption, growth rate, and success at metamorphosis (Mitton *et al.* 1986; Carter 1997; Carter *et al.* 1998). Two common alleles, F and S, segregate at the *ADH* locus. Physiological and enzyme kinetic studies of this reaction revealed biochemical differences among the genotypes (Carter *et al.*, unpublished data). *ADH* enzymes were purified from gilled larvae of each genotype, and the K_{cat}/K_m ratio, a measure of enzyme efficiency, was measured. In the direction of acetaldehyde to ethanol, the ratio was higher in the heterozygote than in either homozygote, and the ratio was higher in *ADH-SS* than in *ADH-FF*. Concentrations of adenosine triphosphate (ATP) were also measured, since ATP concentrations in red blood cells modulate the affinity of haemoglobin for oxygen (Wood *et al.* 1982). The amount of ATP/haemoglobin was higher in *ADH-SS* homozygotes than in *ADH-FF* homozygotes, with heterozygotes having intermediate levels. The relative affinities of haemoglobin for oxygen determine the relative abilities to scavenge oxygen from the water and to deliver oxygen to tissues. *ADH-SS* homozygotes are at a disadvantage in ponds with low oxygen, for their haemoglobin has a low affinity for oxygen, and is inefficient at absorbing oxygen in the gills. However, in ponds with high levels of oxygen, the *ADH-SS* has an advantage, for it has no problem collecting oxygen in the gills, and it is more efficient than other genotypes at releasing oxygen in muscles and other tissues.

Variation at the *ADH* locus is associated with pond oxygen levels and time to metamorphosis (Carter 1997). The frequency of *ADH-SS* homozygotes increases (Fig. 2) with increasing levels of dissolved oxygen in the ponds. The frequency of heterozygotes does not vary with the level of dissolved oxygen. Studies in the field and in the laboratory indicate that *ADH-SS* homozygotes metamorphose more slowly in hypoxic water than in normoxic water, but perform well in supersaturated water. Consequently, *ADH-SS* homozygotes metamorphose in supersaturated ponds in higher relative frequencies than do *ADH-FF* individuals; this difference explains the increase of the *ADH-SS* frequency with increasing oxygen content of the pond (Fig. 2). *ADH-SF* individuals metamorphose in significantly higher than expected relative frequencies in both hypoxic and supersaturated water, so they are likely to comprise a high proportion of breeding adults. This over-representation of *ADH* heterozygotes among breeding adults is sufficient to explain the maintenance of the *ADH* polymorphism under heterozygote advantage (Hartl & Clark 1997).

2.2. Glycerate dehydrogenase in pinyon

The glycerate dehydrogenase (*GLY*) polymorphism in pinyon pine, *Pinus edulis*, exhibits microgeographic variation between starkly contrasting soil types at Sunset Crater, Arizona and between relatively wet and dry sites at Owl Canyon, Colorado (Mopper *et al.* 1991; Cobb *et al.* 1994; Mitton *et al.* 1998). At Sunset Crater, the contrasting soils are normal sandy-loam versus a deep bed of cinders produced by a volcanic eruption. The cinder soil imposes both water and nutrient stresses on plants (Mopper *et al.* 1991). In Owl Canyon, Colorado, relatively dry and moist sites were identified by associated plant communities and the sizes and densities of trees. In replicated comparisons, the frequency of the slow allele (*S*) at the *GLY* locus was higher on cinder soils than on adjacent sandy-loam soils (Cobb *et al.* 1994; Mopper *et al.* 1991) and higher on dry sites than on wet sites (Mitton *et al.* 1998).

A comparison of young and mature trees at Sunset Canyon revealed that genotypic frequencies differed significantly between these age groups, which were interspersed on the lava fields. If the assumption is made that the seedlings of both groups started with similar

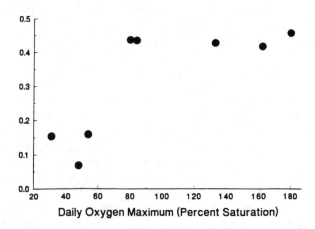

Figure 2: Frequency of the *ADH-SS* in tiger salamanders as a function of oxygen concentration expressed as a percentage of saturation. Each data point represents a different pond near Gothic, Colorado. Spearmans r = 0.74, P < 0.05. From Carter (1997).

frequencies, the difference in genotypic frequencies can be used to estimate relative viabilities. The relative viabilities for *GLY-FF*, *GLY-FS*, and *GLY-SS* was 0.43, 0.62, and 1.00, respectively (Table 3). In an independent study on trees at a nearby site, recent growth rates were estimated with the weight of four year old branches. Growth rates were lowest in *GLY-FF* and highest in *GLY-SS*, so the ranking of genotypes was the same as in studies of viability. The growth rate of *GLY-SS*, estimated by the weights of branches, was twice the growth rate of *GLY-FF*. Thus, both growth rates and viabilities exhibited large differences among genotypes, and both were consistent with the patterns of microgeographic variation reported at Sunset Crater and at Owl Canyon.

In an effort to elucidate the mechanism by which *GLY* genotypes influence survival and growth, trees within one of the dry sites were examined to test the hypothesis that stomatal sizes and densities are heterogeneous among *GLY* genotypes. Stomatal areas were calculated from the mean values for the genotypes, using the formula *area* = πbh, where π is 3.14, and *b* and *h* are half the lengths of the major and minor axes of an ellipse. The stomatal areas of the *GLY-FF* and *GLY-SS* homozygotes were very similar, but the stomatal areas of the *GLY-FS* heterozygotes were 28% greater than the stomatal areas of the homozygotes (Mitton *et al.* 1998). Ratios of the mean lengths to the mean widths revealed heterogeneity in the shape of the stomata among the genotypes (Table 3). A bivariate plot of stomatal lengths and widths (Fig. 3) revealed that the shapes of the *GLY-FS* and *GLY-SS* homozygotes do not overlap. Thus, stomata of the three common genotypes are distinctly different.

How might variation at the *GLY* locus be related to variation in sizes and shapes of stomata? The gene product of the *GLY* locus is an enzyme, and it is unlikely that the enzyme has a direct role in the development of stomata. One of the products of the reaction catalysed by GLY is serine, a precursor to glycine betaine, which accumulates in the cells of both plants and animals in response to desiccation. Perhaps the development of stomata is influenced by the water balance of the pinyon, leading to the development of distinct stomata in the three *GLY* genotypes. Studies are currently underway to test this hypothesis.

2.3. Microsatellite variation and fitness correlates

Microsatellite loci are sequences noted for high numbers of alleles differing in the number of repeats of a simple nucleotide series (see Estoup & Anders, this volume). The variability at microsatellite loci can be summarized with heterozygosity, the number of alleles, and d^2, a measure of the difference in the number of repeats between two alleles at a locus. The value of d^2 for homozygotes is always zero, whereas for a heterozygote with alleles containing, say, 30 and 40 repeats, $d^2 = (30 - 40)^2 = 100$.

Table 3: Viabilities, growth rates, and measurements on stomata for glycerate dehydrogenase genotypes in pinyon pine, *Pinus edulis*. Growth rate is in grams/4 years/branch, and stomatal length and width are 10^{-5} m. All variables are heterogeneous among the glycerate dehydrogenase genotypes. Data extracted from Cobb *et al.* (1994) and Mitton *et al.* (1998).

	Genotypes		
	GLY-FF	*GLY-FS*	*GLY-SS*
Viability	0.43	0.62	1.00
Growth rate	10.0	15.5	20.0
Stomata			
Length	194.82	232.27	217.37
Width	151.45	159.88	132.91
Length/Width	1.28	1.45	1.63

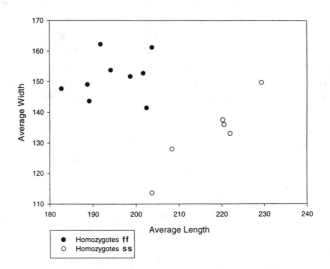

Figure 3: A bivariate scattergram of the lengths and widths of stomata in two glycerate dehydrogenase genotypes in pinyon pine, *Pinus edulis*. Units for length and width are 10^{-5} m. From Mitton *et al.* (1998).

Correlation of multi-locus d^2 and heterozygosity with viability was investigated in two studies on Scottish red deer and Canadian harbour seals. In the first investigation, genetic and biological data for 670 red deer calves born on the Isle of Rum, Scotland, were collected between 1982 and 1996. These data included environmental conditions, status of the mother, the inbreeding coefficient for the calf, and genotypes at nine microsatellite loci (Coulson *et al.* 1998). A similar study of harbour seals produced genetic data on 275 harbour seal pups born on Sable Island, Nova Scotia, in 1994 and 1995. These data included age and condition of the mother, birth date in the pupping season, birth weight, neonatal survival, and genotypes at six microsatellite loci (Coltman *et al.* 1998). In both studies, birth weight and neonatal survival increased with d^2, but not with individual heterozygosity. The authors of both studies argue that, d^2 is a more sensitive measure of the degree of inbreeding than individual heterozygosity. Their reasoning is based on the step-wise model of mutation, where most mutations produce an increase or decrease of one repeat (Weber & Wong 1993: Di Rienzo *et al.* 1994). Therefore, the difference in allele size in a heterozygote (or d^2) can be seen as a measure of the genetic distance between the two uniting gametes (Coulson *et al.* 1998). The genotypes with the lowest values of d^2 are expected to be the most inbred, and thus the positive correlation between d^2 and both birth weight and survival may be caused inbreeding depression.

3. Discordant patterns of geographic variation

Molecular studies of geographic variation have indicated that different sets of markers may indicate different levels and patterns of geographic variation. Protein polymorphisms and DNA markers reveal discordant patterns of geographic variation in deer mice, cod, horseshoe crabs, oysters, lodgepole pine, the closed-cone pines of California, and limber pine (Mitton, 1997). The oyster, *Crassostrea virginica,* example is presented here in detail because it revealed a dramatic difference in the pattern of allozyme and DNA markers, and the authors have presented a plausible hypothesis to explain the discrepancy. Oysters release their gametes into the water, and eggs are fertilized shortly after they enter the water column. Eggs develop quickly into pelagic larvae, which can be carried by currents for weeks, creating the potential of very high levels of gene flow. Allozyme frequencies in oysters exhibit little variation from Maine to Texas, a geographic pattern initially interpreted as evidence for extensive gene flow among populations (Buroker 1983). From these allozyme data, the number of individuals migrating among populations each generation, Nm, was estimated to be approximately 6 (Reeb & Avise 1990). Because the population samples were hundreds of kilometres apart, this estimate indicated that oysters were commonly dispersing hundreds of kilometres. Values of Nm above 1 are generally considered to be capable of overriding genetic drift and homogenising allelic frequencies among populations (Hartl & Clark 1997). Biologists were comfortable with this report of extensive gene flow inferred from homogeneous allelic frequencies, based on predictions from dispersal capacity. In stark contrast to the homogeneity of allozyme frequencies, mtDNA variation has an abrupt discontinuity on the Atlantic coast of Florida, suggesting a barrier to gene flow. This observation was inconsistent with the previous estimate of dispersal distance, for it suggested that oysters were dispersing distances of 1 to 10 kilometres. Was the difference between allozymes and mtDNA due to their different modes of inheritance (biparental versus maternal), or due to other factors?

To resolve this question, data from four anonymous single-copy nuclear RFLPs were collected (Karl & Avise 1992); these markers, like allozymes, reside on nuclear chromosomes and are inherited biparentally. The anonymous RFLPs described the same pattern of geographic variation as did the mtDNA. Thus, the contrasting patterns of geographic variation seen in allozymes and mtDNA could not be attributed to the different modes of inheritance or distance of dispersal. Why would these sets of loci reveal different patterns of geographic variation, and suggest dramatically different levels of gene flow?

A series of experimental studies employing allozymes had revealed natural selection in oysters. Rates of oxygen consumption in oysters were strongly related to genotypes at five allozyme loci (Koehn & Shumway 1982). Under both control and stress conditions, oxygen consumption decreased 50% with the number of heterozygous loci. This observation is relevant to other measures of performance in oysters, since physiologists use resting oxygen consumption to estimate the basal metabolic costs of maintenance. All other things being equal, the genotypes with the lowest basal metabolic rates would be expected to exhibit the highest levels of survival and growth. Consistent with this expectation, survival (Singh 1982; Zouros *et al.* 1983) and growth rate (Singh & Zouros 1978; Zouros *et al.* 1980; Singh 1982; Singh & Green 1984) increase with allozyme heterozygosity in oysters.

After considering alternate hypotheses for the discordant patterns of geographic variation in oysters, Karl and Avise (1992) tentatively concluded that balancing selection acting on enzyme loci caused this set of loci to diverge from the pattern of geographic variation exhibited by the mtDNA and nuclear RFLP's.

4. Sexual selection and the privilege of the heterozygous male

The field of sexual selection has seen dramatic changes in the recent past. Historically, theoreticians expected sexual selection to erode the genetic variability of selected characters (Maynard Smith 1978; Hamilton & Zuk 1982), and for this reason, models of female choice of "good genes" were not considered biologically realistic. However, recent studies of genetic variation have reported that sexually selected characters may retain more genetic variation than other characters (Pomiankowski & Møller 1995; Rowe & Houle 1996). Furthermore, we now appreciate that the choice of a highly heterozygous mate has genetic consequences; the heterozygosity of offspring is correlated with the heterozygosity of their parents (Mitton *et al.* 1993). Perhaps the most important insights have come from molecular studies of sexual selection. Empirical studies of *Colias* butterflies, brine shrimp, and marine snails suggest that heterozygous males enjoy relatively high mating success.

4.1. Colias butterflies

Allozyme genotypes have been used to measure male mating success in natural populations of the sulfur butterflies, *Colias eurytheme* and *C. philodice eriphyle*. The data are most extensive for the phosphoglucose isomerase (*PGI*) locus, for which there are enzyme kinetic data, demographic data, behavioural data, and data on mating success (Watt 1977, 1983; Watt *et al.* 1983, 1985, 1986). Kinetic analyses documented biochemical differences among genotypes and showed that the most common heterozygote is overdominant in the predominant environmental conditions. The heterozygotes have greater viability and fly over a greater range of temperatures than do the homozygotes. But the most remarkable aspect of this story is the relative mating success of the heterozygotes. Because a female uses the sperm from only a single male to fertilize her eggs, inspection of the female's genotype and those of her offspring allows the inference of the paternal genotype. A comparison of the genotypes of males flying in the field with the genotypes revealed by the paternity analysis revealed a strong and consistent male mating advantage for the heterozygotes (Table 4). In *C. eurytheme*, the average frequency of *PGI* heterozygotes in flying males was 46%, but among the males with reproductive success, the average frequency of heterozygotes was 72%. In *C. philodice eriphyle*, the average frequency of

Table 4: The proportion of heterozygous genotypes in a random sample of male *Colias* butterflies (flying) and in males with reproductive success (mating).

Species	Locus	Date	Percentage of Heterozygotes		Probability[c]
			Flying[a]	Mating[b]	
Colias eurytheme	*PGI*	1984	40	70	***
		1985	52	67	*
	PGM	1984	56	74	+
		1985	46	55	NS
	G6PD	1984	46	85	***
		1985	47	72	**
Colias philodice	*PGI*	1984	52	74	***
		1985	56	85	***
	PGM	1984	44	63	**
		1985	47	63	+
	G6PD	1984	33	61	***
		1985	38	52	+
Average			46	69	***

Note: Data from Carter and Watt (1988).
[a]Percentage of males in the field heterozygous for the enzyme
[b]Percentage of males successfully siring broods. These genotypes were inferred from the mother's genotype and the distribution of genotypes in her brood
[c]Probability that the percentages are the same: + = P < .10, * = P < .05, ** = P < .01, *** = P < .001, NS = non significant

PGI heterozygotes in flying males was 54%, but the average frequency of heterozygotes in males with reproductive success was 80%.

Similar differentials of mating success were found (Carter & Watt 1988) with the phosphoglucomutase and the glucose 6 phosphate dehydrogenase polymorphisms in *Colias* (Table 4). At both these loci, the proportions of heterozygous males were higher in males with mating success than in the total sample of males caught in the field. The pattern of heterozygous advantage for male mating success in the three loci examined was relatively consistent across loci, across species, and over years. The frequency of heterozygous males in natural localities ranged from 33 to 56%, but the frequency of heterozygotes in males siring broods was 52 to 85% (Table 4). When the data were combined across years, loci, and species, 46% of the available males were heterozygous, but 69% of the mating success was achieved by the heterozygotes. If these loci are assumed to be independently assorting and additive in their effects, and the relative mating success of the triple heterozygotes is 1.00, then the relative mating success of the triple homozygotes is only 0.38.

4.2. Brine shrimp and snails

Male mating success increased with heterozygosity in laboratory populations of brine shrimp, *Artemia franciscana* (Zapata et al. 1990). Eighty sexually mature virgin females and 160 males were placed in an aquarium, and when a female began to mate, the mating pair was removed. The genotype of each individual was obtained for five allozyme polymorphisms. At single loci, heterozygotes had higher male mating success at two of the loci and lower mating success at one locus. When individual heterozygosity was examined, males' mating success increased with the number of heterozygous loci (Table 5). In comparison to completely homozygous genotypes, which were arbitrarily assigned a fitness of 1.0, individuals heterozygous for three and four loci had fitnesses of 2.99 and 2.55, respectively.

Sexual selection favouring heterozygous males was detected in the marine snail, *Littorina mariae* (Rolán-Alvarez et al. 1995). Snails were collected from the marine alga *Fucus vesiculosus* in the intertidal zone in Muros-Noya Ria, Galicia, Spain. Individuals were characterized as being solitary or copulating, and each individual was scored for nine polymorphic allozyme loci. Reproductive success was estimated as the proportion of copulating individuals for heterozygosity class. Mating success was found to increase with heterozygosity in young males (Table 5).

Table 5: Male mating success as a function of allozyme heterozygosity in the brine shrimp, *Artemia franciscana*, and the marine snail *Littorina mariae*.

| | Individual heterozygosity | | | | |
	0	1	2	3	4
Artemia					
male mating success	1.00	1.39	1.45	2.99	2.55
± standard error		0.19	0.14	0.95	0.25
		*	**	*	**
Littorina					
male mating success	1.00	1.43	1.81	2.30	

Note: * and ** indicate values significantly different from 1.00 at 5% and 1% level, respectively. Extracted from Zapata et al. (1990) and Rolán-Alvarez et al. (1995).

5. Summary

These examples all reveal natural selection with molecular markers. Two examples, *ADH* in tiger salamanders, *GLY* in pinyon pine, present data suggesting that selection is acting directly on those polymorphisms. However, both of the studies are incomplete, so we can not reject the hypothesis that the allozymes are neutral markers in linkage disequilibrium with genes directly influencing the components of fitness. The microsatellite loci in the studies of red deer and harbour seals are almost certainly neutral, but nevertheless they reveal strong selection, probably associated with inbreeding depression.

In the examples presented here, multilocus allozyme heterozygosity is associated with components of fitness in oysters, *Colias* butterflies, brine shrimp, and marine snails. Some biologists contend that associations between multilocus heterozygosity and components of fitness are not important because, on average, they are not very strong, and they are not always detectable. This is a curious criticism; all forms of natural selection are variable in space and time.

Acknowledgments

Pat Carter and Brian Kreiser contributed comments on the manuscript. I wish to acknowledge stimulating discussions with the wonderful diversity of biologists at the conference at Erice.

References

Berry A, Kreitman M (1993) Molecular analysis of an allozyme cline: alcohol dehydrogenase in *Drosophila melanogaster* on the east coast of North America. *Genetics*, **134**, 869-893.

Brandon RN, Burian RM (1984) *Genes, Organisms, Populations: Controversies Over the Units of Selection* MIT Press, Cambridge, Massachussets.

Britten HG (1996) Meta-analysis of the association between multilocus heterozygosity and fitness. *Evolution* **50**, 2158-2164.

Buroker NE, (1983) Population genetics of the American oyster *Crassostrea virginica* along the Atlantic coast and the Gulf of Mexico. *Marine Biology*, **75**, 99-112.

Carter PA (1997) Maintenance of the *Adh* polymorphism in *Ambystoma tigrinum nebulosum* (tiger salamanders). I. Genotypic differences in time to metamorphosis in extreme oxygen environments. *Heredity*, **78**, 101-109.

Carter PA, Watt WB (1988) Adaptation at specific loci. V. Metabolically adjacent enzyme loci may have very distinct experiences of selective pressures. *Genetics*, **119**, 913-924.

Chakraborty R (1981) The distribution of the number of heterozygous loci in an individual in natural populations. *Genetics*, **98**, 461-466.

Cobb NS, Mitton JB, Whitham TG (1994) Genetic variation associated with chronic water and nutrient stress in pinyon pine. *American Journal of Botany*, **81**, 936-940.

Coltman DW, Bowen WD, Wright JM (1998) Birth eight and neonatal survival of harbour seal pups are positively correlated with genetic variation measured by microsatellites. *Proceedings of the Royal Society of London B*, **265**, 803-809.

Coulson TN, Pemberton JM, Albon SD *et al.* (1998) Microsatellites reveal heterosis in red deer. *Proceedings of the Royal Society of London B*, **265**, 489-495.

Darwin C (1859) *On the Origin of Species by Means of Natural Selection, or the Preservation of Favoured Races in the Struggle for Survival.* John Murray, London.

Darwin C (1868) *The Variation of Animals and Plants Under Domestication.* John Murray, London.

DiMichele L, Powers DA (1982a) LDH-B genotype-specific hatching times of *Fundulus heteroclitus* embryos. *Nature*, **296**, 563-565.

DiMichele L, Powers DA (1982b) Physiological basis for swimming endurance differences between *Ldh-B* genotypes of *Fundulus heteroclitus. Science*, **216**, 1014-1016.

Di Rienzo A, Peterson AC, Garza JC *et al.* (1994) Mutational processes of simple sequence repeat loci in human populations. *Proceedings of the National Academy USA,* **91**, 3166-3170.

Dobzhansky TH (1970) *Genetics of the Evolutionary Process.* Columbia University Press, New York.

Dykhuizen DE, DeFramond J, Hartl DL (1984) Selective neutrality of glucose-6-phosphate dehydrogenase allozymes in *Escherichia coli. Molecular Biology and Evolution,* **1**, 162-170.

Eiseley LC (1958) *Darwin's Century. Evolution and the Men Who Discovered It.* Doubleday & Company, Inc.

Endler JA (1986) *Natural Selection in the Wild.* Princeton University Press, Princeton, New Jersey.

Ford EB (1975) *Ecological Genetics.* 4th Edition. Chapman and Hall, London.

Frankel R (1983) *Heterosis: Reappraisal of Theory and Practice.* Springer-Verlag, Berlin.

Frelinger JA (1972) The maintenance of transferrin polymorphisms in pigeons. *Proceedings of the National Academy of Science USA,* **69**, 326-329.

Gillespie JH (1991) *The Causes of Molecular Evolution.* Oxford University Press, New York.

Goldstein DB, Linares AR, Cavalli-Sforza LL, Feldman MW (1995) An evaluation of genetic distances for use with microsatellite loci. *Genetics,* **139**, 463-471.

Gould SJ (1982) *Darwinism and the expansion of evolutionary theory. Science,* **216**, 380-387.

Gyapay G, Morisette J, Vignal A, *et al.* (1994) The 1993-1994 Genethon human genetic linkage map. *Nature Genetics,* **7**, 246-249.

Hall JG, Koehn RK (1983) The evolution of enzyme catalytic efficiency and adaptive inference from steady-state kinetic data. *Evolutionary Biology,* **16**, 53-96.

Hamilton WD (1964) The genetical evolution of social behavior. *Journal of theoretical Biology,* **7**, 1-16.

Hamilton WD, Zuk M (1982) Heritable true fitness and bright birds: a role for parasites. *Science,* **218**, 384-387.

Hartl DL, Clark AG (1997) *Principles of Population Genetics.* Third Edition. Sinauer Associates Inc., Sunderland, MA.

Hilbish TJ, Koehn RK (1985a) Dominance in physiological phenotypes and fitness at an enzyme locus. *Science,* **229**, 52-54.

Hilbish TJ, Koehn RK (1985b) The physiological basis of natural selection at the LAP locus. *Evolution,* **39**, 1302-1317.

Karl SA, Avise JC (1992) Balancing selection at allozyme loci in oysters: implications from nuclear RFLPs. *Science,* **256**, 100-102.

Kimura M (1983) *The Neutral Theory of Molecular Evolution.* Cambridge University Press, Cambridge.

Koehn RK, Diehl WJ, Scott TM (1988) The differential contribution by individual enzymes of glycolysis and protein catabolism to the relationship between heterozygosity and growth rate in the coot clam, *Mulinia lateralis. Genetics,* **118**, 121-130.

Koehn RK, Hilbish TJ (1987) The adaptive importance of genetic variation. *American Scientist,* **75**, 134-140.

Koehn RK, Newell RJE, Immerman F (1980) Maintenance of an aminopeptidase allele frequency cline by natural selection. *Proceedings of the National Academy of Science USA,* **77**, 5385-5389.

Koehn RK, Shumway SE (1982) A genetic/physiological explanation for differential growth rate among individuals of the American oyster, *Crassostrea virginica* (Gmelin). *Marine Biology Letters,* **3**, 35-42.

Koehn RK, Zera AJ, Hall JG (1983) Enzyme polymorphism and natural selection. In: *Evolution of Genes and Proteins,* (eds, Nei M, Koehn RK), pp. 115-136. Sinauer Associates Inc. Sunderland, Massachussets.

Kreitman M, Akashi H (1995) Molecular evidence for natural selection. *Annual Review of Ecology and Systematics,* **26**, 403-422.

Lamkey KR, Staub JE (1998) *Concepts and Breeding of Heterosis in Crop Plants.* CSSA Special Publication Number 25. Crop Science Society of America, Madison, Wisconsin.

Maynard-Smith J (1978) *The Evolution of Sex.* Cambridge University Press, Cambridge.

McDonald JH, Kreitman M. (1991) Adaptive protein evolution at the *Adh* locus in *Drosophila. Nature,* **351**, 652-654.

Michod RE (1982) The theory of kin selection. *Annual Review of Ecology and Systematics,* **13**, 23-55.

Mitton JB (1993a) Theory and data pertinent to the relationship between heterozygosity and fitness.

In: *The Natural History of Inbreeding and Outbreeding,* (ed. Thornhill N), pp. 17-41. University of Chicago Press, Chicago.

Mitton JB (1993b) Enzyme heterozygosity, metabolism, and developmental stability. *Genetica,* **89**, 47-65.

Mitton JB (1997) *Selection in Natural Populations.* Oxford University Press, Oxford.

Mitton JB, Carey C, Kocher TD (1986) The relation of enzyme heterozygosity to standard and active oxygen consumption and body size of tiger salamanders, *Ambystoma tigrinum. Physiological Zoology,* **59**, 574-582.

Mitton JB, Grant MC, Yoshino AM (1998) Glycerate dehydrogenase frequencies in pinyon pine are associated with variation in soil moisture and stomata size. *American Journal of Botany,* in press.

Mitton JB, Pierce BA (1980) The distribution of individual heterozygosity in natural populations. *Genetics*, **95**, 1043-1054.

Mitton JB, Schuster WSF, Cothran EG, De Fries J (1993) The correlation in heterozygosity between parents and their offspring. *Heredity*, **71**, 59-63.

Mopper S, Mitton JB, Whitham TG, Cobb NS, Christensen KM (1991) Genetic differentiation and heterozygosity in pinyon pine associated with resistance to herbivory and environmental stress. *Evolution*, **45**, 989-999.

Nei M (1975) *Molecular Population Genetics and Evolution*. North-Holland, Amsterdam.

Paynter KT, DiMichele L, Hand SC, Powers DA (1991) Metabolic implications of *Ldh-B* genotype during early development in *Fundulus heteroclitus*. *Journal of Experimental Zoology*, **257**, 24-33.

Place AR, Powers DA (1979) Genetic variation and relative catalytic efficiencies: Lactate dehydrogenase B allozymes of *Fundulus heteroclitus*. *Proceedings of the National Academy of Sciences USA*, **76**, 2354-2358.

Pogson GH, Zouros E (1994) Allozyme and RFLP heterozygosities as correlates of growth in the scallop *Placopecten magellanicus*: A test of the associative overdominance hypothesis. *Genetics*, **137**, 221-231.

Pomiankowski A, Møller AP (1995) A resolution of the lek paradox. *Proceedings of the Royal Society of London B*, **260**, 21-29.

Powers DA, Place AR (1978) Biochemical genetics of *Fundulus heteroclitus* (L.). I. Temporal and spatial variation in gene frequencies of *Ldh-B, Mdh-A, Gpi-B*, and *Pgm-A. Biochemical Genetics*, **16**, 593-607.

Powers DA, Schulte PM (1996) A molecular approach to the selectionist/neutralist controversy. In: *Molecular Zoology: Advances, Strategies, and Protocols*, (eds. Ferraris JD, Palumbi SR), pp. 327-352. Wiley-Liss, New York.

Powers DA, Smith M, Gonzalez-Villasenor I *et al.* (1994) A multidisciplinary approach to the selection/neutralist controversy using the model teleost *Fundulus heteroclitus*. In: *Oxford Surveys in Evolutionary Biology*, Volume 9, (eds. Futuyma D, Antonovics), pp. 43-107. Oxford University Press, Oxford.

Reeb CA, Avise JC (1990) A genetic discontinuity in a continuously distributed species: mitochondrial DNA in the American oyster, *Crassostrea virginica. Genetics*, **124**, 397-406

Rolán-Alvarez E, Zapata C, Alvarez G (1995) Multilocus heterozygosity and sexual selection in a natural population of the marine snail *Littorina mariae* (Gastropoda: Prosobranchia). *Heredity*, **75**, 17-25.

Rowe L, Houle D (1996) The lek paradox and the capture of genetic variance by condition dependent traits. *Proceedings of the Royal Society of London B*, **263**, 1415-1421.

Shull GH (1948) What is "Heterosis"? *Genetics*, **33**, 439-446.

Singh SM (1982) Enzyme heterozygosity associated with growth at different developmental stages in oysters. *Canadian Journal of Genetics and Cytology*, **24**, 451-458.

Singh SM, Green RH (1984) Excess of allozyme homozygosity in marine molluscs and its possible biological significance. *Malacologia*, **25**, 569-581.

Singh SM, Zouros E (1978) Genetic variation associated with growth rate in the American oyster (*Crassostrea virginica*). *Evolution*, **32**, 342-353.

Smith DAS (1975) Sexual selection in a wild population of the butterfly *Danaus chrysippus* L. *Science*, **187**, 664-665.

Smith DAS (1980) Heterosis, epistasis and linkage disequilibrium in a wild population of the polymorphic butterfly *Danaus chrysippus* (L.). *Zoolological Journal of the Linnean Society*, **69**, 87-109.

Smith DAS (1981) Heterozygous advantage expressed through sexual selection in a polymorphic African butterfly. *Nature*, **289**, 174-175.

Sober E, Lewontin RC (1982) Artifact, cause, and genic selection. *Philosophy of Science*, **49**, 157-180.

Vrijenhoek RC (1996) Conservation genetics of North American desert fishes. In: *Conservation Genetics: Case Histories from Nature*, (eds. Avise JC, Hamrick JL), pp. 367-397. Chapman and Hall, New York.

Wade MJ (1978) A critical review of the models of group selection. *Quarterly Review of Biology*, **53**, 101-114.

Wallace B (1958) The comparison of observed and calculated zygotic distributions. *Evolution*, **12**, 113-115.

Wallace B (1975) Hard and soft selection revisited. *Evolution*, **29**, 465-473.

Watt WB (1977) Adaptation at specific loci. I. Natural selection in phosphoglucose isomerase of *Colias* butterflies: biochemical and population aspects. *Genetics*, **87**, 177-194.

Watt WB (1983) Adaptation at specific loci. II. Demographic and biochemical elements in the maintenance of the *Colias* PGI polymorphism. *Genetics*, **103**, 691-724.

Watt WB (1992) Eggs, enzymes, and evolution—natural genetic variants change insect fecundity. *Proceedings of the National Academy of Sciences USA*, **89**, 10608-10612.

Watt WB, Carter PA, Blower SM (1985) Adaptation at specific loci. IV. Differential mating success among glycolytic allozyme genotypes of *Colias* butterflies. *Genetics*, **109**, 157-175.

Watt WB, Carter PA, Donohue K (1986) Females' choice of "good genotypes" as mates is promoted by an insect mating system. *Science*, **233**, 1187-1190.

Watt WB, Cassin RC, Swan MS (1983) Adaptation at specific loci. III. Field behaviour and survivorship differences among *Colias Pgi* genotypes are predictable from *in vitro* biochemistry. *Genetics*, **103**, 725-739.

Weber JL, Wong C (1993) Mutation of human short tandem repeats. *Human Molecular Genetics*, **2**, 1123-1128.

Williams GC (1985) A defense of reductionism in evolutionary biology. In: *Oxford Surveys in Evolutionary Biology, Vol. 2*, (eds. Dawkins R, Ridley M), pp. 1-27. Oxford University Press, Oxford.

Wilson DS (1997) Introduction: multilevel selection theory comes of age. *American Naturalist*, **150**, 1-4.

Wood SC, Hoyt RW, Burggren WW (1982) Control of haemoglobin function in the salamander, *Ambystoma tigrinum*. *Molecular Physiology*, **2**, 263-272.

Wright S (1977) *Evolution and Genetics of Populations. Vol. 3. Experimental Results and Evolutionary Deductions*. University of Chicago Press, Chicago.

Zamer WE, Hoffmann, RJ (1989) Allozymes of glucose-6- phosphate isomerase differentially modulate pentose-shunt metabolism in the sea anemone *Metridium senile*. *Proceedings of the National Academy of Science USA*, **86**, 2737-2741.

Zapata C, Gajardo G, Beardmore JA (1990) Multilocus heterozygosity and sexual selection in the brine shrimp *Artemia franciscana*. *Marine Ecology Progress Series*, **62**, 211-217.

Zera AJ, Koehn RK, Hall JG (1983) Allozymes and biochemical adaptation, In: *Comprehensive Insect Physiology, Biochemistry and Pharmacology*, (eds. Kerkut GA, Gilbert LI), pp. 633-674. Pergamon Press, New York.

Zouros E, Foltz DW (1987) The use of allelic isozyme variation for the study of heterosis. In : *Isozymes: Current Topics in Biological and Medical Research, Vol. 13*. (eds. Rattazzi MC, Scandalios JG, Whitt GS) Alan R. Liss, Inc., New York.

Zouros E, Pogson GH (1993) The present status of the relationship between heterozygosity and heterosis. In: *Genetics and Evolution of Aquatic Organisms*, (ed. Beaumont A) pp. 135-146 . Chapman and Hall, London.

Zouros E, Singh SM, Foltz DW, Mallet AL (1983) Post-settlement viability in the American oyster (*Crassostrea virginica*): an overdominant phenotype. *Genetical Research Cambridge*, **41**, 259- 270.

Zouros E, Singh SM, Miles HE (1980) Growth rate in oysters: An overdominant phenotype and possible explanations. *Evolution*, **34**, 856-867.

Advances in Molecular Ecology
G.R. Carvalho (Ed.)
IOS Press, 1998

Molecular Ecology of Hybridization

Loren H. Rieseberg

Biology Department, Indiana University, Bloomington, IN 47405, USA.
e-mail: lriesebe@bio.indiana.edu

Hybridization is an important feature of the evolution of many plant and animal groups. On one hand, it can be viewed as a natural experiment that provides a window on evolutionary processes. On the other hand, it is a significant evolutionary process in its own right that can lead to the origin or merger of species. This chapter reviews the contributions of molecular approaches to our understanding of hybrid zone structure and dynamics, phylogeography, reproductive isolation, introgression, and hybrid speciation. After concepts and terminology are clarified, the potential utility of different kinds of molecular markers for investigating hybridization is reviewed. This is followed by an examination of several models that predict the structure and dynamics of hybrid zones and an exploration of empirical and theoretical studies that test the validity of these models. Finally, I will review how molecular markers have informed our understanding of several consequences of hybridization, such as introgression, hybrid speciation, species extinction, and phylogenetic incongruence.

1. Introduction

Ecological and evolutionary studies of hybridization can largely be divided into two categories: those that employ experimental or natural hybrids to study evolutionary processes and those that study hybridization to infer its role in evolution (Arnold 1992). Both of these approaches are valid. Moreover, due to variation in the frequency and evolutionary consequences of hybridization in different organismal groups, is not surprising that hybridization studies vary widely in emphasis.

Experimental hybridization studies have been used to study the nature of species differences since the 18th century. Although early experiments were somewhat naive, each century has seen technical and theoretical advances that have greatly increased the power of this approach. These advances are exemplified by current utilization of molecular marker-based quantitative genetic studies that can estimate the numbers, effects, locations, and interactions of quantitative trait loci (QTL) that differentiate species (*e.g.* Bradshaw *et al.* 1995; Bachmann & Hombergen 1996).

However, there does appear to be a limit to the resolution that can be achieved by experimental studies due to the small number of generations of recombination that can typically be achieved in the lifetime of an experiment. By contrast, hybrid genotypes resulting from hundreds or thousands of generations of recombination are common in hybrid zones. Also, experimental laboratory studies lack the ecological context characteristic of natural hybrid zones. Thus, Barton & Hewitt (1985), Harrison (1990), and others have argued that hybrid zones provide natural experiments that are not easily duplicated experimentally. In the past decade, considerable efforts have been made to exploit the diversity of genotypes in natural hybrid zones to address questions ranging from genetic architecture (*e.g.* Syzmura & Barton 1991) to host-parasite interactions (*e.g.* Whitham 1989; Fritz *et al.* 1996).

The study of hybridization as an important evolutionary process also has a long history that was initiated by Linnaeus' (1760) contention that new and constant species arose by hybridization. Linnaeus' views were eventually confirmed in both plants and animals (Winge 1917; Gallez & Gottlieb 1982; Dowling & DeMarais 1993), although the process of hybrid speciation was much more complex than ever imagined by Linnaeus. In the early part of the 20th century, it was also speculated that hybridization might play a major role in adaptive evolution (Lotsy 1916; Anderson & Hubrict 1938). The importance of hybridization in adaptive evolution has been difficult to evaluate (Heiser 1973; Rieseberg & Wendel 1993), although Arnold (1997) recently has compiled substantial evidence in favour of a significant role. Other consequences of hybridization that have received attention recently include the genetic assimilation of rare species by more common congeners (Rieseberg & Gerber 1995; Levin *et al.* 1996; Rhymer & Simberloff 1996) and the escape of genetically engineered genes from crop plants into wild populations (Ellstrand 1992).

A common component to major advances in all of these areas of study has been the application of species-specific molecular markers. Molecular markers provide a powerful means for identifying and classifying hybrid genotypes, for characterising patterns of introgression, and for revealing taxa of hybrid origins. The purpose of this chapter is to review the contributions of molecular markers to the study of natural hybridization. After clarifying concepts and terminology, I will discuss the kinds of molecular markers commonly employed by the molecular ecology community and the potential utility of these markers for investigating hybridization phenomena. This is followed by an examination of several models that predict the structure and dynamics of hybrid zones and an exploration of empirical and theoretical studies that test the validity of these models. Finally, I will review how molecular markers have informed our understanding of several consequences of hybridization such as hybrid speciation, introgression, species extinction, and phylogenetic incongruence.

2. Concepts and terminology

Hybridization can have several different meanings for evolutionary biologists. The term can be restricted to organisms formed by cross-fertilization between individuals of different species, or defined more broadly as the offspring between individuals from populations "which are distinguishable on the basis of one or more heritable characters" (Harrison 1990). Similarly, introgression can be narrowly defined as the movement of genes between species mediated by backcrossing or more broadly as the transfer of genes between genetically distinguishable populations. I prefer the broader definitions of hybridization and introgression, since they provide greater flexibility in usage. Nonetheless, my focus in this review will be on hybridization and introgression between species.

A focus on interspecific hybrids requires consideration of species concepts. Unfortunately, the term species has a wide variety of definitions, ranging from concepts based on the ability to interbreed to those based on common descent. Mayr's (1963) biological species concept - "species are groups of interbreeding natural populations which are reproductively isolated from all other such groups" - is perhaps the most widely applied of these. This concept is useful for studies of hybridization and speciation, but if applied stringently the concept would deny species status to most of the hybridising taxa discussed here. Thus, for the purposes of this review, I will refer to biological species as groups of interbreeding populations that are genetically isolated from other such groups, rather than reproductively isolated. By genetic isolation, I mean that the genetic integrity of hybridising species is maintained by selection against foreign alleles or chromosomal segments rather than by avoidance of hybridization. This may seem to be a trivial distinction, but it is clear that most hybrid zones serve as effective barriers to interspecific genetic exchange, even if local introgression is well-documented (Harrison 1990).

3. Molecular markers

Many different kinds of molecular markers have been successfully employed for the study of plant hybridization, ranging from seed proteins and allozymes to arbitrary primer-mediated fingerprinting (Table 1). My comments will be largely limited to DNA polymorphisms, since allozymes are discussed in an earlier chapter.

DNA polymorphisms can be divided into three basic categories based on methodology: restriction fragment length polymorphism (RFLP) analyses, polymerase chain reaction (PCR)-mediated approaches using sequence-characterized primers, and PCR-mediated approaches using arbitrary primers.

The basic theory underlying RFLP analyses is simple. Doubled-stranded DNA is cleaved by restriction endonucleases. The resulting fragments are separated by size using gel electrophoresis. Differences in fragment lengths or RFLPs can be identified that distinguish individuals and/or species. RFLP methods can be applied to almost any DNA sequence, including single-copy and repetitive nuclear genomic sequences, cytoplasmic genomes, and PCR-amplified fragments. It was the application of RFLPs to evolutionary and ecological questions in the late 1970s and early 1980s, in conjunction with the earlier, but extended explosion of allozyme studies, that largely founded the field of molecular ecology.

One of the drawbacks associated with RFLPs was the relatively large amounts of genomic DNA required for successful detection. This was particularly problematic for small or rare organisms. Fortunately, the discovery of PCR in the mid-1980s (Mullis 1990) facilitated the application of molecular approaches to virtually all organisms, regardless of size. Initially, PCR was used to amplify sequence-characterized genomic sequences. Differences in the lengths of these amplified products or their RFLP profiles provided excellent markers for studies of hybridization (e.g. Arnold et al. 1991; Karl & Avise 1993).

Table 1: Characteristics of molecular markers frequently employed in studies of hybridization. Abreviations: AFLPs (amplified fragment length polymorphisms); AP-PCR (arbitrary primer-polymerase chain reaction); DAF (DNA amplification fingerprinting); cpDNA RFLPs (chloroplast DNA restriction fragment length polymorphisms); ISSRs (inter-simple sequence repeats); mtDNA RFLPS (mitochondrial DNA RFLPs); RAPD (random amplified polymorphic DNA); and scnRFLPs (single copy nuclear RFLPs).

Molecular Marker	Number of Independent Markers	Marker Inheritance	Development Effort	Evolutionary Rate
AFLPs	many	dominant	low	moderate
allozymes	30-50	co-dominant	low	slow
AP-PCR	many	dominant	low	moderate
DAF	many	dominant	low	moderate
cpDNA RFLPs	1	usually maternal	low	very slow
ISSRs	many	dominant	low	fast
microsatellite loci	many	co-dominant	high	fast
minisatellite loci	many	dominant[1]	low	very fast[2]
mtDNA RFLPs	1	usually maternal	low	fast
RAPD	many	dominant	low	moderate
scnRFLPs	many	co-dominant	moderate	moderate
nucl. r DNA RFLPs	1-4	co-dominant[3]	low	variable

[1]The inheritance of minisatellites is co-dominant, but they are typically scored as dominant markers because of profile complexity.

[2]Patterns may be too complex for some kinds of hybrid analyses.

[3]Concerted evolution and intragenic recombination can lead to non-Mendelian inheritance.

However, in some instances, levels of polymorphism were low. To enhance detection of polymorphism, recent efforts have focused on the development of primers for hypervariable loci that consist of either large (minisatellite) or small (microsatellite) tandem repeats (Jeffreys 1987; Tautz 1989).

Early uses of PCR required some prior knowledge of the sequence of the target DNA. This represented a problem for organisms where sequence data were lacking. However, this problem was overcome during the early 1990s by the introduction of various methods of arbitrary-primer mediated PCR. These primers can amplify DNA and reveal polymorphisms without prior knowledge of the target DNA sequence. Typically, a single primer of arbitrary sequence is employed in a standard PCR reaction. If the primer binds to sites on different strands of the target DNA that are within about 3-kb of each other, the region between the ends of the priming sites will be amplified. Since this can occur at any number of locations within the genome for any given primer, more than one DNA fragment may result from a single reaction. Products of the reaction are separated by either agarose or acrylamide gel electrophoresis and are visualized by one of several methods, including ethidium bromide staining, silver staining, or by labelling with fluorescent- or radio-labelled nucleotides.

There are several popular versions of arbitrary primer-mediated fingerprinting that vary in terms of primer length, primer composition, annealing temperatures, and assay methods. These include (1) arbitrarily primed-PCR (AP-PCR), which employs primers of 18-20 bp in length (Welsh & McClelland 1990); (2) DNA amplification fingerprinting (DAF) which uses short 5-8 bp primers (Caetano-Anolles *et al.* 1991); and (3) random amplified polymorphic DNA (RAPD) analysis (Williams *et al.* 1990), which employs 10-mer primers. In general, AP-PCR and DAF produce complex profiles that are best resolved on polyacrylamide gels, whereas the simpler RAPD profiles can be resolved on agarose gels.

A similar method that has been introduced recently employs single primers that contain short tandem repeats anchored at the 3' or 5' end by 2-4 arbitrary, degenerate nucleotides (Zietkiewicz *et al.* 1994; Wolfe *et al.* 1997). The markers generated are termed inter-simple sequence repeat markers (ISSRs) and are presumed to amplify regions between microsatellite loci. Although arbitrary primer-mediated fingerprinting methods are extensively employed in molecular ecology including hybridization research, their acceptance has been hampered by their largely dominant mode of inheritance and by questions concerning the reproducibility of results across laboratories.

A recently introduced class of markers, termed amplified fragment length polymorphisms (AFLPs), attempts to combine the favourable attributes of both RFLP and arbitrary primer methods (Vos *et al.* 1995). The method is based on the selective amplification of restriction fragments from digested genomic DNA. As with arbitrary primer methods, only small amounts of DNA are required, and DNA fingerprints can be generated without prior sequence knowledge using a limited number of generic primers. Studies published to date suggest that the AFLP technique is more repeatable between laboratories than other arbitrary primer methods because reaction conditions used for primer annealing are more stringent (Jones *et al.* 1997). Unfortunately, most AFLP loci are dominant, although it is feasible to distinguish between homozygotes and heterozygotes on the basis of band intensity in populations used in mapping studies. Whether this will be possible for genetically variable wild populations is not yet clear.

Given the wealth of available markers, choosing the most appropriate class or classes of markers for a study of hybridization can be difficult. Important considerations include (1) the number of independent species-specific molecular markers that can easily be obtained; (2) the mode of inheritance–markers with biparental codominant inheritance provide twice the information content of either uniparentally inherited cytoplasmic markers or markers with dominant inheritance patterns; (3) the effort and expense of marker development and assays; and (4) evolutionary rates. An ideal class of markers would contain numerous, independent, easily developed loci that exhibit biparental, co-dominant inheritance. The loci would evolve rapidly enough to differentiate species, but slowly enough to allow the detection of ancient hybridization phenomena. Markers that have been or can be mapped genetically are particularly useful, since mapped markers allow the evolutionary dynamics of not only individual markers but entire chromosomal segments to be monitored.

Unfortunately, the `holy grail' of markers has not yet been found, although single-copy nuclear RFLPs (scnRFLPs) come close (Table 1). Instead, most students of hybridization have come to recognize the advantages of employing more than one class of molecular marker. Different classes of markers are likely to vary in mode of inheritance, linkage relationships, and selective pressures, thus revealing different aspects of hybrid zone history and evolutionary dynamics. For example, monitoring of both nuclear and cytoplasmic markers provides an excellent approach for distinguishing between gene flow via pollen or seed dispersal in flowering plants (Arnold *et al.* 1991). Also, the ease and low expense of developing numerous species-specific markers using arbitrary primer methods has tended to favour their application in situations in which large numbers of markers are required (*e.g.* Rieseberg *et al.* 1996a).

Although multiple, independent markers are required for most hybridization studies, complete independence is not always desirable. For example, the complete linkage characteristic of cytoplasmic markers allows relationships among chloroplast DNA (cpDNA) or mitochondrial DNA (mtDNA) haplotypes to be determined. The resulting `gene' trees can be invaluable for inferring historical hybridization events. Linkage among cytoplasmic markers or among nuclear markers also provides a powerful means of distinguishing between hybridization and other evolutionary processes that may produce similar patterns such as convergence or symplesiomorphy (joint retention of ancestral characters). For example, if a putative hybrid species possessed multiple, linked markers of potential parents, the probability that this situation could be attributed to symplesiomorphy or convergence is minimized.

4. Structure and dynamics of hybrid zones

A number of theories or models have been proposed to account for the maintenance, structure, and dynamics of hybrid zones. Although these models are often viewed as being in direct competition, this is not necessarily the case as it seems likely that different rules describe hybrid zones in different organismal groups. Molecular marker studies have played an important role in evaluating these models.

Early zoological workers envisioned two possible outcomes of hybridization: (1) the merger of the hybridising taxa due to extensive introgression or (2) the cessation of hybridization due to the reinforcement of reproductive barriers. By contrast, botanists tended to view hybridization as a creative process often leading to the formation of stable hybrid lineages (Anderson 1949; Stebbins 1950). Although the consequences of hybridization envisioned by botanists and zoologists were vastly different, both groups did agree, at least implicitly, that hybrid zones were ephemeral. This assumption appears to have been widely held until the mid-1970s when a compilation of evidence from empirical hybrid zone studies was used to argue that hybrid zones could be stable for long periods (Moore 1977). Moore suggested that the observed stability was due to a fitness advantage of hybrids in intermediate habitats, often along ecotones. Termed the `bounded hybrid superiority model,' this theory predicts strong correlations between habitat and genotype. The model also assumes that hybrid zones occur along ecotones, leading to the prediction of clinal variation for diagnostic characters (Endler 1977; Moore 1977).

Shortly after the appearance of Moore's (1977) hybrid superiority model, Barton (1979) and Barton & Hewitt (1985) provided mathematical evidence that stable hybrid zones could be maintained by a balance between dispersal of parental individuals into the zone and selection against the hybrids that were produced. In this `dynamic equilibrium´ or `tension zone´ model, hybrids exhibit reduced viability or fertility due to disruptions of co-adapted gene complexes. Thus, selection is independent of the environment, and correlations between habitat and genotype are not predicted. However, like the bounded hybrid superiority model, clinal variation for diagnostic loci is predicted.

Both the bounded hybrid superiority and dynamic equilibrium model predict a clinal structure for hybrid zones. However, in the early 1980s it was recognized that zones may sometimes be mosaic in structure due to adaptation of the parental taxa to patchily distributed habitats (Howard 1986; Harrison 1986). This observation led to the development of the `mosaic hybrid zone model,´ which predicts strong correlations between genotype and habitat. Unlike the bounded hybrid superiority model, hybrids are not assumed to be more fit than the parental species in intermediate habitats. Rather, the hybrid zones are thought to be maintained by a dispersal / selection balance in the same way as envisioned for the dynamic equilibrium model. Thus, clinal variation for diagnostic markers can be predicted on a very local spatial scale and possibly on a very broad geographical scale, but mosaic patterns of variation are predicted at intermediate geographic levels.

Recently, a new model has been proposed, which attempts to incorporate aspects of the three preceding models (Arnold 1997). This `evolutionary novelty´ model is most similar to the mosaic model in that it suggests that both endogenous (environment independent) and exogenous (environment dependent) selection are critical for maintaining hybrid zones. However, it differs from the mosaic model in that hybrids are not predicted to be uniformly less fit than the parental taxa. Rather, hybrid fitness is predicted to be variable and to depend on both hybrid genotype and on habitat. Hybrids are predicted to do particularly well in intermediate or novel habitats, but are not necessarily predicted to perform more poorly than the parents in parental habitats. Like the bounded hybrid superiority and mosaic models, strong correlations between habitat and genotype are predicted in the evolutionary novelty model. However, clinal variation is not necessarily predicted, although clines may be observed in ecotonal habitats or on broad geographical scales.

Analyses of population genetic structure with molecular markers cannot distinguish between all of these models, because they overlap in their predictions. Nonetheless, the geographic structure of hybrid zones and the general importance of habitat selection can be estimated from marker patterns.

In a series of defining reviews on hybrid zones, Barton & Hewitt (1985, 1989) argued that most well-studied hybrid zones meet the expectations of the dynamic equilibrium model. The evidence compiled for this view includes:

- observations that most animal hybrids exhibit at least some sterility or inviability,
- strong linkage disequilibria is observed among loci in most animal hybrid zones,
- coincident clines are often observed for diagnostic loci,
- many animal hybrid zones are uniform and narrow, and in some cases,
- hybrid zones appear to have moved, suggesting that they are environment independent.

Thus, it seems likely that many well-characterized animal hybrid zones do represent tension zones.

Nonetheless, if hybrid zones are viewed on a more global basis, the preponderance of tension zones becomes much less clear. For example, Rieseberg & Ellstrand (1993) reviewed the geographic distribution of species-specific markers in plant hybrid zones and concluded that most plant hybrid zones fail to exhibit the pattern of clinal variation with a monotonic shift in allele frequencies characteristic of tension zones. Rather, plant hybrid zones appear to be mosaic, and taxon-specific molecular markers display an idiosyncratic spatial distribution rather than the concordant patterns predicted for classic tension zones. In addition, numerous studies have documented associations between molecular markers and habitat in plants (*e.g.* Heywood 1986; Cruzan & Arnold 1993, 1994; Hsiao *et al.* 1996), further demonstrating an important role for exogenous selection in maintaining plant hybrid zones. Barton & Hewitt (1989) argue that "clines that are initially obtained by differential adaptation will, as more differences accumulate, develop into tension zones which can be maintained even without the original environmental difference." This is correct, but in most cases environmental differentiation is likely to increase rather than decrease with divergence. A general conclusion that can be drawn from these observations is that environmentally independent tension zones are unlikely to form in most plant groups due to the extraordinarily close link between plants and their environment. Given the higher frequency of hybridization in plants than in most vertebrate or invertebrate species, the majority of hybrid zones are unlikely to represent tension zones.

The importance of the tension zone model in animals also has been questioned (Harrison 1986). Some animal hybrid zones display mosaic genetic structures (*e.g.* Howard 1986; Harrison 1986; Rand & Harrison 1989; MacCallum *et al.* 1998), and habitat preferences are sometimes reported (*e.g.* Rand & Harrison 1989; MacCallum *et al.* 1998). One of the best examples comes from the *Gryllus firmus* X *G. pennsylvanicus* hybrid zone in the northeastern United States. Molecular marker studies suggest clinal variation on a broad geographic scale, but on a local scale, markers exhibit a mosaic distribution (Rand & Harrison 1989). At even finer scales along ecotones, variation is once again clinal in nature. Even paradigmatic examples of tension zones have been questioned by Arnold (1997), who notes that environmental selection provides a reasonable alternative explanation for the concordant clines reported for these zones.

Further discrimination among hybrid zone models will require fitness estimates for hybrid and parental genotypes in both parental and hybrid habitats. Most current estimates are based on greenhouse or laboratory experiments, which do not measure exogenous selection. Nonetheless, these studies indicate that the average viability and fertility of early generation hybrids is typically lower than the parental species, particularly for distantly related taxa (reviewed in Barton & Hewitt 1985; Rieseberg and Carney, unpublished data). This is not surprising, given the co-adapted nature of species genomes (Dobzhansky 1937). However, low average fitness does not preclude the production of later generation hybrid segregates that are as fit or more fit than either parental species. There is substantial empirical evidence for this prediction. First, hybrids often exhibit increased vigour or fecundity. Although this "hybrid vigour" is often partly masked by disharmonious interspecific genomic interactions in early generation hybrids, strong fertility and viability selection will favour the elimination of negative gene combinations and the maintenance of hybrid vigour (Rieseberg *et al.* 1996a). Thus, after just a few generations of selection, fertile hybrid genotypes can be generated that sometimes outperform both parental species. Second, studies that describe fertility, viability, or other fitness parameters in hybrids almost invariably report the presence of a small fraction of hybrid genotypes that are as fit or fitter than parental individuals, even if the hybrids on average exhibit reduced fitness (Heiser 1947; Valentine 1947; Grant 1966a; Reed and Sites 1995; Burke *et al.* 1998).

Although most studies have been restricted to the measurement of endogenous selection, there is a growing body of studies that provide estimates of fitness in natural or manipulated hybrid zones (reviewed in Arnold 1997). In several instances, hybrid fitness appears to be habitat dependent, and in some cases, the average fitness of a particular class or classes of hybrids appears to be equivalent to or to exceed that of their parents, at least for those fitness parameters measured. For example, in big sagebrush hybrid zones, each genotypic class performed best in its own habitat (Wang *et al.* 1997). By contrast, iris hybrids exceeded the parental taxa in vegetative growth in the hybrid habitat and in one of the parental habitats (Emms & Arnold 1997; Burke *et al.* 1998). The big sagebrush example appears to be most consistent with the hybrid superiority model, whereas the iris results seem most consistent with the evolutionary novelty model. Unfortunately, lifetime fitnesses were not estimated in these studies, so it is unclear whether they represent valid exceptions to the general rule of reduced average hybrid fitness. Vegetative growth rates are particularly problematic as a general indicator of hybrid fitness, since hybrid vigour is often observed in even highly sterile individuals.

A possible alternative to studies that attempt to identify and measure important components of fitness in natural hybrid zones would be the use of molecular marker-based parentage studies. By tracking all genotypes in a hybrid population over multiple generations with a large number of molecular markers, it should be possible to estimate parental success or true fitness of all genotypes in a population. Obviously, these data will be most informative if combined with detailed habitat surveys so that interactions between genotype and habitat can be assessed. Such an approach, in which cross-generational genotype x environment interactions are assessed, will probably be required to fully understand hybrid fitness and to reliably discriminate between hybrid zone models.

5. Phylogeography of hybridization

A full understanding of the characteristics of hybrid zones requires some knowledge of the phylogeography of the hybridising species and the nature of the contact event. One important question, which has implications for speciation theory, is whether hybrid zones represent regions of primary versus secondary intergradation (Mayr 1963). Primary intergradation refers to clines that develop between populations that are in continuous contact, whereas secondary integradation refers to clines that result from hybridization between populations that differentiated in allopatry. Although most hybrid zones are assumed to represent examples of secondary intergradation, theoretical work indicates that steep clines can develop along ecotones in the absence of geographical isolation (Slatkin 1973; Endler 1977). Both processes will result in similar patterns of variation, making them difficult to distinguish unless secondary contact is very recent (Harrison 1990). This is unfortunate, since differentiating between primary and secondary contact can provide insights regarding the plausibility and relative importance of parapatric speciation. That is, can barriers to gene exchange arise in the absence of geographic isolation? If reproductive barriers can arise in parapatry, how often does this occur?

Phylogenetic evidence can often be used to distinguish between primary and secondary zones of contact, even if clinal patterns in the hybrid zones are similar. For example, if phylogenetic evidence indicates that the hybridising species are not sister taxa, the zone of contact is almost certainly secondary in origin. This rule is not absolute, however, as sequential instances of parapatric speciation could, given an unlikely series of events, lead to primary intergradation of non-sister taxa. Nonetheless, this basic approach has been used to successfully differentiate between primary and secondary intergradation among both plant and animal species (Thorpe 1984; Beckstrom-Sternberg *et al.* 1991; Brunsfeld *et al.* 1992; Dowling & DeMarais 1993) and should become a routine component of hybrid zone studies.

Biogeographic data also can be used to discriminate between primary and secondary zones of contact. In many cases, range contraction-expansion cycles during the Pleistocene have led to secondary intergradation. This process has been best studied in postglacial Europe, where rapid range expansions have generated hybrid zones in almost every organismal group studied in detail (reviewed in Hewitt 1989). Many of these hybrid zones occur at a common location, providing further evidence for secondary contact due following range expansions. For example, *Bombina* (Arntzen 1978), *Corvus* (Cook 1975), *Mus* (Sage *et al.* 1986), and *Natrix* (Thorpe 1984) hybrid zones occur in roughly the same location in central and northern Europe. In general, accumulating phylogeographic data suggests that most hybrid zones are secondary in origin and corroborates the importance of geographic isolation in speciation. These data also indicate that accurate interpretations of hybrid zone phenomena require allele frequency data from throughout the geographic ranges of the parental species.

6. Hybrid zones and the genetic architecture of reproductive isolation

Hybrid zones provide a means for studying the genetic architecture of reproductive barriers (i.e., the number, location, effects, and interactions of genetic factors that contribute to reproductive isolation). As alluded to in the introduction, the dissection of genetic factors contributing to reproductive isolation is limited in controlled crossing experiments by the small number of generations of recombination that can be obtained in a typical experiment. By contrast, hybrid genotypes resulting from hundreds or thousands of generations of recombination are found in natural hybrid zones. Thus, it becomes theoretically possible to distinguish between the effects of very closely linked genes.

Several different approaches can be used to estimate genetic architecture in natural hybrid zones. One of these is based on cline theory and uses estimates of the width of the region of reduced viability, dispersal rate, patterns of linkage disequilibria, and strength of selection against hybrids to determine gene number (Barton & Hewitt 1985). Application of this approach to well-characterized hybrid zones in *Podisma* (Barton & Hewitt 1981) and *Bombina* (Szymura & Barton 1991) yields gene number estimates of 50-500 in *Podisma* and 26-88 in *Bombina*. These estimates are consistent with the hypothesis that changes at many genes are required for speciation (Fisher 1930) but tell us little about the location, effects, and interactions of specific genes.

Harrison (1990) suggested that patterns of differential introgression could be used to infer the genetic architecture of species barriers. Introgression of genes (and linked markers) contributing to isolation will be retarded, whereas neutral or positively selected chromosomal segments (and linked markers) will introgress at higher frequencies. If the markers have been genetically mapped, the observed patterns of introgression should also make it possible to locate the genes contributing to isolation.

This approach has been employed in both controlled introgression experiments and natural hybrid zones of the wild sunflower species, *Helianthus annuus* and *H. petiolaris* (Rieseberg et al. 1996a; Rieseberg LH & Gardner K unpublished data). Analysis of both the natural and experimental hybrids suggest that many loci scattered throughout the genome contribute to isolation between these species. This approach is illustrated in Figure 1 for one of 17 linkage groups from the three natural hybrid zones. Patterns of introgression were assayed for 139 *H. annuus*-like individuals from the three hybrid zones using 88 mapped *H. petiolaris*-specific markers. The frequencies of introgressed *H. petiolaris* markers can be used to infer the location of loci under selection. For example, Markers 857-1.5, 125-.55, and 181-.79 introgress at significantly lower rates than expected, whereas the frequency of marker 834-1.8 does not differ significantly from expectations (Fig. 1). Presumably, the chromosomal block between markers 857-1.5 and 181-.79 contains one or more genes that contributes to reduced hybrid fitness.

Harrison (1990) further noted that with the availability of mapped molecular markers, it was theoretically possible to determine the genomic locations of quantitative trait loci (QTL) that contribute to reproductive isolation in natural hybrid zones. In contrast to the previous approach, which relies on introgressed marker frequencies to infer the location of loci under selection, this method searches for correlations between the mapped markers and the trait of interest. This approach can therefore be viewed as a kind of marker-based QTL analyses, but in natural hybrid zones rather than in experimental populations.

As far as I know, the only application of this approach has been to the three wild sunflower hybrid zones described above. In this study, associations were calculated between

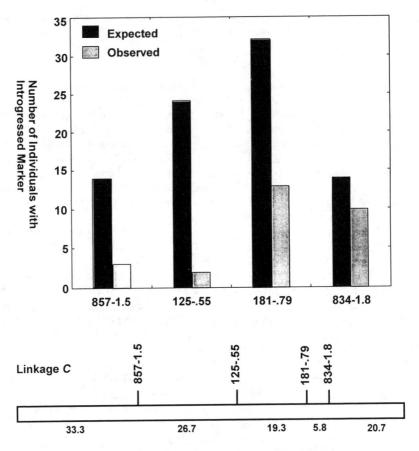

Figure 1: Observed and expected numbers of introgressed markers in 139 *H. annuus*-like individuals from three natural hybrid zones between *Helianthus annuus* and *H. petiolaris* for linkage group *C*, one of 17 linkage groups. This linkage group is collinear (i.e., has the same gene order) in the two species. Molecular markers are shown above, and map distances below, the linkage group. Observed and expected numbers of introgressed markers are given in the bar graph above the linkage group. Markers 857-1.5, 125-.55, 181-.79 introgress at significantly lower rates than expected, whereas the frequency of marker 834-1.8 does not differ significantly from expectations. Expected numbers of introgressed markers are based on overall frequencies of introgression in the seven linkage groups that are collinear between *H. annuus* and *H. petiolaris*. Crossing experiments indicate that average frequencies of marker introgression across these linkage groups are consistent with neutral expectations (Rieseberg et al. 1996a).

pollen viability and 88 molecular markers scattered throughout the sunflower genome. Of these, 56 markers displayed significant associations ($P < 0.01$) compared to less than one expected by chance. This does not mean that 56 loci contribute to reduced fertility since many of the markers associated with fertility are tightly linked. However, it does indicate that fertility has a polygenic basis.

7. Outcomes of hybridization

7.1. Introgression

The most common outcome of hybridization is introgression. Extensive introgression has been well-documented by molecular markers in many groups of organisms, particularly in plants (reviewed in Rieseberg & Wendel 1993) and fish (reviewed in Dowling & Secor 1997). Evolutionary consequences of introgression that have been proposed include increased genetic diversity, transfer of adaptations, origin of adaptations, origin of ecotypes or geographic races, and merger of species (Rieseberg & Wendel 1993). Two of these consequences, the transfer of adaptations and the merger of species, are discussed briefly below.

7.1.1. Transfer of adaptations

In his monograph on introgressive hybridization, Anderson (1949) reasoned that hybrids serve as a "bridge by which groups of genes from one species can invade the germplasm of another." However, there are theoretical difficulties associated with the transfer of adaptations across species barriers. First, alleles contributing to the adaptation of interest must recombine into a new genetic background before they are eliminated by selection against the alleles with which they were initially associated (Barton & Hewitt 1985). If many genes contribute to reduced hybrid fitness, then much of the genome may be resistant to introgression due to linkage. Second, if the adaptation is polygenic, QTL contributing to the trait will become disassociated by recombination in the hybrid zone. Only alleles that are individually favourable are likely to cross the hybrid zone.

Despite these difficulties, numerous possible examples of adaptive trait introgression have been reported in the literature (*e.g.* Heiser 1951; Harlan & deWet 1963; Stutz & Thomas 1964; Heiser 1979; Parsons *et al.* 1993). However, in the majority of examples, it was not possible to distinguish between introgression and alternative explanations for the observed patterns such as convergent evolution or symplesiomorphy. In other studies, neutral markers have been observed to cross hybrid zones (*e.g.* Rieseberg *et al.* 1990; Arnold *et al.* 1991; Parsons *et al.* 1993). Neutral introgression might be viewed as synonymous with adaptive trait introgression since advantageous alleles will cross hybrid zones more readily than neutral markers. However, Rieseberg & Wendel (1993) argued that this conclusion was premature due to the great preponderance of neutral markers relative to favourable ones in hybrid zones.

The most convincing evidence for adaptive trait introgression comes from studies in which introgression of neutral molecular markers and advantageous traits has been examined (Klier *et al.* 1991; Rieseberg *et al.* 1990; Parsons *et al.* 1993). For example, Heiser (1951) provided evidence suggesting that the common sunflower, *H. annuus*, was able to colonize Texas by acquiring advantageous alleles of *H. debilis*, a species already adapted to the area. Rieseberg *et al.* (1990) were able to confirm the introgression of molecular markers between the species. However, because presumably neutral molecular markers rather than genes encoding adaptively significant traits were assayed, Rieseberg *et al.* were cautious in their interpretation of the data, noting that "molecular evidence for introgression does not necessarily prove that the introgression of *H. debilis* into *H. annuus* was in any way adaptive." To determine whether adaptive traits actually have introgressed, my laboratory is currently conducting a QTL analysis of morphological and seed oil characters that differentiate *H. debilis* from allopatric populations of *H. annuus*, but are found in the Texan form of *H. annuus* (jagged leaf serration; speckled stems; basal branching patterns; low ray number; small disks, phyllaries, and seeds; and a higher proportion of saturated seed oils). After the *H. debilis* molecular markers flanking these traits are identified, natural populations of Texan *H. annuus* will be assayed for the flanking *H. debilis* markers. Detection of pairs of flanking markers in Texan *H. annuus* populations will provide strong evidence for the introgressive origin of the morphological traits linked to them.

In a similar study, Parsons *et al.* (1993) documented the movement of plumage characteristics of the golden-collared manakin (*Manacus vitellinus*) into populations that are genetically and morphologically like the white-collared manakin (*M. candei*). Analyses of one mitochondrial and two nuclear markers confirmed the occurrence of hybridization and introgression, although none of the molecular markers moved as far as the golden-collared plumage traits. Parsons *et al.* 1993 argue that positive sexual selection is driving reproductively advantageous traits across the reproductive barrier between these species. Although this does seem to be the most likely explanation, a flanking marker approach such as that described above would remove any doubt as to the origin of golden-collared plumage traits in white-collared populations.

7.1.2. Merger of species

Another possible consequence of introgression is the breakdown of reproductive barriers, which may ultimately lead to the merger of species. If only a small number of loci are under selection, recombination in hybrid zones can lead to the breakdown of linkage disequilibria between premating and postmating barriers or between species-specific phenotypic characters, ecological associations, and the isolating barriers. These recombinant individuals can then serve as a bridge for interspecific gene flow (Stebbins & Daly 1961; Bloom 1976). For example, Bloom and colleagues (Bloom & Lewis 1972; Bloom 1976; Hauber & Bloom 1983) demonstrated that hybridization between two chromosomally divergent *Clarkia* species led to the production of new chromosomal rearrangements that now appear to genetically link populations of the two species. Because the rearrangements are distributed geographically across the hybrid zone, interspecific gene flow can occur with little loss of fertility (Soltis & Bloom 1991).

In many cases, the initial cause of hybridization is natural or human disturbance of the environment, which can disrupt ecological barriers to hybridization (Anderson 1948). Well-studied hybrid zones that were initiated by human-mediated disturbance include plant examples such as wild sunflowers (*Helianthus annuus* / *H. bolanderi*: Stebbins & Daly 1961; Rieseberg *et al.* 1988), irises (*Iris fulva* / *I. hexagona*: Riley 1938; Arnold *et al.* 1990), and yellow and white ladyslippers (*Cypripedium candidum* / *C. pubescens*: Klier *et al.* 1991), as well as animal examples such as blue-wing (*Vermivora pinus*) and golden-winged (*V. chrysoptera*) warblers (Gill 1980) and tree frogs (*Hyla cinerea* / *H. gratiosa*: Schlefer *et al.* 1986). In some instances, these hybrid zones have existed for more than 50 years, suggesting that they may be stable even in the absence of continued habitat disturbance. However, in other situations the cessation of disturbance and recovery of the initial habitat has lead to a cessation of hybridization (Heiser 1979). For example, analysis of three hybrid populations of *Helianthus divaricatus* / *H. microcephalus* over a 42-year period revealed the presence of hybrids throughout this period at one site due to continued removal of large trees (Heiser 1979; Rieseberg unpublished data). By contrast, the original forest habitat has been largely restored at the other two sites, and a single species now occupies these sites.

The merger of species due to introgression appears to be relatively frequent, particularly as a result of human-mediated introductions or translocations (Levin *et al.* 1996; Rhymer & Simberloff 1996). A well-known example involves the multiple introductions of rainbow trout (*Oncorhynchus mykiss*) into endemic cutthroat trout habitats (*O. clarkia*) in the western U.S. Hybridization between the introduced and endemic populations has led to extensive introgression, which is well-documented by both allozyme and mtDNA markers (Allendorf & Leary 1988). Similar results have been reported for introduced (*Cyprinodon variegatus*) and native (*C. Pecosensis*) pupfish populations in the Pecos River drainage (Echelle & Connor 1989), introduced sika deer (*Cervus nippon nippon*) and native red deer (*C. elaphus*) in Scotland (Abernathy 1994), and introduced (*Arbutus unedo*) and native (*A. canarienensis*) arbutus species in the Canary Islands (Salas-Pascual *et al.* 1993).

If one of the hybridising species is rare, the consequences of introgression is more accurately described as genetic assimilation rather than species merger. That is, the more common species simply assimilates the alleles of the rare form with little effect on its own allele frequencies or morphology. Genetic models indicate that this process can occur extremely quickly (Ellstrand & Elam 1993; D. Wolf unpublished data), and numerous examples have been described in both plants (reviewed in Rieseberg 1991; Ellstrand & Elam 1993; Levin *et al.* 1996) and animals (Rhymer & Simberloff 1996). As a result, hybridization is now considered a serious threat to endangered species. In fact, of the 292 North American fishes listed as rare, threatened, or vulnerable in the Red DATA Book published by the International Union for the Conservation of Nature and Natural Resources, 38% are threatened by hybridization (Wilson 1992).

Species that appear to be particularly vulnerable to extinction through hybridization and introgression include relatives of domesticated animals or plants, game relatives, weed relatives, island species, and species endemic to human-occupied habitats for reasons discussed above. The vulnerability of these groups is fairly easy to understand (Rieseberg 1991; Ellstrand & Elam 1993; Levin *et al.* 1996; Rhymer & Simberloff 1996). Almost every crop species is known to be compatible with wild relatives, and crop plants are often grown in sympatry with compatible wild species. This has led to the apparent assimilation of several narrowly endemic wild species by the crop derivatives (Small 1984), the possible conversion of wild ancestors to weeds (reviewed in Levin *et al.* 1996), and the ongoing assimilation of many other wild relatives (McGranahan *et al.* 1988; Ellstrand 1992). Similar threats confront relatives of domesticated animals. For example, 80% of supposedly pure wildcats from northern and western Scotland have traits that are characteristic of domestic cats (Hubbard *et al.* 1992). Relatives of game and weed species also are vulnerable since, as described above for native cutthroat trout populations, they are exposed to frequent introductions of game or weed species.

Island species are threatened by genetic assimilation because of small population size, the general lack of strong genic or chromosomal sterility barriers between congeners, the invasion and colonization of islands by closely related exotics, and the increasing loss and disturbance of habitats due to human activities (Rieseberg 1991). Human disturbance is particularly important on islands because of the small size of species ranges and the importance of ecological barriers to hybridization. In the flora of Hawaii, for example, hybridization is reported in close to 40 genera and 23 plant families (Ellstrand *et al.* 1996). The majority of hybrid combinations involve endemic, often rare species of *Cyrtandra* (67 hybrid combinations), *Dubautia* (24), *Bidens* (10), and *Clermontia* (8). Hybridization has also been reported frequently on the Canary Islands. Threatened plant species include *Argyranthemum coronopifolium* (Brochman 1984), *Lavandula canariensis* (Humphries 1979), *Senecio teneriffae* (Gilmer & Kadereit 1989), and *Arbutus canariensis* (Salas-Pascual *et al.* 1993).

One of best examples of the process of genetic assimilation on islands is the ongoing assimilation of North America's rarest tree, the Catalina Island mahogany (*Cercocarpus traskiae*), by the mountain mahogany (*C. betuloides* var. *blanchae*), a more widespread congener (Rieseberg & Gerber 1995). Catalina mahogany is extremely restricted in distribution, comprising only 11 adult trees from a single canyon on the southwest corner of Santa Catalina Island, one of the Channel Islands off the coast of California. Analyses of the 11 trees with species-specific allozyme, RAPD, and morphological markers revealed that five were hybrids. Moreover, molecular marker analyses revealed that several seedlings were of hybrid origin, suggesting that the process of assimilation is continuing.

7.2. Hybrid speciation

An important question is whether hybridization leads to an overall increase or decrease of biodiversity (Rieseberg & Wendel 1993). If hybridization generally leads to the breakdown of reproductive barriers and the merger of species, then the latter hypothesis would be supported. Alternatively, if hybridization often fosters the formation of entirely new species, then a more creative role for hybridization can be envisioned.

Although Linnaeus argued that new species might form through hybridization, this possibility was largely ignored by Darwin, since by the early 19th century it had been shown that most hybrids were partially or completely sterile and that later generation hybrids reverted back to the parental forms (Darwin 1859). However, a small number of anomalous reports continued to appear of plant hybrids that were constant and fertile and did not segregate back toward the parental species. Later evidence indicated that the constancy of these hybrids resulted from either apomixis or allopolyploidy (Lotsy 1916; Winge 1917). In the early 20th century, it was suggested that hybrid reproduction might also be stabilized in diploid sexual species through `recombinational speciation´ (Müntzing 1930).

Müntzing postulated that the sorting of chromosomal rearrangements in later generation hybrids could, by chance, lead to the formation of new population systems that were homozygous for a unique combination of chromosomal sterility factors. The new hybrid population would be fertile, stable, and at the same ploidal level as its parents, yet partially reproductively isolated from both parental species due to a chromosomal sterility barrier.

Although early authors focused on chromosomal rearrangements (*e.g.* Müntzing 1930, Grant 1958), it is clear that the sorting of genic sterility factors should generate similar results. Thus, current models incorporate both genic and chromosomal sterility factors (Templeton 1981; Rieseberg 1997). Other factors that appear to play a critical role in recombinational speciation include strong natural selection for the most fertile or viable hybrid segregants (Templeton 1981; Rieseberg *et al.* 1996a), rapid chromosomal evolution (Templeton 1981; Rieseberg *et al.* 1995), and the availability of habitats suitable for the establishment of hybrid neospecies (Rieseberg 1991; Arnold 1997).

The feasibility of the recombinational model has been explored experimentally via crossing studies (Stebbins 1957; Grant 1966a, 1966b; Rieseberg *et al.* 1996a). These studies validated the recombinational model by demonstrating that fertile and viable hybrid lineages can be obtained after only a small number of generations (<10) of selfing and/or backcrossing, even if F_1 hybrids were almost completely sterile. Furthermore, the experimentally generated hybrid lineages were often strongly reproductively isolated from the parental species.

Estimating the frequency of homoploid hybrid speciation in nature is more difficult. Fewer than ten cases have been rigorously documented with molecular markers in plants (Rieseberg 1997), and even fewer examples are available for animals (Bullini 1994; Dowling & Secor 1997). However, these low numbers may be an artefact of the difficulty of detecting and documenting homoploid hybrid species, particularly if the hybridization events are ancient. A much larger number of hybrid species has been proposed, and molecular phylogenetic studies continually uncover unexpected cases of ancient hybridization, some of which may have led to speciation (Dowling & Secor 1997; Morgan 1997). Also, hybridization may play an important role as the creative stimulus for speciation in small or peripheral populations (Grant & Grant 1994). Hybridization rates appear to be highest in populations with these characteristics, and hybridization may be more plausible than population bottlenecks for generating the genetic or chromosomal reorganization proposed in founder-effect speciation.

In comparison to allopolyploidy, researchers have expended much less effort toward understanding the mechanistic basis of recombinational speciation. The most detailed studies concern the origin of a wild hybrid sunflower species, *Helianthus anomalus* (Rieseberg *et al.* 1995, 1996a). These studies also illustrate the utility of genetic mapping studies for studying the genomes of both recent and ancient hybrids.

7.2.1. Recombinational speciation in wild sunflowers

As discussed earlier, genetic models suggest that reproductive isolation between a new recombinational species and parental species populations can be facilitated by rapid karyotypic evolution (Grant 1958, Templeton 1981; McCarthy *et al.* 1995). This hypothesis has been tested by comparing genetic linkage maps for *H. anomalus* and its putative parental species, *H. annuus* and *H. petiolaris* (Rieseberg *et al.* 1995). The mapping data revealed extensive chromosomal differentiation between the hybrid and parental genomes. Seven linkage groups in the hybrid genome differed in gene order from both parental species, and three chromosomal breakages, three fusions, and one duplication are required to explain these differences. Rapid chromosomal differentiation does appear to have facilitated reproductive isolation in *H. anomalus*; F_1 hybrids with its putative parental species are partially sterile because of meiotic abnormalities (Chandler *et al.* 1986).

To better understand the genetic processes that accompany or facilitate recombinational speciation, three independent hybrid lineages were synthesized between *H. annuus* and *H. petiolaris* (Rieseberg *et al.* 1996a). Comparison of the genomic composition of the ancient (*H. anomalus*) and synthetic hybrid lineages revealed that all three synthetic hybrid lineages had converged to nearly identical gene combinations, and this set of gene combinations was statistically concordant with that of *H. anomalus*. Similarity in genomic composition between the synthetic and ancient hybrids suggests that deterministic forces such as selection and genetic constraint, rather than stochastic forces, largely govern the formation of recombinational species. Because the synthetic hybrid lineages were generated in the greenhouse, fertility selection probably played a greater role than ecological selection in shaping hybrid genomic composition. This conclusion is supported by the rapid increase in fertility observed in the three synthetic hybrid lineages; average pollen fertility increased from 4% in the F_1 generation to >90% in the fifth-generation hybrids. Congruence in genomic composition also implies that the genomic structure and composition of hybrid species is essentially fixed after a small number of generations of hybridization and remains relatively static thereafter.

To determine if hybrid speciation could indeed occur in a relatively small number of generations, the sizes of parental species chromosome blocks in the *H. anomalus* genome were analysed (Ungerer *et al.* in review). During the evolution of a new hybrid species, parental linkage block sizes are expected to become progressively smaller over time because of recombination. However, continued reductions in block size will be countered by structural fixation of the hybrid genome; subsequent recombination among blocks derived from the same parental species will no longer decrease block size.

To estimate the number of generations of recombination required to achieve the present distribution of parental chromosomal block sizes in the *H. anomalus* genome, observed block sizes were compared with those of a computer-simulated hybrid population (Ungerer *et al.*, unpublished data). This comparison suggests that *H. anomalus* arose extremely rapidly, probably in fewer than 60 generations (Fig. 2).

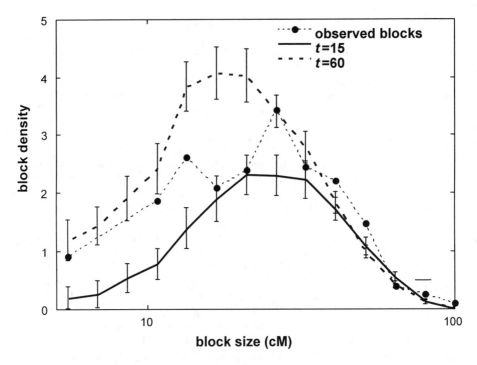

Figure 2: Comparison of frequency spectra of maximum possible parental species block sizes in the *Helianthus anomalus* genome to those of simulation populations after 15 and 60 generations of hybridization. The density of blocks of a particular size is calculated relative to the size of the sampling interval. The increase in area under the curve over time indicates the degree to which the genome is broken up by recombination. A natural log scale was chosen for the x axis because the neutral expectation for the underlying distribution of blocks is linear on this scale.

7.3. Phylogenetic incongruence

Theoretical and empirical studies have demonstrated that incongruence among gene trees or between gene trees and organismal phylogenies can result from a variety of factors, including sampling error, convergence, evolutionary rate heterogeneity, phylogenetic sorting, and hybridization and introgression (Doyle 1992; Avise 1994; Kadereit 1994; Rieseberg *et al.* 1996b; Dowling & Secor 1997). In early studies, phylogenetic incongruence was detected by visual comparisons of trees. However, several quantitative procedures for testing incongruence are now available, of which a likelihood ratio test developed by Hulsenbeck and Bull (1996) is probably most appropriate. In addition, a number of approaches have been proposed for extracting evidence for reticulate evolution directly from parsimony or distance data sets (*e.g.* Bandelt *et al.* 1992; Rieseberg & Morefield, 1995; Jakobsen *et al.* 1997; Maynard Smith & Smith 1998).

In studies of plant phylogeny, hybridization is the explanation most often used to account for incongruence. By contrast, zoologists typically invoke lineage sorting to account for incongruent gene trees among animal taxa (but see Dowling & Secor 1997). This difference in interpretation not only exemplifies the different world view of zoologists and botanists with respect to the frequency and evolutionary significance of hybridization, but it also illustrates the difficulty of differentiating among the many alternative explanations for phylogenetic incongruence.

Two general approaches have been used to test the validity of hybridization as an explanation for phylogenetic incongruence. The first approach uses information from natural history and biogeography to assess the probability of current or past hybridization events. If the allele contributing to phylogenetic incongruence occurs frequently in a sympatric, hybridising congener, then hybridization seems a likely explanation for the observed incongruence (*e.g.* Rieseberg *et al.* 1991; Dowling & DeMarais 1993). By contrast, shared alleles between geographically allopatric species of low vagility seem unlikely to result from hybridization.

A second approach assesses the probability of maintaining highly divergent alleles or haplotypes within a population or species in the absence of interspecific gene flow (*e.g.* Wendel *et al.* 1991; Hanson *et al.* 1996). In the absence of balancing selection, the frequency of transpecific alleles is expected to be low. Thus, high levels of sequence divergence between the native and putatively introgressed allele can be used as evidence for hybridization. Lineage sorting is more difficult to exclude as an explanation if the alleles in question are more similar in sequence.

Application of both approaches to the analysis of gene tree data suggests that hybridization often accounts for incongruence in plants, and has been observed to some degree also in animal taxa. For example, Rieseberg *et al.* (1996b) compiled a list of 89 plant examples of incongruence between cytoplasmic and nuclear trees that are best explained by hybridization, as well as several cases where phylogenetic discordance is attributable to the introgression of nuclear markers. Similar listings are not yet available for animals, although several notable examples are reviewed in Arnold (1997) and Dowling & Secor (1997).

Phylogenetic incongruence can be viewed in two ways by the evolutionist. For students of hybridization, phylogenetic incongruence provides a valuable 'footprint' of past hybridization events and can validate the importance of hybridization throughout the history of the group under investigation. On the other hand, it can hamper the efforts of phylogeneticists to reconstruct organismal phylogeny. Since most methods of phylogenetic reconstruction assume hierarchical rather than reticulate patterns of evolution, these methods cannot generate a correct phylogeny for groups with taxa of hybrid origin. Furthermore, it has been suggested that the presence of hybrids may distort hypothesized relationships among related nonhybrid taxa, and thus possibly limit the utility of standard phylogenetic approaches in hybridising groups of organisms.

Fortunately, empirical tests of the effects of hybrids on phylogenetic trees do not confirm these predictions, except under certain conditions. The most comprehensive studies have been conducted in the Central American species of the genus *Aphelandra* (McDade 1990, 1992, 1997). McDade generated F_1 hybrids between species in this group. Using a detailed morphological data set, she then conducted a series of phylogenetic analyses to test the impact of hybrids on phylogenetic trees. When hybrids between closely related species were included in the phylogenetic analyses, there were typically only minor changes in topology (Fig. 3). However, the inclusion of hybrids between distantly related species did result in the predicted breakdown in cladistic structure and major topological changes (Fig. 3).

Frequent observations of incongruent gene trees also have important implications for the interpretation of gene trees, for sampling strategies employed in phylogenetic studies, and for combining data sets in phylogenetic studies. For example, perhaps due in part to the high frequency of phylogenetic incongruence in studies of both plant and animal species, most systematists now recognize the distinction between gene and species trees and typically employ more than one gene for phylogenetic analyses. Unfortunately, the implications of these data in terms of the need for more extensive population sampling have been largely disregarded in molecular phylogenetic studies. Likewise, the emphasis for combining data sets in phylogenetic analysis has been on searching for character incongruence, whereas the high frequency of reticulation suggests that incongruence in species placement due to hybridization may be a more critical consideration when combining data sets.

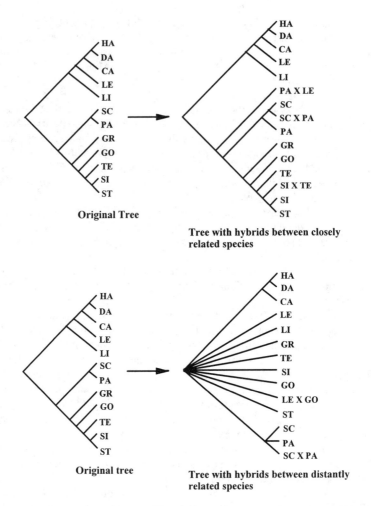

Figure 3: Cladograms of Central American *Aphelandra* species. Modified from McDade (1992).

8. Conclusions and future directions

Analyses of hybridization phenomena has been aided by recent technical and theoretical developments. These include (1) the availability of an almost unlimited supply of molecular markers, (2) the ease with which linkage relationships among markers can be determined, (3) the surprising power of gene trees to detect ancient hybridization events, and (4) theoretical models that provide both a greater understanding of the evolutionary dynamics and outcomes of hybridization events and a means for extracting the maximum information content from empirical data sets.

Future advances are difficult to predict. Clearly the use of genetic mapping approaches to analyse the genomes of both recent and ancient hybrids and to map QTL contributing to reproductive isolation will make valuable contributions. Just as important as these genetic investigations will be experimental ecological studies that provide information concerning the spatial distribution, fitnesses, mating patterns, and selective pressures on different hybrid genotypes in hybrid zones. Of particular value will be lifetime fitness estimates of hybrids based on marker-assisted parentage methods.

However, studies that combine experimental ecological and map-based genetic approaches will be most informative. Of particular promise is the use of mapping data to precisely characterize and/or reconstruct hybrid genotypes on a chromosome by chromosome or trait by trait basis. This will provide a new rigour and precision to both population genetic and field ecological studies that has not been possible in the past. Experiments that fully exploit these capabilities should allow us to test hybrid zone models rigorously, as well as to much more accurately estimate the roles of hybridization and introgression in adaptive evolution and in the formation of new species.

References

Abernathy K (1994) The establishment of a hybrid zone between red and sika deer (genus *Cervus*). *Molecular Ecology*, **3**, 551-562.

Allendorf FW, Leary RF (1988) Conservation and distribution of genetic variation in a polytypic species, the cutthroat trout. *Conservation Biology*, **2**, 170-184.

Anderson E (1948) Hybridization of the habitat. *Evolution*, **2**, 1-9.

Anderson E (1949) *Introgressive Hybridization.* John Wiley, New York.

Anderson E, Hubricht L (1938) Hybridization in *Tradescantia* III. The evidence for introgressive hybridization. *American Journal of Botany*, **25**, 396-402.

Arnold ML (1992) Natural hybridization as an evolutionary process. *Annual Review of Ecology and Systematics*, **23**, 237-261.

Arnold ML (1997) *Natural Hybridization and Evolution.* Oxford University Press, Oxford.

Arnold ML, Buckner CM, Robinson JJ (1991) Pollen-mediated introgression and hybrid speciation in Louisiana irises. *Proceedings of the National Academy of Sciences USA*, **88**, 1398-1402.

Arnold ML, Hamrick JL, Bennett BD (1990) Allozyme variation in Louisiana irises: a test for introgression and hybrid speciation. *Heredity*, **84**, 297-306.

Arntzen JW (1978) Some hypotheses on postglacial migrations of the fire bellied toad *Bombina bombina* (L) and the yellow bellied toad *Bombina variegata* (L). *Journal of Biogeography*, **5**, 339-395.

Avise JC (1994) *Molecular Markers, Natural History, and Evolution.* Chapman & Hall, New York.

Bachmann K, Hombergen EJ (1996) Mapping genes for phenotypic variation in *Microseris* (Lactuceae) with molecular markers. In: *Proceedings of the International Compositae Conference, Kew, 1994. Vol. 2. Biology and Utilization.* (eds. Caligari PDS, Hind DJN), pp. 23-43. Royal Botanic Gardens, Kew, UK.

Bandelt HJ (1992) Split decomposition: A new and useful approach to phylogenetic analysis of distance data. *Molecular Phylogenetics and Evolution*, **1**, 242-252.

Barton NH (1979) The dynamics of hybrid zones. *Heredity*, **43**, 341-359.

Barton NH, Hewitt GM (1981) The genetic basis of hybrid inviability in the grasshopper *Podisma pedestris*. *Heredity*, **47**, 367-383.

Barton NH, Hewitt GM (1985) Analysis of hybrid zones. *Annual Review of Ecology and Systematics*, **16**, 113-148.

Barton NH, Hewitt GM (1989) Adaptation, speciation and hybrid zones. *Nature*, **341**, 497-503.

Beckstrom-Sternberg S, Rieseberg LH, Doan K (1991) Gene lineage analysis of populations of *Helianthus niveus* and *H. petiolaris*. *Plant Systematics and Evolution*, **175**, 125-138.

Bloom WL (1976) Multivariate analysis of the introgressive replacement of *Clarkia nitens* by *Clarkia speciosa* subsp. *polynatha*. *Evolution*, **20**, 412-424.

Bloom WL, Lewis H (1972) Interchanges and interpopulational gene exchange in *Clarkia speciosa*. *Chromosomes Today*, **3**, 268-284.

Bradshaw HD, Wilbert SM, Otto KG, Schemske DW (1995) Genetic mapping of floral traits associated with reproductive isolation in monkeyflowers (*Mimulus*). *Nature*, **376**, 762-765.

Brochmann C (1984) Hybridization and distribution of *Argranthemum coronopifolium* (Asteraceae-Anthemideae) in the Canary Islands. *Nordic Journal of Botany*, **4**, 729-736.

Brunsfeld SJ, Soltis DE, Soltis PS (1992) Evolutionary patterns and processes in *Salix* sect. *Longifoliae*: Evidence from chloroplast DNA. *Systematic Botany*, **17**, 239-256.

Bullini L (1994) Origin and evolution of animal hybrid species. *Trends in Ecology and Evolution*, **9**, 422-426.

Burke JM, Carney SE, Arnold ML (1998) Hybrid fitness in Louisiana irises: analysis of parental and F_1 performance. *Evolution*, **51**, 37-43.

Caetano-Anolles G, Bassam GJ, Gresshof PM (1991) High resolution DNA amplification fingerprinting using very short arbitrary oligonucleotide primers. *Biotechnology*, **9**, 553-556.

Chandler JM, Jan C, Beard BH (1986) Chromosomal differentiation among the annual *Helianthus* species. *Systematic Botany*, **11**, 353-371.
Cook A (1975) Changes in the carrion/hooded crow hybrid zone and the possible importance of climate. *Bird Study*, **22**, 165-168.
Cruzan MB, Arnold ML (1993) Ecological and genetic associations in an *Iris* hybrid zone. *Evolution*, **47**, 1432-1445.
Cruzan MB, Arnold ML (1994) Assortative mating and natural selection in an *Iris* hybrid zone. *Evolution*, **48**, 1946-1958.
Darwin C (1859) *On the Origin of Species by Means of Natural Selection, or the Preservation of Favoured Races in the Struggle for Life*. John Murray, London.
Dobzhansky TH (1937) *Genetics and the Origin of Species*. Columbia University Press, New York.
Dowling TE, DeMarais BD (1993) Evolutionary significance of introgressive hybridization in cyprinid fishes. *Nature*, **362**, 444-446.
Dowling TE, Secor CL (1997) The role of hybridization and introgression in the diversification of animals. *Annual Review of Ecology and Systematics*, **28**, 593-620.
Doyle JJ (1992) Gene trees and species trees: molecular systematics as one-character taxonomy. *Systematic Botany*, **17**, 144-163.
Echelle AA, Connor PJ (1989) Rapid, geographically extensive genetic introgression after secondary contact between two pupfish species (*Cyprinodon*, Cyprinodontidae). *Evolution*, **43**, 717-727.
Ellstrand NC (1992) Gene flow by pollen: implication for plant conservation genetics. *Oikos*, **63**, 77-86.
Ellstrand NC, Elam DR (1993) Population genetic consequences of small population size: implications for plant conservation. *Annual Review of Ecology and Systematics*, **24**, 217-242.
Ellstrand NC, Whitkus R, Rieseberg LH (1996) Distribution of spontaneous plant hybrids. *Proceedings of the National Academy of Sciences USA*, **93**, 5090-5093.
Emms SK, Arnold ML (1997) The effect of habitat on parental and hybrid fitness: reciprocal transplant experiments with Louisiana irises. *Evolution*, **51**, 1112-1119.
Endler JA (1977) *Geographic Variation, Speciation, and Clines*. Princeton University Press, Princeton, NJ.
Fisher RA (1930) *The Genetical Theory of Natural Selection*. Oxford University Press, Oxford.
Fritz RS, Roche BM, Brunsfeld SJ, Orians CM (1996) Interspecific and temporal variation in herbivore responses to hybrid willows. *Oecologia*, **108**, 121-129.
Gallez GP, Gottlieb, LD (1982) Genetic evidence for the hybrid origin of the diploid plant *Stephanomeria diegensis*. *Evolution*, **36**, 1158-1167.
Gill FB (1980) Historical aspects of hybridization between blue-winged and golden-winged warblers. *Auk*, **104**, 444-449.
Gilmer K, Kadereit JW (1989) The biology and affinities of *Senecio teneriffae* Schultz Bip., an annual endemic from the Canary Islands. *Botanische Jahrbuch*, **11**, 263-273.
Grant PR, Grant BR (1994) Phenotypic and genetic effects of hybridization in Darwin's finches. *Evolution*, **48**, 297-316.
Grant V (1958) The regulation of recombination in plants. *Cold Spring Harbor Symposium in Quantitative Biology*, **23**, 337-363.
Grant V (1966a) Selection for vigor and fertility in the progeny of a highly sterile species hybrid in *Gilia*. *Genetics*, **53**, 757-775.
Grant V (1966b) The origin of a new species of *Gilia* in a hybridization experiment. *Genetics*, **54**, 1189-1199.
Hanson MA, Gaut BS, Stec AO, Fuerstenberg SI, Goodman MM, Coe EH, Doebley JF (1996) Evolution of anthocyanin biosynthesis in maize kernels: the role of regulatory and enzymatic loci. *Genetics*, **143**, 1395-1407.
Harrison RG (1986) Pattern and process in a narrow hybrid zone. *Heredity*, **56**, 337-349.
Harrison RG (1990) Hybrid zones: windows on evolutionary process. *Oxford Surveys in Evolutionary Biology*, 7, 69-128.
Harlan JR, de Wet JMJ (1963) The compilospecies concept. *Evolution*, **17**, 497-501.
Hauber DP, Bloom WL (1983) Stability of a chromosomal hybrid zone in *Clarkia nitens* and *C. speciosa* ssp. *polyantha* complex (Onagraceae). *American Journal of Botany*, **70**, 1454-1459.
Heiser CB (1947) Hybridization between the sunflower species *Helianthus annuus* and *H. petiolaris*. *Evolution*, **1**, 249-262.
Heiser CB (1951) Hybridization in the annual sunflowers: *Helianthus annuus* X *H. debilis* var. cucumerifolius. *Evolution*, **5**, 42-51.
Heiser CB (1973) Introgression re-examined. *Botanical Review*, **39**, 347-366.
Heiser CB (1979) Hybrid populations of *Helianthus divaricatus* and *H. microcephalus* after 22 years. *Taxon*, **28**, 71-75.
Hewitt GM (1989) The subdivision of species by hybrid zones. In: *Speciation and its Consequences* (eds. Otte D, Endler JA), pp. 85-110. Sinauer Associates, Inc., Sunderland, MA.

Heywood JS (1986) Clinal variation associated with edaphic ecotones in hybrid populations of *Gaillardia pulchella*. *Evolution*, **40**, 1132-1140.

Howard DJ (1986) A zone of overlap and hybridization between two ground crickets. *Evolution*, **40**, 34-43.

Hsiao J-Y, Wang B-S, Rieseberg LH (1996) Microgeographic allozyme variation in Yushan cane (*Yushania niitakayamensis*; Poaceae). *Plant Species Biology*, **11**, 207-212.

Hubbard AL, McOrist S, Jones TW, Boid R, Easterbee N (1992) Is survival of European wildcats *Felis silvestris* in Britain threatened by interbreeding with domestic cats? *Biological Conservation*, **61**, 203-208.

Hulsenbeck JP, Bull JJ (1996) A likelihood ratio test to detect conflicting phylogenetic signal. *Systematic Biology*, **45**, 92-98.

Humphries CJ (1979) Endemism and evolution in Macronesia. In: *Plants and Islands.* (ed. Bramwell D), pp. 171-179. Academic Press, London.

Jakobsen IB, Wilson SR, Easteal S (1997) The partition matrix: Exploring variable phylogenetic signals along nucleotide sequence alignments. *Molecular Biology and Evolution* **14**, 474-484.

Jeffreys AJ (1987) Highly variable minsatellites and DNA fingerprints. *Biochemical Society Transactions*, **15**, 309-317.

Jones CJ, Edwards KJ, Castaglione S *et al.* (1997) Reproducibility testing of RAPD, AFLP and SSR markers in plants by a network of European laboratories. *Molecular Breeding*, **3**, 381-390.

Kadereit JW (1994) Molecules and morphology, phylogenetics and genetics. *Botanica Acta*, **107**, 369-373.

Karl SA, Avise JC (1993) PCR-based assays of Mendelian polymorphisms from anonymous single-copy nuclear DNA: techniques and applications for population genetics. *Molecular Biology and Evolution*, **10**, 342-361.

Klier K, Leoschke MJ, Wendel JF (1991) Hybridization and introgression in white and yellow ladyslipper orchids (*Cypripedium candidum* and *C. pubescens*). *Journal of Heredity*, **82**, 305-319.

Levin DA, Francisco-Ortega J, Jansen RK (1996) Hybridization and the extinction of rare species. *Conservation Biology*, **10**, 10-16.

Linné C (1760) Disquisitio de sexu plantarum, ab Academia Imperiali Scientiarum Petropolitana praemio ornata. *Amoenitates Academicae*, **10**, 100-131.

Lotsy JP (1916) *Evolution by Means of Hybridization.* M. Nijhoff, The Netherlands.

Mayr E (1963) *Animal species and evolution.* Harvard University Press, Cambridge, MA.

MacCallum CJ, Nürnberger B, Barton NH, Syzmura JM (1998) Habitat preference in a *Bombina* hybrid zone in Croatia. *Evolution*, **52**, 227-239.

Maynard Smith J, Smith NH (1998) Detecting recombination from gene trees. *Molecular Biology and Evolution*, **15**, 590-599.

McCarthy EM, Asmussen MA, Anderson WW (1995) A theoretical assessment of recombinational speciation. *Heredity*, **74**, 502-509.

McDade L (1990) Hybrids and phylogenetic systematics. I. Patterns of character expression in hybrids and their implications for cladistic analysis. *Evolution*, **44**, 1685-1700.

McDade L (1992) Hybrids and phylogenetic systematics. I. The impact of hybrids on cladistic analysis. *Evolution*, **46**, 1329-1346.

McDade L (1997) Hybrids and phylogenetic systematics. I. Comparison with distance methods. *Systematic Botany*, **22**, 669-683.

McGranahan GH, Hansen J, Shaw DV (1988) Inter- and intraspecific variation in the California black walnuts. *Journal of the American Horticultural Society*, **113**, 760-765.

Moore WS (1977) An evaluation of narrow hybrid zones in vertebrates. *Quarterly Review of Biology*, **52**, 263-267.

Morgan DR (1997) Reticulate evolution in *Machaeranthera* (Asteraceae). *Systematic Botany*, **22**, 599-616.

Mullis KB (1990) The unusual origin of the polymerase chain reaction. *Scientific American*, **262**, 56-65.

Müntzing A (1930) Outlines to a genetic monograph of the genus *Galeopsis*. *Hereditas*, **13**, 185-341.

Parsons TJ, Olson SL, Braun MJ (1993) Unidirectional spread of secondary sexual plumage traits across an avian hybrid zone. *Science*, **260**, 1643-1646.

Rand DM, Harrison RG (1989) Ecological genetics of a mosaic hybrid zone: mitochondrial, nuclear, and reproductive differentiation of crickets by soil type. *Evolution*, **43**, 432-449.

Reed KM, Sites JW Jr (1995) Female fecundity in a hybrid zone between two chromosome races of the *Sceloporus grammicus* complex (Sauria, Phrynosomatidae). *Evolution*, **49**, 61-69.

Rhymer JM, Simberloff D (1996) Extinction by hybridization and introgression. *Annual Review of Ecology and Systematics*, **27**, 83-109.

Rieseberg LH (1991) Homoploid reticulate evolution in *Helianthus*: evidence from ribosomal genes. *American Journal of Botany*, **78**, 1218-1237.

Rieseberg LH (1997) Hybrid origins of plant species. *Annual Review of Ecology and Systematics*, **27**, 359-389.

Rieseberg LH, Beckstrom-Sternberg S, Doan K (1990) *Helianthus annuus* ssp. *texanus* has chloroplast DNA and nuclear ribosomal RNA genes of *Helianthus debilis* ssp. *cucumerifolius*. *Proceedings of the National Academy of Sciences USA*, **87**, 593-597.

Rieseberg LH, Soltis DE, Palmer JD (1988) A molecular re-examination of introgression between *Helianthus annuus* and *H. bolanderi*. *Evolution*, **42**, 227-238.

Rieseberg LH, Beckstrom-Sternberg S, Liston A, Arias D (1991) Phylogenetic and systematic inferences from chloroplast DNA and isozyme variation in *Helianthus* sect. *Helianthus*. *Systematic Botany*, **16**, 50-76.

Rieseberg LH, Ellstrand NC (1993) What can morphological and molecular markers tell us about plant hybridization? *Critical Reviews in Plant Science*, **12**, 213-241.

Rieseberg LH, Wendel J (1993) Introgression and its consequences in plants. In: *Hybrid Zones and the Evolutionary Process*, (ed. Harrison R), pp. 70-109. Oxford University Press, New York.

Rieseberg LH, Gerber D (1995) Hybridization in the Catalina mahogany: RAPD evidence. *Conservation Biology*, **9**, 199-203.

Rieseberg LH, Morefield JD (1995) Character expression, phylogenetic reconstruction, and the detection of reticulate evolution. *Monographs in Systematic Botany from the Missouri Botanical Garden* **53**, 333-354.

Rieseberg LH, Van Fossen C, Desrochers A (1995) Hybrid speciation accompanied by genomic reorganization in wild sunflowers. *Nature*, **375**, 313-316.

Rieseberg LH, Sinervo B, Linder CR, Ungerer MC, Arias DM (1996a) Role of gene interactions in hybrid speciation: evidence from ancient and experimental hybrids. *Science*, **272**, 741-745.

Rieseberg LH, Whitton J, Linder R (1996b) Molecular marker discordance in plant hybrid zones and phylogenetic trees. *Acta Botanica Neerlandica*, **45**, 243-262.

Riley HP (1938) A character analysis of colonies of *Iris fulva*, *Iris hexagona* var. *giganticaerulea* and natural hybrids. *American Journal of Botany*, **25**, 727-728.

Roberts HF (1929) *Plant Hybridization before Mendel*. Princeton University Press, Princeton, NJ.

Sage RD, Heyneman D, Lim K-C, Wilson AC (1986) Wormy mice in a hybrid zone. *Nature*, **324**, 60-63.

Salas-Pascual M, Acebes-Ginoves JR, Del Arco-Aguilar (1993) *Arbutus* X *androsterilis*, a new interspecific hybrid between *A. canariensis* and *A. unedo* from the Canary Islands. *Taxon*, **42**, 789-792.

Schlefer EK, Romano MA, Guttman SI, Ruth SB (1986) Effects of twenty years of hybridization in a disturbed habitat on *Hyla cinerea* and *Hyla gratiosa*. *Journal of Herpetology*, **20**, 210-221.

Slatkin M (1973) Gene flow and selection in a cline. *Genetics*, **75**, 733-756.

Small E (1984) Hybridization in the domesticated-weed-wild complex. In: *Plant Biosystematics* (ed. Grant WF), pp. 195-210. Academic Press, New York.

Soltis PS, Bloom WL (1991) Allozymic differentiation between *Clarkia nitens* and *Clarkia speciosa* (Onagraceae). *Systematic Botany*, **16**, 399-406.

Stebbins GL (1950) *Variation and Evolution in Plants*. Columbia University Press, New York.

Stebbins GL (1957) The hybrid origin of microspecies in the *Elymus glaucus* complex. *Cytologia Supplemental Volume*, **36**, 336-340.

Stebbins GL, Daly GK (1961) Changes in the variation of a hybrid population of *Helianthus* over an eight-year period. *Evolution*, **15**, 60-71.

Stutz HC, Thomas LK (1964) Hybridization and introgresssion in *Cowania* and *Purshia*. *Evolution*, **18**, 183-195.

Syzmura JM, Barton NH (1991) The genetic structure of the hybrid zone between the fire-bellied toads *Bombina bombina* and *B. variegata*: comparisons between transects and between loci. *Evolution*, **45**, 237-291.

Tautz D (1989) Hypervariability of simple sequences as a general source for polymorphic DNA markers. *Nucleic Acids Research*, **17**, 6463-6471,

Templeton AR (1981) Mechanisms of speciation–a population genetic approach. *Annual Review of Ecology and Systematics*, **12**, 23-48.

Thorpe RS (1984) Primary and secondary transition zones in speciation and population differentiation: A phylogenetic analysis of range expansion. *Evolution*, **38**, 233-243.

Valentine DH (1947) Studies in British Primulas. Hybridization between primrose and oxlip (*Primula vulgaris* Huds. and *P. elatior* Schreb.). *New Phytologist*, **46**, 229-253.

Vos P, Hogers R, Bleeker M *et al.* (1995) AFLP: a new technique for DNA fingerprinting. *Nucleic Acids Research*, **23**, 4407-4414.

Wang H, McArthur ED, Sanderson SC, Graham JH, Freeman DC (1997) Narrow hybrid zone between two subspecies of big sagebrush (*Artemesia tridentata*): Asteraceae. IV: reciprocal transplant experiments. *Evolution*, **51**, 95-102.

Welsh J, McClelland M (1990) Fingerprinting genomes using PCR with arbitrary primers. *Nucleic Acids Research*, **18**, 7213-7218.

Wendel JF, Stewart JM, Rettig JH (1991) Molecular evidence for homoploid reticulate evolution among Australian species of *Gossypium*. *Evolution*, **45**, 694-711.

Whitham TG (1989) Plant hybrid zones as sinks for pests. *Science*, **244**, 1490-1493.

Williams JGK, Kubelik AR, Livak KJ, Rafalsky JA, Tingey SV (1990) DNA polymorphisms amplified by arbitrary primers are useful as genetic markers. *Nucleic Acids Research,* **18**, 6531-6535.

Wilson EO (1992) *The Diversity of Life.* Harvard University Press, Cambridge, MA.

Winge Ö (1917) The chromosomes: their number and general importance. *Comptes Rendus des Travaux du Labortoire Carlsberg,* **13**, 131-275.

Wolfe AD, Xiang Q-Y, Kephart SR (1997) Old wine in new skin–reassessing hybridization in *Penstemon* using microsatellite markers. *American Journal of Botany,* **84**, 245-246.

Zietkiewicz E, Rafalski A, Labuda D (1994) Genome fingerprinting by simple sequence repeat (SSR)-anchored polymerase chain reaction amplification. *Genomics,* **20**, 176-183.

Advances in Molecular Ecology
G.R. Carvalho (Ed.)
IOS Press, 1998

Variable Environments and Evolutionary Diversification in Inland Waters

Paul D.N. Hebert

Department of Zoology, University of Guelph, Guelph,
Ontario, N1G 2W1, Canada. e-mail: phebert@uoguelph.ca

Molecular analyses are providing the first comprehensive insights concerning the temporal patterning of diversification for many groups of organisms. Molecular studies on the life of inland waters have shown that phenotypic stasis is much more common than expected. In fact, both phylogeographic and phylogenetic analyses suggest that rates of morphological divergence are ordinarily slow despite a population structure conducive to genetic differentiation and speciation. However, rapid bursts of morphological divergence have occurred in some assemblages of aquatic organisms suggesting that restraints on diversification are occasionally ruptured. Variation in the physical environment appears to impact both molecular and morphological evolution by altering mutation rates and by exposing, through genotype by environment (GxE) interactions, otherwise cryptic variation to selection. Experimental studies have established that environmental variables play an important role in modulating mutation rates and recent studies confirm that these impacts alter rates of molecular evolution in natural populations. There is also evidence that extreme environments play a role in accelerating morphological change. For example, among biota from modern inland waters, rapid morphological divergence is most prevalent in lineages which have colonized unusually deep waters. Their phenotypic transformations suggest the importance of hydrostatic pressures in altering phenotypic arrays through GxE interactions, setting the stage for a rapid response to selection. Both the fossil record and molecular studies also suggest that many groups of organisms showed a burst of morphological divergence soon after their origin. Although causal factors are difficult to probe, evidence of an accelerated rate of molecular evolution coincident with the origin of lineages suggests that morphological transitions were favoured by environmental perturbations which may have operated on a planetary scale.

1. Introduction

Biological factors are thought to play a primary role in explaining the striking disparities in rates of molecular and morphological evolution among taxa (Stanley 1985; Li 1997). Rates of molecular evolution have often been linked to variables such as generation length and metabolism, while bursts of morphological diversification have been attributed to relaxed competition and predation. This chapter examines an alternate possibility - that variability in the physical environment plays an important role in establishing the pace of both morphological and molecular change. The potential impacts of some environmental variables, such as UV or radioisotopes, upon mutation rates is obvious, but there may be more pervasive environmental effects on gene replication. Such impacts might influence rates of phenotypic transitions if the supply of mutations is a rate-limiting step in evolution. The physical environment can also increase the amount of phenotypic variation available for selective processing by altering the expression of genes, exposing previously neutral polymorphisms to selection. Waddington (1953) coined the term genetic assimilation to describe situations in which environmental variability enabled otherwise cryptic genetic diversity to impact the external phenotype, allowing selection to subsequently alter the genetic composition of populations. Although the study of genotype-environment interactions has attracted substantial interest (Via & Lande 1985; Gillespie & Turelli 1989; Fry *et al.* 1996), the general role of environmental variability in altering the reaction norm of genotypes and accelerating the response to selection has not been critically investigated.

The first section of this chapter explores the factors which modulate rates of molecular evolution, and establishes that environmental effects are strong in some settings. The next section examines the patterning of morphological transitions in aquatic life from three perspectives. The first case study exploits phylogeographic investigations to examine the duration of past episodes of gene pool fragmentation in the component populations of single species and the phenotypic response to these bouts of isolation. The other two case studies expand the time horizon, examining the situation dependence of morphological transitions in the fauna of inland waters in both space and time. The chapter concludes with an effort to place these results in a broader context, by examining the general role of environmental change in spurring molecular and morphological divergence.

Molecular studies have played a key role in setting the stage for this analysis by enabling the first general perspective on the generation of biological diversity. Inferences concerning rates of morphological divergence are no longer restricted to lineages with comprehensive fossil records. Instead, molecular approaches are enabling evolutionary biologists to mine taxonomic territories which were barren for paleontological prospectors.

2. Varied rates of molecular evolution - analytical artefacts and biological effects

Comparisons of the extent of sequence divergence among species have revealed striking variation in rates of molecular evolution among genes. These gene by gene differences are most conspicuously linked to functionality with the highest rates of change in the most functionally trivial segments of DNA (Li 1997; Yang & Nielsen 1998). The presence of such rate heterogeneity is a useful analytical attribute because, through judicious selection of genes, it is possible to study both ancient and recent events (Ayala 1997). However, rate variation is not only apparent in comparisons among genes; it is also evident in studies of homologous genes (Britten 1986). One of the commonest forms of such rate variation arises as an analytical artifact. Many studies show an apparent reduction in rates of sequence change with time, an effect which arises as a consequence of multiple hits at substitutional hotspots. When rates of sequence divergence are compared over very different time scales, these differences can be large. For example, rates of nucleotide substitution in mitochondrial 12S rDNA show a 40-fold reduction (2.00% versus 0.045%) if one compares sequence divergence over an interval of a few million years (Brower 1994) versus hundreds of million years (Lynch & Jarrell 1993). Similarly superoxide dismutase shows a 3-fold reduction in its rate of evolution as one compares taxa with divergence times rising from 100 to 500 million years (Fitch & Ayala 1994; Ayala 1997).

Other rate heterogeneity derives from biological factors (Table 1). Variation in the number of rounds of DNA replication per unit of time influences the rate of sequence change. Hence, organisms with short generation intervals typically have faster rates of molecular evolution than those with long lifespans (Hafner *et al.* 1994). For example, rates of synonymous substitutions are twice as fast in *Drosophila* as in rats, and 10 times as fast as in primates (Moriyama 1987; Kisakibaru & Matsuda 1995). Similarly, the symbiotic

Table 1: Factors influencing rates of mutation and molecular evolution at a particular gene locus

Biological	Genetic	Environmental
Generation Length	Mutator Genes	Stress
Rounds of DNA replication	Shifting nucleotide usage	Transcriptional activity
Metabolic rate		Mutagenic agents
Demographics		Salinity, thermal regimes

bacterium *Buchnera* shows a rate of 16S rDNA sequence divergence 36 times faster than that of its insect host (Moran *et al.* 1993, 1995), but only slight rate acceleration in comparison to free-living bacteria (Ochman & Wilson 1987; Moran 1996). Measures of generation length are an insufficient tool for the standardization of rates of molecular evolution for multicellular organisms, because they ignore the cycles of DNA replication which intervene between the generation of a zygote and its own synthesis of gametes (Miyata *et al.* 1987). This effect is not trivial as there are often more than 100 such cycles of cell division and variation even exists between the sexes, because of the greater number of cell divisions during spermatogenesis than oogenesis (Shimmin *et al.* 1993). For example, the sperm produced by a 30 year old human male represent some 400 cycles of cell division, while the number of cell divisions that generate an egg is 24, regardless of female age (Vogel & Motulsky 1997). The impact of cell cycle variation on rates of molecular evolution is evidenced by the 2-10 fold elevation of mutation rates in male versus female gametes for a range of vertebrates (Chang *et al.* 1994; Huang *et al.* 1997; Ellegren & Fridolfsson 1997).

Even after the impacts of multiple hits and varying generation lengths are considered, residual variation in rates of molecular evolution remains. Some of this variation may derive from unrecognized diversity in the number of rounds of DNA replication, but there is evidence that other factors also modulate molecular evolution. Modest increases in rates of nucleotide substitution in bacteria (Moran *et al.* 1995) and *Drosophila* (De Salle & Templeton 1988) have been linked to the role of founder effects in facilitating the fixation of weakly deleterious mutations and raising rates of evolution above those apparent in lineages where only neutral substitutions prevail. There is also increasing evidence that variation in the incidence of errors per cycle of replication plays an important role in determining rate variation (Martin & Palumbi 1993; Magnasco & Thaler 1996). For example, rates of sequence change in the mitochondrial DNA of homeotherms are generally higher than those in poikilotherms, perhaps reflecting increased oxidative damage (Martin & Palumbi 1993; Rand 1994).

2.1. Rate heterogeneity and instantaneous calibrations

Heterogeneity in rates of sequence divergence compromises both the accuracy of efforts to date the origins of lineages or adaptations and the recovery of true phylogenetic relationships (Yang 1996). Because of these impacts, substantial efforts need to be directed towards the calibration of rates of sequence divergence (Bromham *et al.* 1996, Mindell & Thacker 1996). There is cause for optimism as it does appear that shifts in rates of molecular evolution ordinarily involve systemic changes rather than gene by gene variation (Muse & Gaut 1997). There are also a substantial number of opportunities for conventional approaches to calibration, exploiting organisms with either a detailed fossil record or a known history of vicariance (Rambaut & Bromham 1998). The broader study of these cases should provide a better sense of the extent of rate variation among lineages and the factors which modulate it, often making it possible to narrow the uncertainty in rates of molecular evolution. There are, however, many organisms in which it will be impossible to critically calibrate rates of molecular evolution using conventional approaches because of their lack of a fossil record or a known vicariance history. However, even these organisms can be studied by abandoning the usual approach to calibration, which involves quantifying the extent of sequence divergence among lineages accumulated over millions of years, and instead examining rates of molecular evolution over just a single generation. There is one drawback to such instantaneous calibrations - the amount of DNA which must be screened for diversity is formidable. For example, with a mutation rate of 10^{-9} per nucleotide, only a single mutation would be detected by screening 10^6 copies of a gene which was 10^3 bp in length. However, because of new approaches to mutation detection, this constraint is becoming less serious (Dianzani *et al.* 1993; Gorelick *et al.* 1996).

The first efforts at instantaneous calibrations, involving the study of D-loop sequence diversity in human mitochondrial DNA, have revealed two surprises. Firstly mothers and their offspring did not always share the same dominant sequence (Howell *et al.* 1996; Parsons *et al.* 1997). Instead, females effectively homoplasmic for one genotype occasionally produced offspring homoplasmic for a different genotype, suggesting stringent mitochondrial bottlenecking during oogenesis. The studies have also revealed an unexpectedly high incidence of sequence changes with these genealogical estimates being about 20 times higher than those expected from conventional calibrations (250% versus 11.9%/site/my). Interestingly the genealogical results are closely congruent with those derived using a coalescent approach (Lundstrom *et al.* 1992). The divergence between evolutionary estimates and those derived from the genealogical and coalescence approaches can be explained if newly arisen mutants are unstable, destined to quickly revert back to their original state, or if they are deleterious, slated for selective elimination. Nonetheless these ephemeral variants may play a significant role in explaining the patterning of sequence divergence over short intervals. The results are, for example, provoking a re-examination of the age of modern human lineages (Gibbons 1998).

2.2. The modulation of mutation rates

The genealogical approach to calibration reinforces the linkage between rates of mutation and molecular evolution. The work suggests that a more detailed understanding of the extent and causes of variation in mutation rates is likely to significantly extend our understanding of the origins of variation in rates of molecular evolution (Table 1). The genetic control of mutation rates has long been recognized, but it was traditionally assumed that rates were stabilized at low and relatively invariant levels (Leigh 1970; 1973). Recent work on microbial systems has revealed a considerably more dynamic situation with complex genetic and environmental effects. Natural bacterial populations are polymorphic for mutator genes of varying potency, with those of greatest effect (10^3 increase) knocking out parts of the DNA repair system (Leclerc *et al.* 1996; Matic *et al.* 1997). Novel or variable environments favour genes producing a substantial increase in mutation rates (Chao & Cox 1983; Sniegowski *et al.* 1997). Similar disfunctional repair systems occur in other organisms, including humans, but mutator genes only reach appreciable frequencies in asexual lineages, where they benefit from their linkage to newly arisen favourable mutations (Taddei *et al.* 1997). This constraint suggests that selection for mutator genes and the resultant shifts in mutation rates are unlikely to provide a general explanation for divergent rates of molecular evolution.

Aside from varied mutation rates derived from differing efficiencies of DNA repair and replication, mutation pressures linked to altered nucleotide usage can also produce shifts in rates of molecular evolution (Sueoka 1988; 1993). One of the most striking examples of this effect is provided by the convergence in nucleotide composition of plasmids to that of their host (Lawrence & Ochman 1997). Shifts in nucleotide usage have, however, also been implicated as causal agents in the varied rates of molecular evolution of some eukaryotes. For example, dipterans show a 20-fold increase in their rates of 18S and 28S rDNA evolution in comparison to other insects (Friedrich & Tautz 1997). This rise in evolutionary rates occurred briefly in the early evolution of dipterans when A-T content rose in both nuclear and mitochondrial genomes. However, once this shift was complete, rates of nucleotide transition slowed so that comparisons among the member taxa of modern dipteran lineages reveal no rate acceleration. Given the genomic-wide nature of this A-T increase, there was undoubtedly a transient burst of molecular evolution in all genes, but the evidence of this acceleration is only now apparent in very slowly evolving genes (De Rijk *et al.* 1995) where its signature has not been muted by subsequent sequence divergence.

2.3. Environmental effects on mutation rates

The impact of environmental factors on mutation rates is not restricted to indirect effects achieved through the alteration of gene frequencies at mutator loci, since mutation rates are also altered through genotype x environment interactions (Table 1). For example, bacterial colonies show a general elevation in their mutation rates when nutritionally stressed (Cairns *et al.* 1988; Foster 1997) and up to 500-fold variation in mutation rates have been reported in human cell lines in response to varying nutrient levels. It is not clear if these increased mutation rates are simply an inadvertent consequence of damage resulting from starvation or if they represent a more carefully orchestrated response of the genome (Bridges 1997). Other mutagenic responses to environmental variation are more obviously co-ordinated. The SOS response in bacteria is induced by single strand breaks and not only leads to their repair, but also to a rise in general mutation rates (Walker 1995). Other mechanisms lead to targeted mutagenesis (Thaler 1994). Actively transcribed genes are mutated more frequently than those, which are repressed, a result deriving from the greater susceptibility of single, compared to double, stranded DNA to damage (Davis 1989). As a result of this effect, mutagens typically cause a 10-30 times higher incidence of mutations in transcriptionally active genes than in those which are repressed (Wright 1997). Differences in spontaneous mutation rates between repressed and active genes show a similar range of variation. Work on the mitochondrial genome has produced conflicting results with evidence of the expected elevation of mutation rates in single stranded DNA apparent in fish but not in mammals (Bielawski & Gold 1996; Nedbal & Flynn 1998).

The transcriptional focusing of mutational activity provides a powerful mechanism for elevating rates of mutation in specific genes or gene assemblages. For example, in both *Escherichia coli* and yeast, amino acid starvation elicits the stringent response, which leads to the depression of a battery of amino acid biosynthetic enzymes (Datta & Jinks-Robertson 1995). Under these conditions, mutation rates at these loci show a substantial increase (Wright 1997). The inducibility of many genes in multicellular organisms sets the stage for similar transcriptional focusing and environment-dependent variation in their mutation rates.

Aside from variation in the mutation rates of homologous genes deriving from diversity in repair systems or varied transcriptional activity, there is an array of other potential environmental effects. Differential exposure to mutagenic agents, ranging from UV light to allelochemicals, represents one obvious potential cause of genomic-wide shifts in mutation rates (Halliwell & Gutteridge 1989; Hartman *et al.* 1991; Brash *et al.* 1991). However, other more subtle effects may also exist. For example, since the functioning of enzymatic proteins, including DNA repair systems, is influenced by salt concentrations, shifts in the salinity of marine or inland waters might alter mutation rates (Lanyi 1974). Varied cycles of aridity might similarly lead to shifts in the mutation rates of organisms with desiccation resistant lifestages, because DNA damage accumulates during periods of crytobiosis (Levin 1990; Mattimore & Battista 1996).

The existing information suggests that environmental effects on mutation rates could readily account for the 10-50-fold variation in rates of sequence change known to occur among homologous genes in different lineages, but much more work is required to verify this fact. If environmental factors do play a key role in governing the incidence of mutations, linkages should also be apparent between environmental conditions and rates of molecular evolution. Although the search for such associations has only begun, evidence of such linkages is becoming apparent (Lutzoni & Pagel 1997; Bleiweiss 1998).

2.4. Environmental effects on molecular evolution: aquatic case studies

One interesting exploration of rate heterogeneity in aquatic organisms has involved foraminiferans. Because of their calcareous shells, these protists have an excellent fossil record enabling calibrations of their rates of evolution (Kennett and Srinivasan 1983). Most foraminiferans are benthic, but a few lineages have made a transition to the plankton and it is the contrast in rates of molecular evolution between these two groups which is of particular significance. The planktonic lineages, which have arisen since the Cretaceous, are partitioned into 4 different families (Vargas *et al.* 1997). Evolutionary rates of 18S rDNA in the benthic lineages and one family of planktonic foraminiferans are comparable to those in other organisms, but three other planktonic families show extreme rate acceleration. Two of these families show rates of 18S rDNA divergence that are nearly 100x higher than those of their benthic counterparts, while the remaining family shows a 20-fold acceleration (Vargas *et al.* 1997; Pawlowski *et al.* 1997). This rate acceleration has been linked to their higher exposure to UV light. Many benthic forms are also exposed to high levels of light as they occur in intertidal areas, but they produce a solid calcareous shell, pierced only by tiny pores, which protects the nucleus from solar exposure. The sole family of planktonic foraminiferans which shares this shell morphology, the Candeinidae, is also the only planktonic family which has not shown rate acceleration. The other families of planktonic foraminiferans produce shells which provide much less protection from solar radiation, and the two families with the most rapid rates of divergence have honeycomb-like shells.

While planktonic foraminiferans show exceptional rate acceleration, other groups appear to show a similar response to solar exposure. Echinoderms have an excellent fossil record and three-fold variation in rates of sequence divergence at 28S rDNA has been identified among different lineages. In this group, deep-water species and those which are buried in the substrate show slower rates of sequence divergence than those from shallow waters, and it has been suggested that this difference is due to their varied UV exposure (Smith *et al.* 1992).

In other cases detailed fossil records are unavailable, but phylogenetic data provide convincing evidence for rate variation. The problematic phylogenetic position of the anostracan crustacean *Artemia* based on analyses of 18S rDNA sequence divergence derives from its exceptionally rapid rate of evolution (Maley & Marshall 1998). Members of this genus, which occur only in hypersaline waters, appear to show rate acceleration in many genes. For example, divergence time estimates, based on usual globin calibrations, suggest that subunits of the 9 domain haemoglobin in *Artemia salina* arose more than 700 million years ago, an estimate which is clearly too early since this gene array is a derived character in anostracans (Trotman *et al.* 1994). In other cases, such as the Na-K pump gene, which shows greater divergence between two species of *Artemia* than all vertebrates (Iwabe *et al.* 1996), it is tempting to link rate acceleration to selection. However, even in this case, most nucleotide substitutions are synonymous, suggesting that mutation rates are elevated. Freshwater anostracans show much more typical rates of sequence divergence than *Artemia* indicating that rate acceleration is not a general property of anostracans. Moreover, rate acceleration is apparent in varied crustacean lineages from salt lakes, a result suggesting that high salt concentrations impair DNA repair enzyme activity and set the stage for rapid molecular evolution (Hebert *et al.*, unpublished data).

These three studies provide evidence of strong environmental impacts on rates of molecular evolution. There is a need to investigate the frequency of such rate diversity in a broader range of lineages and environments. Even if such effects are currently rare, they may have been more general in the past. The earth has experienced major shifts in thermal regime, the atmosphere dramatic shifts in gas concentrations and the oceans marked shifts in salinity (Conway Morris 1995); these planetary perturbations could have provoked shifts in rates of molecular evolution across broad assemblages of organisms.

3. Varied rates of morphological divergence: an overview

The variation in rates of morphological divergence among lineages is even more pronounced than that evident at the molecular level (Stanley 1985). Despite apparently similar exposures to mutation and selection, some lineages have shown morphological stasis for hundreds of millions of years, while others have shown rapid change. One of the most significant problems for evolutionary biology lies in gaining a deeper understanding of the factors responsible for this heterogeneity. Molecular studies have not provided a simple explanation for phenotypic stability; the gene pools of living fossils have substantial genetic variation and their rates of molecular evolution appear normal (Avise *et al.* 1994 but see Omland 1997). Although stasis has routinely been explained by invoking normalizing selection, a critical assessment of its role is difficult. As Kauffman (1993) notes, there is a need for a much more thorough understanding of the incidence of stasis and the settings in which it occurs. In the past, cases of stasis were recognized through reference to fossils, a serious constraint given the poor record for most groups. Molecular studies are now making it possible to gain a much better sense of the past velocities of morphological change in lineages which lack a fossil record. The following three case studies (3.1.1.- 3.1.3.) exploit molecular analyses to explore the situational and taxonomic dependence of morphological transitions in the life of inland waters.

3.1. Phylogeographic patterns and rates of morphological divergence in aquatic life

Phylogeographic studies focus on examination of the geographic patterning of gene frequencies in single species which has arisen as a result of the relatively recent interplay of vicariance and dispersal events (Avise 1994; Hewitt 1996). These studies enable the recognition of past episodes of population fragmentation and, when coupled with assumptions concerning rates of molecular evolution, permit both the estimation of the age of lineages which comprise a taxon and provide a sense of their rates of morphological transition.

Phylogeographic studies on aquatic life have now been sufficiently intensive to enable examination of the prevalence of past range fragmentation in species with differing vicariance histories and dispersal regimes. Aquatic organisms show striking divergence in their dispersal syndromes with some species employing active dispersal, while other rely on the passive dispersal of desiccation resistant stages. The apparent effectiveness of this latter mode of dispersal has been invoked to explain the phenotypic uniformity of such organisms across their broad geographic ranges (Darwin 1859). Some researchers have envisaged a virtual rain of dispersal stages ensuring genetic continuity on a global scale (Mayr 1963). Genetic studies have forced a re-examination of this conclusion since, in case after case, analysis has revealed that such lineages consist of cryptic taxa showing enough genetic divergence to suggest their reproductive isolation for millions of years. The results indicate that the morphological similarity of passively dispersed organisms from protists to crustaceans is not a product of gene pool cohesion, but instead reflects their slow rates of morphological divergence (Nanney 1982, Taylor *et al.* 1998a).

Work on actively dispersed organisms has provided evidence of similar episodes of past range fragmentation, although the divergence times are less. Studies on the Holarctic fish fauna have shown that most species include two or more genetically divergent lineages (Bernatchez & Wilson 1998). The pattern of secondary contact between the isolates appears linked to vicariance history. In glaciated regions, the positioning of phylogeographic boundaries varies among species and the secondary admixture of lineages is common. By contrast, in areas which remained ice-free throughout the Pleistocene, lineages show little secondary contact and there is a high degree of concordance in the phylogeographic patterns of different species (Avise 1994). These phylogeographic studies have produced information that is of use in probing rates of morphological transition. Lineages of northern fish species seem to have originated as a consequence of range fragmentation during Pleistocene glaciations, although the extent of divergence suggests that their origins often antedate the last advance, indicating that populations experienced cyclic retreats to certain refugial areas (Bernatchez & Wilson 1998). By comparison fish in the southern regions of North America typically show greater sequence diversity among their component lineages, suggesting longer histories of habitat occupancy.

Although many cases where populations have been isolated for brief intervals have undoubtedly been overlooked because the genetic imprint of such isolation is so subtle, phylogeographic studies indicate that most aquatic organisms have experienced periods of range fragmentation that severed gene flow and allowed regional divergence. Few species conform to a human model of dispersal from a single group of populations in the last 200,000 years. Instead most aquatic taxa include regional populations with sequence divergences suggesting their isolation for intervals ranging from a few hundred thousand to more than a million years.

The morphological divergence among population groups revealed through phylogeographic analysis is generally small. Lineages of North American freshwater fishes with genetic differences suggesting their isolation for periods of less than 0.5 million years have rarely been accorded taxonomic status in prior morphological studies. On the other hand, lineages with divergences suggesting more than a million years of isolation often represent clades which were recognized as distinct subspecies. The results of genetic studies on passively dispersed organisms, ranging from protists to crustaceans, indicate that morphological stasis has sometimes been sustained for many millions of years (Nanney 1982, Colbourne *et al.* 1997). Collectively these studies suggest that morphological change among lineages from inland waters is typically slow. However, phylogeographic studies, by their nature, undoubtedly provide a downwardly biased perspective on rates of morphological transitions. Since these studies examine the patterning of genetic divergence in populations thought to be members of a single species, they exclude cases where rapid morphological transitions resulted in the formation of a new species or higher taxon. For this reason, there is a need to examine the patterning of genetic divergence from a broader taxonomic perspective.

3.1.1. Morphological transitions in inland waters

Molecular studies on the life of inland waters have an important role to play in efforts to examine the factors which influence rates of morphological innovation. Not only are population boundaries well defined, but habitat age is often precisely known, setting an upper limit to the time available for the divergence of resident species. The isolation of these habitats sets the stage for gene pool fragmentation and founder effects which have long been thought to accelerate evolutionary progress (Wright 1978). Moreover, the clearly defined differences in selective regime between intermittent and permanent aquatic habitats would seem to provide an outstanding venue for disruptive selection. Intermittent habitats often lack visual predators, have detritus-based food webs and require desiccation resistant stages, while organisms in permanent waters regularly confront visual predators, exploit phytoplankton-based food webs and persist without diapause.

Despite these expectations of rapid divergence, the rates of morphological diversification in the life from most inland waters have been slow. Lineages of terrestrial plants which have invaded inland waters have shown little diversification, with most families containing just a single genus (Barrett & Graham 1997). The same phylogenetic restraint is shown among the plankton of inland waters, with many families including either a single genus or a small number of weakly defined lineages. Benthic organisms show higher taxonomic diversity, but even their morphological diversity is restrained. For example, freshwater gastropods have explored a much smaller segment of molluscan morphospace than their marine or terrestrial counterparts (Hubendick 1952).

The puzzling lack of diversification in most freshwater environments is reinforced when one examines life in the world's largest lakes (Martens *et al.* 1994). Most of the ten million lakes on earth occur in relatively small, shallow basins, but some lakes are much larger and deeper (Fig. 1). Aside from their unusual physical attributes, these lakes differ in another important way from their smaller counterparts - they are much older (Martens 1997). While most small bodies of water occupy basins which have originated in the last 10,000 years,

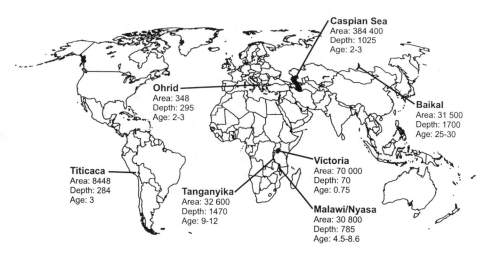

Figure 1: The surface area (km^2), maximum depth (m) and age (My) of 7 lake basins with endemic species flocks.

large lakes occupy basins whose ages range from 0.5-30 million years. From a biological perspective the most distinctive aspect of these lakes is the frequent occurrence of endemic species flocks which appear to have originated through intralacustrine speciation. The development of such species flocks was initially regarded as problematic, but it has gradually been accepted that these habitats are large enough, structurally complex enough, and old enough to have enabled the slow accumulation of this diversity (Fryer 1991). Although more work is needed, recent studies have complicated this neat neo-Darwinian explanation for the extraordinary diversity in these lakes. It is now clear that both the species flocks and the lakes are often much younger than the basins they occupy.

The haplochromine cichlids of the African rift lakes represent the most intensively studied example of these radiations (Greenwood 1974; McCune 1997). The haplochromines from Lake Victoria appear to include at least 400 species and have developed in a lake basin which is about 0.5 million years old. However, many of the component species in this flock appear to have originated much more recently, since the lake itself refilled just 12,400 years ago after an arid phase (Johnson *et al.* 1996). The recent origins of this assemblage have been verified by studies showing less than 0.5% sequence divergence in cytochrome B among its members (Meyer *et al.* 1994). The species flock in Lake Victoria is younger than most of the phylogeographic subgroups of single fish species found in temperate North America! Genetic studies suggest that the haplochromine flocks in Lakes Tanganyika and Malawi have arisen over a longer interval, perhaps 2-3 million years. However, some groups, such as the 80 species of rock cichlids in Lake Malawi have likely originated much more recently because they are habitat specialists which occupy areas that were dry until 1860 (Owen *et al.* 1990). This pattern of rapid diversification is also apparent in Lake Baikal where 20 endemic species of cottoids have diversified in the last 2-4 million years into fish which are so morphologically divergent that they have been placed in three different families (Slobodyanyuk *et al.* 1995; Hunt *et al.* 1997).

Aside from fish, a broad range of benthic invertebrates has also diversified in the ancient lakes. The radiation of 260 species of gammarid amphipods in Lake Baikal is most spectacular, but lesser radiations are known in prosobranch molluscs, turbellarian flatworms, and both ostracod and copepod crustaceans. Genetic studies on these groups have been very limited, but allozyme and cytogenetic work suggest that the Baikal amphipods show little genetic divergence (Yampolsky *et al.* 1994).

The occurrence of explosive radiations in long-lived lakes is not unique to modern environments as there is evidence of similar radiations in the past. The fossil record shows that freshwater ostracods are usually more morphologically conservative than their marine counterparts, but there are some cases of explosive diversification in paleo-ancient lakes (Bate & Robinson 1978). The genus *Cypridea* diversified into more than 150 species in the inland waters of western Europe over a 30 million year interval in the Jurassic. Similarly Lake Steinheim, which persisted for a few hundred thousand years following its origin through a meteorite impact in the Miocene, was only 4 km in diameter, but was the site of an endemic radiation of gastropods (Gorthner & Meier-Brook 1985, Reif 1985).

The restriction of these adaptive radiations to long-lived lakes has focussed attention on the importance of time as the arbiter of diversification. As a result, it is paradoxical that evidence is now accumulating which suggests that the faunal assemblages are much younger than the lake basins they occupy. If cichlid swarms have diversified in just a few hundred years in the rift lakes, why are similar radiations absent from lakes in glaciated areas that are 10,000 years old? Species flocks have also failed to develop in intermittent lakes or rivers, even when the water course or basin is ancient, such as Lake Eyre which apparently originated about 2 million years ago. Although elements of its fauna may have persisted for this long interval, as their diapausing stages survive dry periods, they have not diversified. Conversely the oceans, despite their long persistence, have not provoked the same rapid diversification of life seen in long-lived lakes. For example, more than 250 species pairs of fish, crabs and echinoderms have shown very limited morphological divergence since closure of the Isthmus of Panama some 3 million years ago (Vrba 1980). These patterns suggest that ancient lakes have other unique characteristics, aside from age, which foster diversification.

Researchers studying the faunas of these ancient lakes have emphasized that only a small proportion of the resident lineages has formed species flocks (Sturmbauer & Meyer 1992). This observation has motivated the search for speciation syndromes - factors which predispose organisms to rapidly diverge. This search has suggested that diversification is restricted largely to benthic organisms which both brood their young and possess limited dispersal abilities, setting the stage for allopatric divergence in single lake basins (Cohen & Johnston 1987). Other workers have suggested a critical role for lake depth in provoking radiations, noting that most young habitats are less than 10 m in depth, while ancient lakes typically exceed 500 m. The potential importance of depth in promoting diversification is reinforced by the fact that taxa found in the nearshore zone and surface waters of ancient lakes have failed to diversify, whereas most deepwater taxa are endemic. For example, the gill-bearing prosobranch molluscs, which inhabit deepwaters, invariably show higher endemicity than the air-breathing pulmonates which are typically restricted to shallow waters (Boss 1978; Michel 1994).

Although some workers have suggested the importance of water depth in promoting diversification, no mechanistic explanation for this pattern has been proposed. However, there is a biochemical basis for the impact of depth on evolutionary diversification which lies in the fundamental laws governing the free energy changes which accompany chemical reactions ($\Delta G = \Delta H - T\Delta S + P\Delta V$). The net free energy change (ΔG) associated with all chemical reactions is impacted by the chemical energy shift or enthalpy (ΔH), the change in entropy (ΔS) and by the interaction between pressure (P) and volume (V) changes associated with the reaction (Somero 1990). Temperature increases accelerate enzyme reactions because they increase entropy, diminishing the free energy change. In terrestrial environments the impact of volume changes linked to reactions is invariably small because atmospheric pressure is low. However, in aquatic environments hydrostatic pressures increase rapidly with depth so this term gains importance. In contrast to increasing temperature which leads to a general acceleration in reactions, increases in pressure accelerate those reactions which lead to a volume decrease and slow those involving an increase. This varied pressure response sets the stage for the disruption of biochemical pathways and the fracturing of character canalization. Although the effects of hydrostatic pressure have not been examined from an organismic perspective, physiological studies have examined the impacts upon the kinetic behaviour of enzymes. This work has shown that the kinetic properties of enzymes from species typically restricted to shallow waters are often strongly impacted by hydrostatic pressures with up to a 50% shift in K_m values and V_{max} activities at pressures equivalent to those at 50 m depth. Adaptation to pressure effects is possible and enzymes isolated from deepwater marine organisms are protected from these effects as a result of amino acid reconfigurations (Somero 1992). Since the vast majority of inland waters are shallow, freshwater organisms are adapted to life at low pressures. When such forms colonize deep lakes, the stage is set for the generation of much novel phenotypic diversity, enabling the selective transformation of populations, leading to rapid anagenetic change. Pressure effects might also act as agents in cladogenesis by provoking depth-dependent morphological reconfigurations which could act to deter gene exchange and serve as a basis for the evolution of reproductive isolation. It is worth emphasizing that since oceanic life has a long history of exposure to deepwater environments, bursts of evolutionary diversification would only be expected in marine lineages which have made a recent depth transition.

3.1.2. Species flocks beyond ancient lakes

It should be possible to ascertain the relative importance of biological attributes and depth in provoking flock formation by examining the evolutionary response of lineages in a broader geographic context. If depth plays a key role in unleashing phenotypic diversification, then lineages showing species flocks in deep lakes should show little diversification in other surface waters. On the other hand, if biological attributes play a lead role, one expects these groups to show similar proliferation in other environments. The results of such analyses show that some lineages which have formed flocks in large lakes have also diversified in other surface waters. The cichlid fishes are one example of a lineage which has shown rapid speciation in many settings, but this group is not unique. For example, the ostracod genus *Candona*, which is represented by a large number of endemic species in both Lakes Baikal and Ohrid, is also the most specious genus of ostracods in other freshwater habitats across the Holarctic (Martens 1994). However, other lineages show a different pattern. Forty seven species of *Cytherissa* occur in Lake Baikal, but only one widely distributed species occurs in balance of the Holarctic. Similarly the hyallelid amphipods are represented by at least 28 species in Lake Titicaca, but only a few species with broad distributions occur in North America (Dejoux 1992). This idiosyncratic commitment to diversification is puzzling enough to suggest the need for more detailed studies on these groups.

Hyallela azteca is a species which has long been regarded as the ultimate amphipod generalist. It not only ranges from the tropics to the arctic, but occupies virtually every freshwater habitat including ponds, lakes, streams and rivers (Pennak 1989). Individuals show variation in size and reproductive behaviour but this has been linked to phenotypic plasticity induced by environmental variables (Strong 1972; Wellbourn 1995). Genetic studies have now shown that the situation is more complex. A survey of populations in one small region of North America revealed the presence of 6 clades, showing substantial genetic divergence (Witt & Hebert, unpublished data). Divergence in one mitochondrial gene, cytochrome oxidase I (COI), exceeded 30% among most pairs of these taxa, indicating that *H. azteca* is a species complex which likely includes a large number of deeply diverged species. Despite their limited morphological divergence, several species in this complex co-occur in most habitats without hybridization.

This result is in one sense unexciting, as it provides just one more example of a common message; the taxonomic diversity of aquatic invertebrates has been seriously underestimated (Knowlton 1993). However, viewed more parochially, the limited morphological divergence among members of the *azteca* complex is important simply because the assemblage shows so much less morphological diversity than the allied species flock in Lake Titicaca. However, to confirm that the pace of morphological diversification has been accelerated in Titicaca it is critical to compare the age of the species flock in this lake with that of the *azteca* complex. Resolution of this issue is currently constrained by the lack of comprehensive genetic information. However, as Lake Titicaca is less than 3 million years of age, it is likely that the species flock within its boundaries will show far less COI diversity than already detected in the *azteca* complex, indicating its relatively rapid morphological diversification.

A similar situation involving mysid crustaceans has been studied in more detail. A single species of *Mysis* is present in lakes across North America, and three other species occur in Eurasia (Väniöla 1995). Populations of these four species show little morphological diversity, despite their marked genetic divergence. Populations of five marine species show a similar pattern. By contrast the three species of *Mysis* in the deep waters of the Caspian, show extremely limited genetic divergence, but marked morphological divergence.

The results of these studies provide a surprising view of evolution. The phenotypic stasis of lineages in most inland waters is not a consequence of gene pool cohesion or limited genetic divergence. Instead lineages have shown little morphological change despite massive genetic restructuring. By contrast, lineages in large lakes show striking morphological change, but limited genetic differentiation. The discovery of lineages showing substantial morphological divergence despite limited genetic change coincides with both neo-Darwinian expectations and the success of artificial selection in creating phenotypic novelty. However, the frozen phenotypes of lineages showing marked genetic divergence is less expected and suggests the value of studies which examine the nature of character state evolution in lineages showing this pattern of constrained diversification.

3.1.3. Evolutionary restraint and relaxation in the Cladocera

Molecular studies are providing the first temporal perspective on the origins of morphological diversity in many groups of organisms. Recent work of this type has, for example, provided new details on the evolutionary trajectories of the cladoceran crustaceans, one of the dominant groups of the zooplankton in inland waters. The limited fossil record for these organisms suggests that some extant genera were present in the Mesozoic, but it has long been assumed that many modern species arose in a burst of diversification after the Pleistocene (Brooks 1957).

Genetic studies on *Daphnia*, the best known cladoceran genus, have revealed a much more leisurely pace of differentiation. Sequence divergence of 12S rDNA indicates that the daphniids of North America and Australia can be assigned to four different subgenera, which show enough divergence to suggest they arose more than 100 million years ago (Colbourne & Hebert 1997; Hebert *et al.*, unpublished data). Each of these subgenera includes a number of component species which are themselves divisible into species complexes. Again, the extent of sequence divergence among the individual complexes in a subgenus suggests their origin in the late Mesozoic. This work indicates that the genus *Daphnia* consists of a number of ancient lineages which have shown little morphological diversification since the Mesozoic except the recurrent loss or gain of specific traits. The overriding message is one of character state convergence and the predictability of morphological trajectories in particular environmental settings (Colbourne & Hebert 1997; Colbourne *et al.* 1997).

Although a broader taxonomic survey is required, the limited information on other cladoceran genera suggests similar phenotypic stasis. For example, the genus *Holopedium* has long been thought to include only a single species, but genetic studies indicate that it includes two deeply divergent lineages (Hebert & Finston 1997). Although these clades appear to have originated at least 20 million years ago, the morphological differences between them are subtle. Given the limited phenotypic divergence over much of the Cenozoic, but the broad morphological diversity among genera and families of cladocerans, it is apparent that there was a burst of diversification in the past.

The origins of the Cladocera have long been shrouded in uncertainty but molecular studies are providing new insights. This clade was first erected in the 19th Century, but Fryer (1987) concluded from morphological studies that it was an artificial amalgm of distantly related lineages. Cladocerans do show far more striking morphological variation than any other group of the zooplankton (Fig. 2). Species show varied feeding behaviour; some are predatory, others are herbivores. They vary in habitat occupancy; some species are planktonic, others are benthic. They show varying reproductive behaviour; one genus retains naupliar stages, while other taxa employ direct development. As a result of their extreme morphological and life history diversity, Fryer (1987) partitioned the group into four orders.

Recent molecular studies (Taylor *et al.*, unpublished data) challenge this conclusion and provide convincing evidence that the cladocerans are monophyletic, showing that cyclestheriids, a family of conchostracan crustaceans, are the mother of all cladocerans. These organisms share several derived features with the Cladocera, but possesses far more pairs of thoracic limbs suggesting the importance of homeotic mutations in cladoceran origins. However, what special set of circumstances allowed the rise and diversification of cladocerans? It has been suggested that the origin in teleost fishes in the early Mesozoic provoked the phenotypic reconfiguration of the plankton (Lynch & Kerfoot 1987). Certainly prior to their evolution, the oceans were populated by large-bodied planktonic crustaceans which today occur only in habitats whose ephemerality prevents their colonization by fish. The rise of teleosts may have provided a *raison d'être* for the

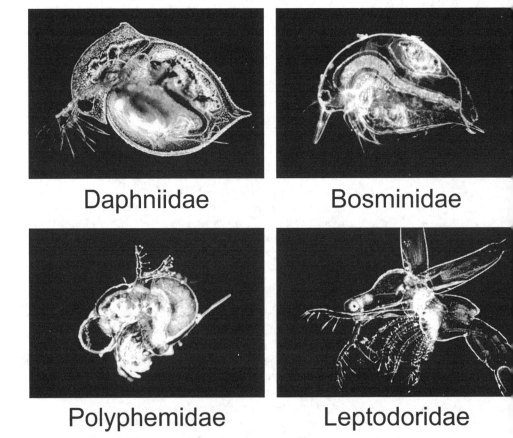

Figure 2: Phenotypic diversity among 4 of 11 cladoceran families.

radiation of small-bodied plankton, but it does not explain why the nascent cladocerans showed such remarkable fluidity in shape, segmentation patterns and life cycles. Conversely it fails to explain why cladoceran phenotypes crystallized so rapidly and why there has been such limited exploration of new phenotypes since this time.

3.2. The patterning and pace of evolutionary diversification in inland waters

Although these three case studies (3.1.1. - 3.1.3.) cannot provide a general overview of evolutionary change in inland waters, they jointly suggest a pattern of evolutionary transitions that is not easily reconciled with gradualistic models of diversification. Many lineages appear trapped in an iterative pattern of character state loss and acquisition which results in little morphological change over long periods of time, while other lineages show bursts of differentiation. For example, the phylogeographic analyses provided evidence of past episodes of population subdivision linked to either range fragmentation or limited dispersal abilities. Although estimated intervals of separation often exceeded a million years, morphological divergence among isolates was restrained, suggesting that morphological transitions are ordinarily slow. Studies of species assemblages from inland waters showed that morphological similarity was often strong among taxa showing marked genetic divergence, reinforcing the evidence for slow morphological transitions. By contrast, surprisingly rapid morphological change was apparent in some species assemblages from the world's largest lakes. Although the divergence in shallow water cichlids demands an alternate explanation, the focusing of this diversification in deepwater taxa suggests that hydrostatic pressure disrupts phenotypic canalization, exposing novel phenotypic variants to selection and setting the stage for the rapid transmogrification of lineages with little genetic divergence. The examination of evolutionary trajectories in the cladoceran crustaceans reinforces the situation dependence of morphological transitions. Following early explosive diversification, phenotypic transitions in this group slowed. The possible linkage between this brief phase of morphological innovation and shifts in predation regime fails to provide a satisfying explanation for either the degree of innovation or its abrupt cessation. Considered jointly, these case studies provide evidence for a more strongly episodic pattern of diversification than expected under gradualistic models of evolution.

4. Morphological transitions - a paleontological perspective

As molecular studies increasingly make it possible to gain an historical perspective on the origins of modern life, both the need and opportunities for the integration of neontology and paleontology strengthen. One of the most important goals of this alliance must be to extend understanding of the factors responsible for the remarkably spasmodic nature of evolutionary diversification. Certainly the fossil record has revealed that the origins of biological diversity have been saltatory. The stunning diversification of Cambrian life in just 10 million years (Bowring et al. 1993) was preceded by the near morphological stasis of life for perhaps a billion years (Schopf 1994 but see Conway Morris 1998). Even since the Cambrian, evolutionary rates have been far from uniform. The fossil record provides compelling evidence of major collapses in biodiversity every 100 million years or so, followed by the rapid diversification of some lineages. As evidence mounts that these events were provoked by major physical crises, their occurrence is less problematic, because they can be linked to episodic shifts in selection regimes (Alvarez et al. 1980; Pope et al. 1994; Kroll et al. 1996). However, the fossil record provides evidence of other evolutionary patterns which are less easily explained. The pattern of punctuated equilibrium in which brief bursts of morphological divergence follow long intervals of stasis is now well established but has no simple explanation. The pattern of co-ordinated stasis, in which whole communities of organisms show little change for long intervals followed by a bout of rapid diversification is even more problematic (Brett *et al.* 1996). The classic example of coordinated stasis involves a diverse marine assemblage of corals, trilobites, echinoderms and brachiopods which occurred for a 60 million year interval in the mid-Paleozoic (Brett & Baird 1995). Over this time, members of the assemblage showed 14 intervals of near-stasis for periods ranging from 3 to 7 million years, each followed by brief bursts of morphological divergence. Although it has been suggested that co-ordinated stasis results when communities are so tightly integrated that they resist invasion and evolutionary innovation, the lack of such intense cohesion in modern species assemblages suggests the need to investigate other explanations.

Given that stasis rules, what are the exceptional circumstances which provoke lineages to launch into morphological reconfigurations? The fossil record suggests the importance of physical regimes, as evolutionary innovation seems to be focused in physically variable, species-poor environments. For example, evolutionary innovation in marine environments has been centered in variable nearshore areas rather than in stable offshore basins, a surprising result because offshore areas have much higher species diversity (Jablonski *et al.* 1983). There is evidence of a similar bias on land - the key elements of the modern flora appear to have arisen in the early Tertiary in polar regions rather than at mid- or low latitudes (Hickey *et al.* 1983). These observations have led to the suggestion that environmental variability enhances the likelihood of large evolutionary changes. If physical factors do play an important role in modulating rates of phenotypic change, then environmental shifts on a planetary scale might be expected to launch phenotypic reconfigurations on a broad taxonomic scale. The sporadic but community-wide morphological reconfigurations evident in studies of coordinated stasis might reflect the common response to episodes of such environmental change.

5. Morphological transitions - a neontological perspective

As evolutionary biologists increasingly employ molecular analyses to investigate the origins of modern life, evidence for the prevalence of lineages showing phenotypic stasis builds. Darwin (1859) noted that life in inland waters shows little geographic diversification, but erred in attributing this similarity to unrestrained migration. Instead it arises because morphology rarely shifts even when gene flow is severed. The phenotypic restraint which has characterized cladocerans since shortly after their origin is rife in organisms from protists (Nanney 1982) to vertebrates. For example, 26 species of *Plethodon* salamanders have originated over a 60 million year period, but show very limited morphological diversity despite a population structure conducive to founder effects and selective divergence (Wake *et al.* 1983). Although stasis is often linked to normalizing selection, this explanation loses its vitality when phenotypic stability persists despite exposure to striking environmental variation. Yet the fossil record and molecular studies of modern life show stasis in lineages exposed to divergent environments and shifting biotic regimes.

The patterning of evolutionary innovation in aquatic environments poses a particularly serious difficulty for invocations of stabilizing selection as an explanation for stasis. Not only is phenotypic stasis rampant in aquatic life, but it is difficult to suggest that stabilizing selection operates on continental scales, while diversifying selection operates in single habitats. Yet such must be the case if one is to explain the patterning of diversification in the life of inland waters. The phenotypic congruence among members of the *Hyallela azteca* complex in North and South America requires stabilizing selection across varying salinity gradients, predation regimes, climatic conditions, habitat permanency and both latitudinal and elevational gradients, while diversifying selection must be invoked to explain the swarm of hyallelids in Lake Titicaca.

The central role of selection in spurring bursts of evolutionary innovation is widely accepted, but the testability of this proposition is limited because rapid morphological change has not been linked to a specific shift in selection regime. Increases in rates of evolutionary diversification have sometimes been linked to an increased intensity of selection, as in the supposed role of fish predation in provoking cladoceran diversification. However, in many other cases, relaxed selection has been invoked to explain the radiations apparent on archipelagoes and following faunal collapses (Mayr 1963). Since both reductions and increases in selection intensity are thought to provoke radiations, why stasis? Prior efforts to account for heterogeneity in rates of evolutionary diversification have often given little attention to the possibility that shifts in evolutionary innovation are driven by bursts of mutation. Yet there is a general sense that the supply of advantageous mutations is often an important rate limiting step in both molecular and morphological evolution (Hill 1982; Lande 1988; Li 1997).

6. The environment and evolution

Models of evolution tend to view the environment as a passive sieve accepting or rejecting phenotypic diversity generated by a random mutational process. However, the study of factors influencing mutation rates suggests that the environment may take a much more proactive role, modulating the rate of introduction of variation and even influencing the sorts of mutation which occur through mechanisms such as transcriptional focussing (Davis 1989, Thaler 1994). If mutations play a rate-limiting step in morphological evolution, then bursts of phenotypic diversification might be provoked by shifts in the incidence of mutations.

Given environmental influences on mutation rates, it is worth enquiring if past planetary perturbations have played a role in producing past bursts of evolutionary diversification. Studies which are probing rates of evolutionary diversification in random segments of the genome may prove useful to test this hypothesis, since they should enable a search for episodic shifts in rates of molecular evolution. The occurrence of such rate variation should be evidenced by discordance between the dates of origin of taxa obtained from the fossil record and from studies of molecular evolution. If past environmental conditions provoked a burst of mutations, then extrapolations based on current rates of molecular evolution should overestimate the age of clades. Evidence of such discordance is building. The fossil record suggests that both birds and mammals diversified very rapidly at the end of the Cretaceous (Feduccia 1995) but molecular data, employing deep Cenozoic calibrations, suggest that many of the component lineages of these vertebrate groups originated some 100 million years earlier (Janke *et al.* 1994; Hedges *et al.* 1996; Cooper & Penny 1997; Kumar & Hedges 1998). There is also evidence for a similar discrepancy concerning the timing of diversification of animal phyla. The fossil record provides convincing evidence that divergence occurred from 540-530 million years ago, while molecular data suggest an origin some 1400 million years ago (Wray *et al.* 1996; but see Ayala *et al.* 1998). These discrepancies may reflect the incompleteness of the fossil record, but this seems unlikely given, for example, the intensive studies on Mesozoic vertebrates. These discrepancies would disappear if there was a 100-fold elevation in mutation rates for a million year period, or a briefer more intense shift in mutation rates, near the Cretaceous and Cambrian boundaries. There is evidence that environmental conditions were very unstable for at least 500,000 years at the Mesozoic/Cenozoic boundary (Conway Morris 1995). If further evidence supports the episodic nature of molecular evolution in these cases, it will be important to ascertain both the generality of these effects on other lineages and their impacts on rates of phenotypic change. Although molecular and morphological evolution are often viewed as being decoupled, Omland (1997) has presented evidence to suggest a correspondence in their rates.

Aside from its potential role in accelerating evolutionary divergence through impacts on mutation rates, environmental variation can influence evolutionary rates by altering the phenotypic arrays available for selective processing through GxE effects. Phenotypic plasticity induced by the environment is often viewed as sheltering the need for genetic change (Wake *et al.* 1983) and this is true for responses which involve alternate canalized states. Predator-mediated shape changes which provide protection from predation provide a clear example of this effect (Tollrian 1995). However, environmental variability can also disrupt canalization, exposing otherwise cryptic variation to selection. First recognized by Waddington (1953), this process can enable swift changes in character states by exploiting the novel phenotypic expression of pre-existing variation. The rapid diversification of life in deep lakes is perhaps most easily explained by the broad impacts of hydrostatic pressure in disrupting character canalization. If further studies confirm this effect, the impacts of GxE interactions on rates of evolutionary progress will need to be examined in other settings. Exposure to unusual thermal regimes or distinctive chemical challenges might similarly disrupt canalization, setting the stage for rapid morphological change.

7. Future studies

This chapter has made it clear that there is a need to gain a deeper understanding of the patterning of morphological divergence through time. Has divergence ordinarily occurred in brief pulses as suggested by the fossil record and some molecular studies or do most lineages show evidence of gradualistic change? This question can be answered by mapping character states on molecular phylogenies. The detection of deep genetic divergences among lineages showing little morphological differentiation coupled with a starburst origin of taxa showing marked morphological divergence would suggest episodic evolution. If such patterns prove common, and existing data suggest they are, efforts should be directed towards ascertaining if episodic evolution derives from bursts of mutation or from shifts in the selective processing of a constant pool of variation. The possible involvement of the physical environment in provoking episodic shifts in mutation rate can be examined in two fashions. There is firstly a need for experimental studies which exploit recent advances in screening DNA diversity to examine the impacts of physical variables such as salinity, U.V. light and hydrostatic pressure on rates of mutation. Experimental perturbations might extend beyond those encountered in modern environments to test organismic responses to paleoenvironmental challenges such as elevated oxygen and methane levels and transient pressure shocks. There is also a need for efforts to both identify cases of heterogeneity in rates of molecular evolution among closely allied lineages and to ascertain their linkage, if any, to environmental variables. Aside from extending knowledge of the factors which influence rates of molecular diversification, there is a need for more information concerning the processes which govern rates of morphological diversification. The growing evidence for morphological stasis in the life of inland waters makes it clear that new molecular taxonomies will need to be forged for many groups. Because such work is unlikely to be carried out in a comprehensive fashion, a few groups should be targeted for the intensive analysis needed to examine the relationship between morphological and genetic divergence. Aside from descriptive studies, there is a need for experimental work which examines the influence of environmental variables on the selective processing of variation. For example, studies on aquatic lineages might test the impact of pressure changes on phenotypic arrays. Efforts should also be launched to gain a deeper mechanistic understanding of the genetic basis for morphological diversity through collaborations with developmental biologists. Through the fusion of more detailed insights concerning the factors modulating the introduction of new genetic diversity and the processes determining its phenotypic impact, it should be possible to advance understanding of the origins of phenotypic diversity in aquatic life.

Acknowledgements

Research grants from NSERC have supported both the assembly of this chapter and my laboratory's work on aquatic organisms. I thank J. Witt, L. Weider and two anonymous reviewers for their helpful critiques of an earlier version of this chapter.

References

Alvarez L, Alvarez W, Azaro F, Michel HV (1980) Extraterrestrial cause for the Cretaceous-Tertiary extinction. *Science, 208*, 1095-1108.

Avise JC (1994) *Molecular Markers, Natural History and Evolution.* Chapman and Hall, New York.

Avise JC, Nelson WS, Sugita H (1994) A speciational history of "living fossils": molecular evolutionary patterns in horseshoe crabs. *Evolution, 48*, 1986-2002.

Ayala FJ (1997) Vagaries of the molecular clock. *Proceedings of the National Academy of Sciences USA, 94*, 7776-7783.

Ayala FJ, Rzhetsky A, Ayala FJ (1998) Origin of the metazoan phyla: molecular clocks confirm paleontological estimates. *Proceedings of the National Academy of Sciences USA, 95*, 606-611.

Barrett SCH, Graham SW (1997) Adaptive radiation in the aquatic plant family Pontederiaceae: insights from phylogenetic analysis. In: *Molecular Evolution and Adaptive Radiation,* (eds. Givnish TJ, Systma KJ), pp. 225-258. Cambridge University Press, Cambridge.

Bate R, Robinson E (1978) *A Stratigraphical Index of British Ostracoda.* Steel House Press, Liverpool.

Bernatchez L, Wilson CC (1998) Comparative phylogeography of Nearctic and Palearctic fishes. *Molecular Ecology, 7*, 431-452.

Bielawski JP, Gold JR (1996) Unequal synonymous substitution rates within and between two protein-coding mitochondrial genes. *Molecular Biology and Evolution, 13*, 889-892.

Bleiweiss R (1998) Slow rates of molecular evolution in high-elevation hummingbirds. *Proceedings of the National Academy of Science USA, 95*, 612-616.

Boss KJ (1978) On the evolution of gastropods in ancient lakes.   In: *Pulmonates Vol. 2A Systematics, Evolution and Ecology,* (eds. Fretter V, Peake J), pp 385-428. Academic Press, London.

Bowring SA, Gotzinger JP, Isachsen CE, Knoll AH, Pelechaty SM, Kolosov P (1993) Calibrating rates of early Cambrian evolution. *Science, 261*, 1293-1298.

Brash DE, Rudolph JA, Simon JA, Lin A, McKenna GJ, Baden HP, Halperin AJ, Ponten J (1991) A role for sunlight in cancer: UV-induced p53 mutations in squamous cell carcinoma. *Proceedings of the National Academy of Sciences USA, 88*, 10124-10128.

Brett CE, Baird GC (1995) Co-ordinated stasis and evolutionary ecology of Silurian to Middle Devonion faunas in the Appalachian Basin. In: *New Approaches to Speciation in the Fossil Record,* (eds. Erwin DH, Anstey RL), pp 285-315. Columbia University Press.

Brett CE, Ivany LC, Schopf KM (1996) Co-ordinated stasis: an overview. *Palaeogeography, Palaeoclimatology and Palaeoecology, 127*, 1-20.

Bridges BA (1997) Hypermutation under stress. *Nature, 387*, 557-558.

Britten RJ (1986) Rates of DNA sequence evolution differ between taxonomic groups. *Science, 231*, 1393-1398.

Bromham L, Rambaut A, Harvey PH (1996) Determinants of rate variation in mammalian DNA sequence evolution. *Journal of Molecular Evolution,* **43**, 610-621.

Brooks JL (1957) The systematics of North American *Daphnia. Memoirs of the Connecticut Academy of Sciences,* **13**, 1-180.

Brower AVZ (1994) Rapid morphological radiation and convergence among races of the butterfly *Heliconius erato* inferred from patterns of mitochondrial DNA evolution. *Proceedings of the National Academy of Sciences USA,* **91**, 6491-6495.

Cairns J, Overbaugh J, Miller S (1988) The origin of mutants. *Nature,* **335**, 142-145.

Chang BH-J, Shimmin LC, Shyue S-K, Hewett-Emmett D, Li W-H (1994) Weak male-driven molecular evolution in rodents. *Proceedings of the National Academy of Sciences USA,* **91**, 827-831.

Chao L, Cox FC (1983) Competition between high and low mutating strains of *Escherichia coli. Evolution,* **37**, 125-134.

Cohen AS, Johnston MR (1987) Speciation in brooding and poorly dispersing lacustrine organisms. *Palaios,* **2**, 426-435.

Colbourne JK, Hebert PDN (1996) The systematics of North American *Daphnia* (Crustacea: Anomopoda): a molecular phylogenetic approach. *Philosophical Transactions of the Royal Society, B,* **351**, 349-360.

Colbourne JK, Hebert PDN, Taylor DJ (1997) Evolutionary origins of phenotypic diversity in *Daphnia.* In: *Molecular Evolution and Adaptive Radiation,* (eds. Givnish TJ, Systma KJ), pp. 163-189. Cambridge University Press, Cambridge.

Conway Morris S (1995) Ecology in deep time. *Trends in Ecology and Evolution,* **10**, 290-294.

Conway Morris S (1998) The evolution of diversity in ancient ecosystems: a review. *Philosophical Transactions of the Royal Society, B,* **353**, 327-346.

Cooper A, Penny D (1997) Mass survival of birds across the Cretaceous - Tertiary boundary: molecular evidence. *Science,* **275**, 1109-1113.

Coulter GW (1994) Speciation and fluctuating environments, with reference to ancient East African lakes. *Archiv fr Hydrobiologie Beihefte Ergebnisse der Limnologie,* **44**, 127-137.

Darwin C (1859) *On the Origin of Species by Means of Natural Selection.* John Murray, London.

Datta A, Jinks-Robertson S (1995) Association of increased spontaneous mutation rates with high levels of transcription in yeast. *Science,* **268**, 1616-1619.

Davis BD (1989) Transcriptional bias: a non-Lamarkian mechanism for substrate-induced mutations. *Proceedings of the National Academy of Sciences USA,* **86**, 5005-5009.

Dejoux C (1992) The Amphipoda. In: *Lake Titicaca,* (eds. Dejoux C, Iltis A), pp. 346-356. Kluwer, Netherlands.

De Rijk PY, Van De Peer Y, Van Den Broeck I, De Wachter R (1995) Evolution according to large ribosomal subunit RNA. *Journal of Molecular Evolution,* **41**, 366-375.

De Salle R, Templeton AR (1988) Founder effects and the rate of mitochondrial DNA evolution in Hawaiian *Drosophila. Evolution,* **42**, 1076-1084.

Dianzani I, Camaschella C, Ponzone A, Cotton RGH (1993) Dilemmas and progress in mutation detection. *Trends in Genetics,* **9**, 403-405.

Ellegren H, Fridolfsson A-K (1997) Male-driven evolution of DNA sequences in birds. *Nature Genetics,* **17**, 182-184.

Feduccia A (1995) Explosive evolution in Tertiary birds and mammals. *Science,* **267**, 637-638.

Fitch WM, Ayala FJ (1994) The superoxide dismutase molecular clock revisited. *Proceedings of the National Academy of Sciences USA,* **91**, 6802-6807.

Foster PL (1997) Nonadaptive mutations occur on the F episomes during adaptive mutation conditions in *Escherichia coli. Journal of Bacteriology,* **179**, 1550-1554.

Friedrich M, Tautz D (1997) An episodic change of rDNA nucleotide substitution rate has occurred during the emergence of the insect order Diptera. *Molecular Biology and Evolution,* **14**, 644-653.

Fry JD, Heinsohn SL, Mackay TFC (1996) The contribution of new mutations to genotype-environment interaction for fitness in *Drosophila melanogaster. Evolution,* **50**, 2316-2327.

Fryer G (1987) A new classification of the branchiopod Crustacea. *Zoological Journal of the Linnean Society,* **91**, 357-383.

Fryer G (1991) Comparative aspects of adaptive radiation and speciation in Lake Baikal and the great rift lakes of Africa. *Hydrobiologia,* **211**, 137-146.

Gibbons A (1998) Calibrating the mitochondrial clock. *Science,* **279**, 28-29.

Gillespie JH, Turelli M (1989) Genotype-environment interactions and the maintenance of polygenic variation. *Genetics,* **121**, 129-138.

Gorelick NJ, Tindall KR, Glickman BW (1996) Introduction: state of the art in transgenic animals in mutation research. *Environmental and Molecular Mutagenesis,* **8**, 295-298.

Gorthner A, Meier-Brook C (1985) The Steinheim Basin as a paleo-ancient lake. In: *Lecture Notes in Earth Sciences 1.Sedimentary and Evolutionary Cycles*, (eds. Bayer U, Seilacher A), pp. 322-334. Springer-Verlag, Berlin.

Greenwood PH (1974) The cichlid fishes of Lake Victoria, East Africa: the biology and evolution of a species flock. *Bulletin of the British Museum (Natural History), Zoology Supplement*, **6**, 1-134.

Hafner MS, Sudman PD, Villablanca FX, Spradling TA, Demastes JW, Nadler SA (1994) Disparate rates of molecular evolution in cospeciating hosts and parasites. *Science*, **265**, 1087-1090.

Halliwell B, Gutteridge JM (1989) *Free Radicals in Biology and Medicine*. Clarendon Press, Oxford.

Hartman Z, Hartman PE, McDermott WL (1991) Mutagenicity of cool white fluorescent light for *Salmonella*. *Mutation Research*, **260**, 25-38.

Hebert PDN, Finston TL (1997) Taxon diversity in the genus *Holopedium* (Crustacea: Cladocera) from the lakes of eastern North America. *Canadian Journal of Fisheries and Aquatic Sciences*, **54**, 1928-1936.

Hedges SB, Parker PH, Sibley CG, Kumar S (1996) Continental breakup and the ordinal diversification of birds and mammals. *Nature*, **381**, 226-229.

Hewitt G (1996) Some genetic consequences of ice ages, and their role in divergence and speciation. *Biological Journal of Linnean Society*, **58**, 247-276.

Hickey LJ, West RM, Dawson MR, Choi DK (1983) Arctic terrestrial biota: paleomagnetic evidence of age disparity with mid-northern latitudes during the late Cretaceous and early Tertiary. *Science*, **221**, 1153-1156.

Hill WB (1982) Predictions of response to artificial selection from new mutations. *Genetical Research*, **40**, 255-278.

Howell N, Kubacka I, Mackey DA (1996) How rapidly does the human mitochondrial genome evolve. *American Journal of Human Genetics*, **59**, 501-509.

Huang W, Chang BH-J, Gu X, Hewett-Emmett D, Li W-H (1997) Sex differences in mutation rate in higher primates estimated from AMG intron sequences. *Journal of Molecular Evolution*, **44**, 463-465.

Hubendick B (1952) On the evolution of the so-called thallasoid molluscs of Lake Tanganyika. *Arkiv Zoology Stockholm*, **3**, 319-323.

Hunt DM, Fitzgibbon J, Slobadyanyuk SJ, Bowmaker JK, Dulai KS (1997) Molecular evidence of the cottoid fish endemic to Lake Baikal deduced from nuclear DNA evidence. *Molecular Phylogenetics and Evolution*, **8**, 415-422.

Iwabe N, Kuma K, Takashi T (1996) Evolution of gene families and relationship with organismal evolution: rapid divergence of tissue-specific genes in the early evolution of chordates. *Molecular Biology and Evolution*, **13**, 483-493.

Jablonski D, Sepkowski JJ Jr, Boltjer DJ, Sheehan PM (1983) Onshore-offshore patterns in the evolution of Phanerozoic shelf communities. *Science*, **222**, 1123-1125.

Janke A, Feldmaier-Fuchs G, Kelley Thomas W, von Haeseler A, Paaba S (1994) The marsupial mitochondrial genome and the evolution of placental mammals. *Genetics*, **137**, 243-256.

Johnson, TC, Scholz CA, Talbot MR, Kelts K, Ricketts RD, Ngobi G, Bening K, Ssemmanda I, McGill JW (1996) Late Pleistocene dessication of Lake Victoria and rapid evolution of cichlid fishes. *Science*, **273**, 1091-1093.

Kauffman SA (1993) *The Origins of Order*. Oxford University Press, Oxford.

Kennett JP, Srinivasan MS (1983) *Neogene Planktonic Foraminifera, a Phylogenetic Atlas*. Hutchinson Ross, Strousdberg, Pa.

Kerfoot WC, Lynch M (1987) Branchiopod communities: associations with planktivorous fish in space and time. In: *Predation: Direct and Indirect Impact on Aquatic Communities*, (eds. Kerfoot WC, Sih A), pp. 367-378. University Press of New England, Hanover.

Kisakibaru Y, Matsuda H (1995) Nucleotide substitution type dependence of generation time effect of molecular evolution. *Japanese Journal of Genetics*, **70**, 373-386.

Knowlton N (1993) Sibling species in the sea. *Annual Review of Ecology and Systematics*, **24**, 189-216.

Kroll AH, Bambach RK, Canfield DE, Grotzinger JP (1996) Comparative earth history and late Permian mass extinction. *Science*, **273**, 452-458.

Kumar S, Hedges SB (1998) A molecular timescale for vertebrate evolution. *Nature*, **392**, 917-920.

Lande R (1988) Quantitative genetics and evolutionary theory. In: *Proceedings of the Second International Conference on Quantitative Genetics*. (eds. Weir B, Eisen EJ, Goodman MM, Namkoon G), pp.71-84. Sinauer Associates, Sunderland, Mass.

Lanyi JK (1974) Salt-dependent properties of proteins from extremely halophilic bacteria. *Bacteriology Reviews*, **38**, 272-290.

Lawrence JG, Ochman H (1997) Amelioration of bacterial genomes: rates of change and exchange. *Journal of Molecular Evolution*, **44**, 383-397.

LeClerc JE, Li B, Payne WL, Cebula TA (1996) High mutation frequencies among *Escherichia coli* and *Salmonella* pathogens. *Science*, **274**, 1208-1211.

Leigh EG (1970) Natural selection and mutability. *American Naturalist*, **104**, 301-305.

Leigh EG (1973) The evolution of mutation rates. *Genetics*, **73**, 1-18.

Levin DA (1990) The seed bank as a source of genetic novelty in plants. *American Naturalist*, **135**, 563-572.

Li W-H (1997) *Molecular Evolution*. Sinauer Associates, Sunderland, Mass.

Lundstrom R, Tavaré S, Ward RH (1992) Estimating substitution rates from molecular data using the coalescent. *Proceedings of the National Academy of Sciences USA*, **89**, 5961-5965.

Lutzoni F, Pagel M (1997) Accelerated evolution as a consequence of transitions to mutualism. *Proceedings of the National Academy of Science USA*, **94**, 11422-11427.

Lynch M, Jarrell PE (1993) A method of calibrating molecular clocks and its application to animal mitochondrial DNA. *Genetics*, **135**, 1197-1208.

Magnasco MO, Thaler DS (1996) Changing the pace of evolution. *Physics Letters A*, **221**, 287-292.

Maley LE, Marshall CR (1998) The coming of age of molecular systematics. *Science*, **279**, 505.

Martens K (1994) Ostracod speciation in ancient lakes: a review. *Archiv fr Hydrobiologie Beihefte Ergebnisse der Limnologie* , **44**, 203-222.

Martens K (1997) Speciation in ancient lakes. *Trends in Ecology and Evolution*, **12**, 177-182.

Martens K, Coulter G, Goddeeris B (1994) Speciation in ancient lakes - 40 years after Brooks. *Archiv fr Hydrobiologie Beihefte Ergebnisse der Limnologie*, **44**, 75-96.

Martin AP, Palumbi SR (1993) Body size, metabolic rate, generation time and the molecular clock. *Proceedings of the National Academy of Science USA*, **90**, 4087-4091.

Matic I, Rodman M, Taddei F, Picard B, Doit C, Birgen E, Denamur E, Elion J (1997) Highly variable mutation rates in commensal and pathogenic *Escherichia coli*. *Science*, **277**, 1833-1834.

Mattimore,V, Battista JR (1996) Radioresistance of *Deinococcus radiodurans*: functions necessary to survive ionizing radiation are also necessary to survive prolonged desiccation. *Journal of Bacteriology*, **178**, 633-637.

Mayr E (1963) *Animal Species and Evolution*. Belknap Press, Harvard.

McCune AR (1997) How fast is speciation? Molecular, geological and phylogenetic evidence from adaptive radiations of fishes. In: *Molecular Evolution and Adaptive Radiation*, (eds. Givnish TJ, Systma KJ), pp. 583-610. Cambridge University Press, Cambridge.

Meyer A, Montero C, Spreinat A (1994) Evolutionary history of the cichlid fish species flocks of the East African great lakes inferred from molecular phylogenetic data. *Archiv fr Hydrobiologie Beihefte Ergebnisse der Limnologie*, **44**, 407-423.

Michel E (1994) Why snails radiate: a review of gastropod evolution in long-lived lakes, both recent and fossil. *Archiv fr Hydrobiologie Beihefte Ergebnisse der Limnologie*, **44**, 285-317.

Mindell DP, Thacker CE (1996) Rates of molecular evolution: phylogenetic issues and applications. *Annual Review of Ecology and Systematics*, **27**, 279-305.

Miyata T, Hayoshida H, Kuma K, Mitsuyasu K, Yasunga T (1987) Male driven molecular evolution: a model and nucleotide sequence analysis. *Cold Spring Harbour Symposia in Quantitative Biology*, **52**, 863-867.

Moran NA (1996) Accelerated evolution and Muller's ratchet in endosymbiotic bacteria. *Proceedings of the National Academy of Science USA*, **93**, 2873-2878.

Moran NA, Munson MA, Baumann P, Ishikawa H (1993) A molecular clock in endosymbiotic bacteria is calibrated using the insect hosts. *Proceedings of the Royal Society London, B*, **253**, 167-171.

Moran NA, van Dohlen CD, Baumann P (1995) Faster evolutionary rates in endosymbiotic bacteria than in cospeciating insect hosts. *Journal of Molecular Evolution*, **41**, 727-731.

Moriyama EN (1987) Higher rates of nucleotide substition in *Drosophila* than in mammals. *Japanese Journal of Genetics*, **62**, 139-147.

Muse SV, Gaut BS (1997) Comparing patterns of nucleotide substitution rates among chloroplast loci using the relative ratio test. *Genetics*, **146**, 393-399.

Nanney DL (1982) Genes and phenes in *Tetrahymena*. *Bioscience*, **32**, 783-788.

Nedbal MA, Flynn JJ (1998) Do the combined effects of the asymmetric process of replication and DNA damage from oxygen radicals produce a mutation rate signature in the mitochondrial genome? *Molecular Biology and Evolution*, **15**, 219-223.

Ochman H, Wilson AC (1987) Evolution in bacteria: evidence for a universal substitution rate in cellular genomes. *Journal of Molecular Evolution*, **26**, 74-86.

Omland KE (1997) Correlated rates of molecular and morphological evolution. *Evolution*, **51**, 1381-1393.

Owen RB, Crossley R, Johnson TC, *et al.* (1990) Major low levels of Lake Malawi and their implications for speciation rates in cichlid fishes. *Proceedings of the Royal Society of London, B*, **240**, 519-523.

Parsons TJ, Muniec DS, Sullivan K *et al.* (1997) A high observed substitution rate in the human mitochondrial DNA control region. *Nature Genetics*, **15**, 363-368.

Pawlowski J, Bolivar I, Fahrni JF, de Vargas C, Gouy M, Zaninetti L (1997) Extreme differences in rates of molecular evolution of Foraminifera revealed by comparison of ribosomal DNA sequences and the fossil record. *Molecular Biology and Evolution*, **14**, 498-505.

Pennak RW (1989) *Freshwater Invertebrates of the United States*. 3rd Ed. Wiley & Sons, New York.

Pope KO, Baines KH, Ocampo AC, Ivanov BA (1994) Impact winter and the Cretaceous/Tertiary extinctions: results of a Chicxulub asteroid impact model. *Earth Planetary Science Letters*, **128**, 719-725.

Rambaut A, Bromham L (1998) Estimating divergence dates from molecular sequences. *Molecular Biology and Evolution,* **15**, 442-448.

Rand DM (1994) Thermal habit, metabolic rate and the evolution of mitochondrial DNA. *Trends in Ecology and Evolution*, **9**, 125-131.

Reif W-E (1985) Endemic evolution of *Gryraulus kleini* in the Steinheim Basin (Planorbid snails, Miocene, Southern Germany). In: *Lecture Notes in Earth Sciences 1. Sedimentary and Evolutionary Cycles*, (eds. Bayer U, Seilacher A), pp. 256-294. Springer-Verlag, Berlin.

Schopf JW (1994) Disparate rates, differing fates: tempo and mode of evolution changed from the Precambrian to the Phanerozoic. *Proceedings of the National Academy of Science USA*, **91**, 6735-6742.

Shimmin LC, Chang BH-J, Li W-H (1993) Male-driven evolution of DNA sequences. *Nature*, **362**, 745-747.

Slobodyanyuk SJ, Kinlchik ME, Pavlova ME, Belikov SI, Novitsky AL (1995) The evolutionary relationships of two families of cottoid fishes in Lake Baikal (Eastern Siberia) as suggested by analysis of mitochondrial DNA. *Journal of Molecular Evolution*, **40**, 392-399.

Smith AB, Lafay B, Christen R (1992) Comparative variation of morphological and molecular evolution through geologic time: 28S ribosomal RNA versus morphology in echinoids. *Philosophical Transactions of the Royal Society of London, B*, **338**, 365-382.

Sniegowski PD, Gerrish PJ, Lenski RE (1997) Evolution of high mutation rates in experimental populations of *E. coli*. *Nature*, **387**, 703-705.

Somero GN (1990) Life at low volume change: hydrostatic pressure as a selective factor in the aquatic environment. *American Zoologist*, **30**, 123-135.

Somero GN (1992) Adaptations to high hydrostatic pressure. *Annual Review of Physiology*, **54**, 557-577.

Stanley SM (1985) Rates of evolution. *Paleobiology*, **11**, 13-26.

Strong DR (1972) Life history variation among populations of an amphipod (*Hyallela azteca*). *Ecology*, **53**, 1103-1111.

Sturmbauer C, Meyer A (1992) Genetic divergence, speciation and morphological stasis in a lineage of African cichlid fishes. *Nature*, **358**, 578-582.

Sueoka N (1988) Directional mutation pressure and neutral molecular evolution. *Proceedings of the National Academy of Science USA*, **85**, 2653-2657.

Sueoka N (1993) Directional mutation pressure, mutator mutations, and the dynamics of molecular evolution. *Journal of Molecular Evolution*, **37**, 137-153.

Taddei F, Rodman M, Maynard-Smith J, Toupance B, Gouyan PH, Godelle B (1997) Role of mutator alleles in adaptive evolution. *Nature*, **387**, 700-702.

Taylor DJ, Finston TL, Hebert PDN (1998a) Biogeography of a widespread freshwater crustacean: pseudocongruence and cryptic endemism in the North American *Daphnia laevis* complex. *Evolution*, in press.

Thaler DS (1994) The evolution of genetic intelligence. *Science*, **264**, 224-225.

Tollrian R (1995) Predator-induced morphological defenses: costs, life history shifts, and maternal effects in *Daphnia pulex*. *Ecology*, **76**, 1691-1705.

Trotman CNA, Manning AM, Bray JA, Jellie AM, Moens L, Tate WP (1994) Interdomain linkage in the polymeric hemoglobin molecule of *Artemia*. *Journal of Molecular Evolution*, **38**, 628-636.

Vinla R (1995) Origin and recent endemic divergence of a Caspian *Mysis* species flock with affinities to the "glacial relict" crustaceans in boreal lakes. *Evolution*, **49**, 1215-1223.

Vargas de C, Zaninett L, Hilbrecht H, Pawlowski J (1997) Phylogeny and rates of molecular evolution of planktonic Foraminifera: SSU rDNA sequences compared to the fossil record. *Journal of Molecular Evolution*, **45**, 285-294.

Via S, Lande R (1985) Genotype-environment interactions and the evolution of phenotypic plasticity. *Evolution*, **39**, 505-523.

Vogel F, Motulsky A (1997) *Human Genetics: Problems and Approaches*. 3rd Edition. Springer Verlag, Berlin.

Vrba ES (1980) Evolution, species and fossils: how does life evolve? *South African Journal of Science*, **76**, 61-84.

Waddington CH (1953) Genetic assimilation of an acquired character. *Evolution*, **7**, 118-126.

Wake DB, Roth G, Wake MH (1983) On the problem of stasis in organismal evolution. *Journal of Theoretical Biology*, **101**, 211-224.

Walker GC (1995) SOS-regulated proteins in translesion DNA synthesis and mutagenesis. *Trends in Biochemical Sciences*, **20**, 416-420.

Wellbourn GA (1995) Predator community composition and patterns of variation in life history and morphology among *Hyallela* (Amphipoda) populations in southeast Michigan. *American Midland Naturalist*, **133**, 322-332.

Wray GA, Levinton JS, Shapiro LH (1996) Molecular evidence for deep Precambrian divergences among metazoan phyla. *Science*, **274**, 568-573.

Wright BE (1997) Does selective gene activation direct evolution.? *Federation of European Biochemical Societies Letters,* **402**, 4-8.

Wright S (1978) *Evolution and Genetics of Populations Vol. 4. Variability within and among populations.* University of Chicago Press, Chicago.

Yampolsky L Yu, Kamaltynov RM, Ebert D, Filatov DA, Chernykh VI (1994) Variation of allozyme loci in endemic gammarids of Lake Baikal. *Biological Journal of the Linnean Society*, **53**, 309-323.

Yang ZH (1996) Among-site variation and its impact on phylogenetic analyses. *Trends in Ecology and Evolution*, **11**, 367-372.

Yang ZH, Nielsen R (1998) Synonymous and nonsynonymous rate variation in nuclear genes of mammals. *Journal of Molecular Evolution*, **46**, 409-418.

Advances in Molecular Ecology
G.R. Carvalho (Ed.)
IOS Press, 1998

A Guide to Software Packages for Data Analysis in Molecular Ecology

Andrew Schnabel[1], Peter Beerli[2], Arnaud Estoup[3], David Hillis[4]

[1]*Department of Biological Sciences, Indiana University South Bend, South Bend, Indiana 46615 USA. e-mail: aschnabe@iusb.edu*

[2]*Department of Genetics, University of Washington, Seattle, Washington 98195 USA. e-mail: beerli@genetics. washington.edu*

[3]*Laboratoire de Modélisation et de Biologie Evolutive, 488 rue croix Lavit, URBL-INRA, 34090 Montpellier, France. e-mail: estoup@zavez02.ensam.inra.fr*

[4]*Department of Zoology and Institute of Cellular and Molecular Biology, University of Texas, Austin, Texas 78712 USA. e-mail: hillis@bull.zo.utexas.edu*

We briefly discuss software packages for the analysis of molecular ecological data, focusing on three levels of analysis: parentage and relatedness, population genetic structure, and phylogeny reconstruction. For the first two levels of analysis, we have gathered lists of some of the packages that we consider to be the most useful and user-friendly. For each package, we provide information on names of authors, date of latest update, compatible operating systems, types of data handled and analyses supported, availability, and literature citations. For software packages dealing with phylogeny reconstruction, we refer the reader to specific literature and website sources where this information has already been compiled

1. Introduction

Molecular ecologists use protein or DNA markers to address questions about interactions between organisms and their biotic and abiotic environments. These studies often result in the generation of large and complex molecular data sets, and one of the challenges facing many workers is how to analyse those data properly. In this chapter, we present summary information on several of the numerous computer software packages for the analysis of genetic relationships among individuals, populations, and species. We do not claim that this information is complete, or perfectly up-to-date, because new programs and updates of older programs are appearing almost monthly. Although some overlap will inevitably exist between different levels of analysis, we have chosen to divide the summary into three areas: parentage and relatedness, population genetic structure and gene flow, and phylogeny reconstruction.

2. Relationships among individuals: parentage and relatedness

Our understanding of social systems, mating behaviours, correlates of reproductive success, and dispersal patterns in natural populations depends on the possibility of genetically differentiating individuals, assigning both male and female parentage to individual progeny, and estimating with sufficiently high precision the genetic relatedness between groups or pairs of interacting individuals (Queller & Goodnight 1989; Cruzan 1998; Parker *et al.* 1998; Estoup, this volume). Studies of plant populations often use parentage analyses to address questions of outcrossing rates, effective pollen dispersal, and variation in male fertility, but rarely is the focus on genetic relatedness per se (Schnabel, this volume). On the other hand, in animal studies, relatedness and parentage are linked through studies of altruistic behaviour, social and genetic mating systems, and kin selection (Hughes 1998). Although polymorphic genetic markers have been used for a long time in cases when pedigree information must be ascertained, as in animal breeding selection programs or in human paternity analysis, the advent of molecular markers with high levels of polymorphism has opened new perspectives for studies of parentage and relatedness in natural populations (Queller *et al.* 1993; Avise 1994; Estoup *et al.* 1994; Morin *et al.* 1994; Blouin *et al.* 1996; Taylor *et al.* 1997; Aldrich & Hamrick 1998; Hughes 1998; Parker *et al.* 1998; Prodöhl *et al.* 1998).

Compared with the number of software packages available for higher levels of analyses (see below), very few programs are available for the analysis of parentage or for the estimation of genetic relatedness (Appendix 1). Written specifically for plants, the set of programs by Ritland (1990) is the most widely used package for the analysis of outcrossing rates. More detailed parentage analyses are possible with POLLENFLOW (JD Nason, unpublished), which combines paternity exclusion analyses with the fractional paternity model of Devlin *et al.* (1988) and the maximum-likelihood models of Roeder *et al.* (1989) and Devlin & Ellstrand (1990), such that the user is able to obtain estimates both of pollen gene flow into the study population and relative fertilities of all possible male parents (Schnabel, this volume). A similar approach to parentage inference is taken in CERVUS (Marshall *et al.* 1998), which implements the likelihood models of Thompson (1975, 1976) and Meagher (1986). A very simple approach is taken by Danzmann (1997) in PROBMAX, which calculates probabilities that individuals are the offspring of specific parental pairs. The probability values indicate the number of loci sampled for each progeny that conform to Mendelian expectations for the pair of parents being tested. Finally, two well-developed programs are available for the estimation of relatedness based on the models of Queller and Goodnight (1989). The package KINSHIP tests hypotheses of pedigree relationships between pairs of individuals, and RELATEDNESS uses a regression technique to measure relatedness between groups of individuals.

3. Relationships among populations: population genetic structure and gene flow

Many questions asked by molecular ecologists require that they conduct a survey of genetic diversity across several populations of a species. Such surveys estimate how much genetic variation a particular species maintains within its populations for a particular set of molecular markers (e.g., allozymes) and how that variation is partitioned among populations. Based on these data, inferences can be made about effective population sizes, natural selection, patterns of mating and dispersal, gene flow, and biogeographical history of the populations (e.g., Gentile & Sbordoni 1998; Godt & Hamrick 1998; Gonzalez *et al.* 1998; Xu *et al.* 1998). Hundreds of surveys of population genetic structure can be found in the literature, most of which prior to 1990 used either allozymes or mitochondrial DNA restriction sites (Hamrick & Godt 1989; Avise 1994). In the past decade, however, a large and rapidly growing number of studies have used a wider variety of molecular markers, such as DNA sequences, RAPDs, AFLPs, and microsatellites (e.g., Arden & Lambert 1997; Fischer & Matthies 1998; Paetkau *et al.* 1998; Winfield *et al.* 1998).

Given this great abundance of studies, it is not surprising that the number of available software packages for the analysis of population genetic structure is also large. Most of the early programs were written with allozymes in mind, and several of the currently available packages are still limited in the types of data that can be handled. In contrast to software for phylogenetic reconstruction (see below), there is no single source either in print or as a website that brings all of this information together. In collecting this diverse array of programs, we found that many of the more user-friendly programs (e.g., ARLEQUIN, GDA, GENEPOP, GENETIX, POPGENE, TFPGA) had much overlap in the analyses they perform (Appendix 2). First, several packages calculate basic statistics of genetic variation, such as the proportion of polymorphic loci, the average number of alleles per locus, and heterozygosity. Those programs that handle a wider variety of data types also calculate statistics such as nucleotide diversity. Second, many packages will conduct tests for Hardy-Weinberg equilibrium. Third, most of the programs we report will estimate patterns of genetic structuring using the hierarchical approach of Wright and/or Cockerham and Weir. A smaller proportion of the programs also include methods for analysing microsatellite data using R_{ST} (e.g., ARLEQUIN, FSTAT, GENEPOP, RSTCALC) or Analysis of Molecular Variance (AMOVA in ARLEQUIN). Fourth, a several of the programs will calculate one or more pairwise genetic distance measures (e.g., Nei's distance, Rogers distance), and will analyse those distances using some sort of clustering algorithm (e.g., UPGMA or neighbour joining). Last, several of the programs will estimate the level of linkage disequilibrium between loci. Although a number of home-grown programs for Macintosh computers must certainly exist, the large majority of packages we found were written for either a DOS or Windows platform. On a final note, the best available program for analysing genetic structure within hybrid zones appears to be ANALYSE by Barton & Baird (1998).

All of the programs in Appendix 2 work within a traditional Wrightian framework of geographic structuring and estimation of gene diversity statistics based on allele frequencies. The introduction of coalesence theory by Kingman (1982) created new methods for analysing population data (Hudson 1990; Beerli, this volume). Coalescence theory focuses on the sampled gene copies and looks backward in time to calculate the probability that two randomly chosen gene copies in the sample have a common ancestor t time units in the past. This process is driven only by the effective population size, N_e, and mutation rate. Kingman (1982) showed that the time when all lineages coalesced for a sample of 2, 4, and infinite gene copies is $2N_e$, $3N_e$, and $4N_e$, respectively. This Kingman coalescence process can be easily extended to incorporate other population parameters like population size, growth rate, recombination rate, and migration rates (Hudson 1990). Beerli (this volume) and Wakeley (1998) have shown that approaches based on coalescence theory are superior to approaches based on allele frequencies.

Two main groups of programs exist for coalescence analysis (Appendix 3), those that use segregating sites in the sample and those that integrate over all possible genealogies. In the sofware package SITES (Hey & Wakeley 1997), the coalescent is used to generate expectations for the number of segregating sites in a sample of sequences, and these expecetations are subsequently used to estimate population parameters. Most other programs listed in Appendix 3 integrate over all possible genealogies (*e.g.* MIGRATE). These programs are very computer intensive, but they use all possible information in the data, such as the history of mutation events. They also can be applied to several different types of molecular data other than sequence data. The general approach is to find the maximum likelihood of the population parameters, where the likelihood function is defined as the sum of probabilities over all possible genealogies. For each of these genealogies, one calculates the probability given the parameters and given the sampled data (Beerli, this volume).

4. Relationships among species: phylogeny reconstruction

The field of molecular systematics has become an increasingly important part of ecological studies during the past two decades. During that time, the number of computer programs for data preparation (e.g., entering and aligning DNA sequences), phylogenetic inference, tree comparisons, and other associated analyses has mushroomed to the point of being beyond the scope of any paper or website. For those readers considering phylogenetic analysis for the first time, we recommend reading Hillis (this volume) and the volume, *Molecular Systematics* (Hillis *et al.* 1996), within which Swofford *et al.* (1996) present an extensive list of software programs for the analysis of phylogenetic and population genetic data. Because that publication is now nearly 3 years old, some of the information may be out of date, but nonetheless it represents a good starting point. Alternatively, we advise visiting the website of the J. Felsenstein laboratory at the University of Washington (http://evolution.genetics.washington.edu). At that website, one can find descriptions of approximately 120 phylogeny packages that are arranged by (i) method of phylogenetic inference; (ii) computer systems on which they work; (iii) most recent listings; and (iv) those most recently updated.

Acknowledgements

We thank all those people who sent us information about their programs and all those who maintain websites with information about their own and other people's software.

References

Aldrich PR, Hamrick JL (1998) Reproductive dominance of pasture trees in a fragmented tropical forest mosaic. *Science*, **281**, 103-105.
Ardern SL, Lambert DM (1997) Is the black robin in genetic peril? *Molecular Ecology*, **6**, 21-28.
Avise, JC (1994) *Molecular Markers, Natural History and Evolution*, Chapman & Hall, London UK.
Bahlo M, Griffiths RC (1998) Inference from gene trees in a subdivided population. *Theoretical Population Biology*, in press.
Barton NH, Baird SJE (1998) Analyse 2.0. Edinburgh: http://helios.bto.ed.ac.uk/ evolgen/index.html.
Belkhir K, Borsa P, Goudet J, Chikhi L, Bonhomme F, (1998) GENETIX, logiciel sous Windows™ pour la génétique des populations. Laboratoire Génome et Populations, CNRS UPR 9060, Université de Montpellier II, Montpellier France.
Blouin MS, Parsons M, Lacaille V, Lotz S (1996) Use of microsatellite loci to classify individuals by relatedness. *Molecular Ecology*, **5**, 393-401.
Cornuet JM, Luikart G (1997) Description and power analysis of two tests for detecting recent population bottlenecks from allele frequency data. *Genetics*, **144**, 2001-2014.
Cruzan MB (1998) Genetic markers in plant evolutionary ecology. *Ecology*, **79**, 400-412.
Danzmann RG (1997) PROBMAX: A computer program for assigning unknown parentage in pedigree analysis from known genotypic pools of parents and progeny. *Journal of Heredity*, **88**, 333.
Devlin B, Ellstrand NC (1990) The development and application of a refined method for estimating gene flow from angiosperm paternity analysis. *Evolution*, **44**, 248-259.
Devlin B, Roeder K, Ellstrand NC (1988) Fractional paternity assignment, theoretical development and comparison to other methods. *Theoretical and Applied Genetics*, **76**, 369-380.
Estoup A, Solignac M, Cornuet JM (1994). Precise assessment of the number of patrilines and of genetic relatedness in honey bee colonies. *Proceedings of the Royal Society of London, B*, **258**, 1-7.
Fischer M, Matthies D (1998) RAPD variation in relation to population size and plant fitness in the rare *Gentianella germanica* (Gentianaceae). *American Journal of Botany*, **85**, 811-820.
Garnier-Gere P, Dillmann C (1992) A computer program for testing pairwise linkage disequilibrium in subdivided populations. *Journal of Heredity*, **83**, 239.
Gentile G, Sbordoni V (1998) Indirect methods to estimate gene flow in cave and surface populations of *Androniscus dentiger* (Isopoda: Oniscidea). *Evolution*, **52**, 432-442.

Godt MJW, Hamrick JL (1998) Allozyme diversity in the endangered pitcher plant *Sarracenia rubra* ssp. *alabamensis* (Sarraceniaceae) and its close relative *S. rubra* ssp. *rubra*. *American Journal of Botany*, **85**, 802-810.

Gonzalez S, Maldonado JE, Leonard JA *et al.* (1998) Conservation genetics of the endangered Pampas deer (*Ozotoceros bezoarticus*). *Molecular Ecology*, **7**, 47-56.

Goodman SJ (1997) Rst Calc: a collection of computer programs for calculating estimates of genetic differentiation from microsatellite data and determining their significance. *Molecular Ecology*, **6**, 881-885.

Goudet J (1995) Fstat version 1.2: a computer program to calculate Fstatistics. *Journal of Heredity*, **86**, 485-486.

Griffiths RC, Tavaré S (1994) Sampling theory for neutral alleles in a varing environment. *Philosophical Transactions of the Royal Society London, B*, **344**, 403-410.

Griffiths RC, Tavaré S (1996) Computational methods for the coalescent. In: *Progress in Population Genetics and Human Evolution* (eds. Donnelly P, Tavaré S). IMA Volumes in Mathematics and its Applications. Springer Verlag, Berlin.

Hamrick JL, Godt MJW (1989) Allozyme diversity in plant species. In: *Plant Population Genetics, Breeding and Genetic Resources* (eds. Brown AHD, Clegg MT, Kahler AL, Weir BS), pp. 43-63. Sinauer, Sunderland, MA.

Hey J, Wakeley J (1997) A coalescent estimator of the population recombination rate. *Genetics*, **145**, 833-846.

Hillis DM, Moritz C, Mable BK (1996) *Molecular Systematics 2nd ed.* Sinauer, Sunderland, MA.

Hudson RR (1990) Gene genealogies and the coalescent process. *Oxford Surveys in Evolutionary Biology*, **7**, 1-44.

Hughes C (1998) Integrating molecular techniques with field methods in studies of social behavior: a revolution results. *Ecology*, **79**, 383-399.

Kingman J (1982) The coalescent. *Stochastic Processes and their Applications*, **13**, 235-248.

Kuhner MK, Yamato J, Felsenstein, J (1995) Estimating effective population size and mutation rate from sequence data using Metropolis-Hastings sampling. *Genetics* , **140**, 421-430.

Kuhner MK, Yamato J, Felsenstein J (1998) Maximum likelihood estimation of population growth rates based on the coalescent. *Genetics*, **149**, 429-439.

Marshall TC, Slate J, Kruuk LEB, Pemberton JM (1998) Statistical confidence for likelihood-based paternity inference in natural populations. *Molecular Ecology*, **7**, 639-655.

Meagher, TR (1986) Analysis of paternity within a natural population of *Chamaelirium luteum*. I. Identification of most-likely male parents. *The American Naturalist*, **128**, 199-215.

Morin PA, Wallis J, Moore JJ, Woodruff DS (1994) Paternity exclusion in a community of wild chimpanzees using hypervariable simple sequence repeats. *Molecular Ecology*, **5**, 469-478.

Paetkau D, Waits LP, Clarkson PL *et al.* (1998) Variation in genetic diversity across the range of North American brown bears. *Conservation Biology*, **12**, 418-429.

Parker PG, Snow AA, Schug MD, Booton GC, Fuerst PA (1998) What molecules can tell us about populations: choosing and using a molecular marker. *Ecology*, **79**, 361-382.

Prodöhl P A, Loughry WJ, McDonough CM, Nelson WS, Thompson EA, Avise JC (1998) Genetic maternity and paternity in a local population of armadillo assessed by microsatellite DNA markers and field data. *The American Naturalist*, **151**, 7-19.

Queller CR, Goodnight KF (1989) Estimating relatedness using genetic markers. *Evolution*, **43**, 258-259.

Queller CR, Strassmann JE, Hughes CR (1993) Microsatellites and kinship. *Trends in Evolution and Ecology*, **8**, 285-288.

Rannala B, Hartigan JA (1996) Estimating gene flow in island populations. *Genetical Research*, **67**, 147-158.

Rannala B, Mountain JL (1997) Detecting immigration by using multilocus genotypes. *Proceedings of the National Academy of Sciences USA*, **94**, 9197-9201.

Raymond M, Rousset F (1995a) GENEPOP (version 1.2): population genetics software for exact tests and ecumenicism. *Journal of Heredity*, **86**, 248-249.

Raymond M, Rousset F (1995b) An exact test for population differentiation. *Evolution*, **49**, 1280-1283.

Ritland K (1990) A series of FORTRAN computer programs for estimating plant mating systems. *Journal of Heredity*, **81**, 235-237.

Roeder K, Devlin B, Lindsay BG (1989) Application of maximum likelihood methods to population genetic data for the estimation of individual fertilities. *Biometrics*, **45**, 363-379.

Rozas J, Rozas R (1995) DnaSP, DNA sequence polymorphism: an interactive program for estimating population genetics parameters from DNA sequence data. *Computer Applications in Bioscience*, **11**, 621-625.

Rozas J, Rozas R (1997) DnaSP version 2.0: a novel software package for extensive molecular population genetics analysis. *Computer Applications in Bioscience*, **13**, 307-311.

Schneider S, Kueffer JM, Roessli D, Excoffier L (1997) Arlequin ver. 1.1: A software for population genetic data analysis. Genetics and Biometry Laboratory, University of Geneva, Switzerland.

Sork VL, Campbell D, Dyer R *et al.* (1998) Proceedings from a Workshop on Gene Flow in Fragmented, Managed, and Continuous Populations. National Center for Ecological Analysis and Synthesis, Santa Barbara, California. Research Paper No. 3. Available at http://www.nceas.ucsb.edu/papers/geneflow/

Swofford DL, Olsen GJ, Waddell PJ, Hillis DM (1996) Phylogenetic inference. In: *Molecular Systematics*, *2nd ed.* (eds. Hillis DM, Moritz C, Mable BK), pp. 407-514. Sinauer, Sunderland, MA.

Taylor AC, Horsup A, Johnson CN, Sunnucks P, Sherwin B (1997) Relatedness structure detected by microsatellite analysis and attempted pedigree reconstruction in an endangered marsupial, the northern hairy-nosed wombat *Lasiorhinus krefftii*. *Molecular Ecology*, 6, 9-19.

Thompson, EA (1975) The estimation of pairwise relationships. *Annals of Human Genetics*, **39**, 173-188.

Thompson, EA (1976) Inference of genealogical structure. *Social Science Information*, **15**, 477-526.

Tufto J,Engen S, Hindar K (1996) Inferring patterns of migration from gene frequencies under equilibrium conditions. *Genetics*, **144**, 1911-1921.

Yeh FC, Yang RC, Boyle TJB, Ye ZH, Mao JX (1997) POPGENE, the user-friendly shareware for population genetic analysis. Molecular Biology and Biotechnology Centre, University of Alberta, Canada.

Yeh FC, Boyle TJB (1997) Population genetic analysis of co-dominant and dominant markers and quantitative traits. *Belgian Journal of Botany*, **129**, 157.

Wakeley J (1998) Segregating sites in Wright's island model. *Journal of Theoretical Population Biology*, **53**, 166-174.

Wakeley J, Hey J (1997) Estimating ancestral population parameters. *Genetics*, **145**, 847-855.

Weir, B (1996) *Genetic Data Analysis*. Sinauer, Sunderland, MA.

Winfield MO, Arnold GM, Cooper F *et al.* (1998) A study of genetic diversity in *Populus nigra* ssp. *betulifolia* in the Upper Severn Area of the UK using AFLP markers. *Molecular Ecology*, 7, 3-11.

Xu J, Kerrigan RW, Sonnenberg AS, Callac P, Horgen PA, Anderson JB (1998) Mitochondrial DNA variation in natural populations of the mushroom *Agaricus bisporus*. *Molecular Ecology*, 7, 19-34.

Appendix 1: List of software packages for the study of parentage and relatedness using molecular markers.

Package name, latest update (author)	Operating system	Types of data handled	Analyses supported	Availability, literature citation
CERVUS v. 1.0, 17/6/98 (T Marshall)	Windows95	Diploid, codominant markers	Uses a most-likely approach to parentage inference and estimates confidence in parentage of most likely parents. Can be used to calculate allele frequencies, run simulations to determine critical values of likelihood ratios and analyse parentage in populations of animals and plants. A simulation system can estimate the resolving power of a series of single-locus marker systems for parentage inference.	Freeware from http://helios.bto.ed.ac.uk/evolgen/index.html Marshall *et al.* (1998)
KINSHIP v. 1.2, (KF Goodnight, DC Queller, T Posnansky)	MacOS (PowerPC and 68K)	Diploid, codominant markers	Performs maximum likelihood tests of pedigree relationships between pairs of individuals in a population. The user enters two hypothetical pedigree relationships, a primary hypothesis and a null hypothesis, and the program calculates likelihood ratios comparing the two hypotheses for all possible pairs in the data set. Includes a simulation procedure to determine the statistical significance of results. Also calculates pairwise relatedness statistics.	Freeware from http://www.bioc.rice.edu/~kfg/GSoft.html Queller & Goodnight (1989)
MLT (K Ritland)	DOS	Diploid or tetraploid, codominant markers	A set of programs that finds maximum-likelihood estimates of outcrossing rates for plant populations. Also estimates parental gene frequencies and inbreeding coefficients. Special programs within the package can handle autotetraploids and ferns.	Freeware by contacting the author at ritland@unixg.ubc.ca Ritland (1990)

Appendix 1: Continued

Package name, latest update (author)	Operating system	Types of data handled	Analyses supported	Availability, literature citation
POLLENFLOW v. 1.0, 26/3/98 (JD Nason)	MacOS (PowerPC and 68K)	Diploid, codominant markers	Implements two different models. First, a paternity exclusion-based model estimates total rate of pollen immigration from a single external source into a defined local population. Second, a likelihood-based model estimates relative male fertility within a population as well as pollen immigration from one or more external sources. Male fertility estimates are adjusted to eliminate biases due to cryptic gene flow.	Freeware by contacting the author at john-nason@uiowa.edu Sork *et al.* (1998)
PROBMAX, 17/11/97 (RG Danzmann)	DOS	Codominant and dominant/ recessive diploid markers	Ascertains the parentage of individuals when genotypic data on both parents and progeny are available. Also includes PROBMAXG, which generates possible progeny genotypes from the parental mixtures to test whether a given set of genetic markers will be able to discriminate all progeny back to parental sets, and PROBMAXN, which allows testing of possible parent/progeny assignments if null alleles segregating at some markers are suspected.	Freeware by anonymous ftp to 131.104.50.2 (password = danzmann) or contact the author at rdanzman@ uoguelph.ca Danzmann (1997)
RELATEDNESS v. 5.0.4, 29/6/1998 (KF Goodnight, DC Queller)	MacOS (PowerPC and 68K)	Diploid, codominant markers	Estimates genetic relatedness between demographically-defined groups of individuals using a regression measure of relatedness. Calculates symmetrical and asymmetrical relatedness and jackknife standard errors. Allows up to 32 demographic variables in defining those individuals to be used in calculating the relatedness statistic.	Freeware from http://www.bioc.rice .edu/~kfg/GSoft. html Queller & Goodnight (1989)

Appendix 2: List of software packages that will analyse geographically structured populations using traditional estimators based on gene frequencies.

Package name, latest update (author)	Operating system	Types of data handled	Analyses supported	Availability, literature citation
ANALYSE v. 2.0, 5/98 (SJE Baird, NH Barton)	MacOS (PowerPC)	Diploid and haploid genetic markers, quantitative trait values, spatial coordinates (1 and 2 dimensions), environmental variables	Likelihood analysis of data from hybrid zones. Performs three types of analyses: general data handling (e.g., selecting subsets of the data satisfying particular criteria), analysis of random fluctuations in genotype frequency (e.g., estimating Fst, Fis, and standardised linkage disequilibrium), and analysis of a set of multilocus clines (e.g., estimating variation between clines).	Freeware from http://helios.bto.ed.ac.uk/evolgen/index.html Barton & Baird (1998)
ARLEQUIN v. 1.1, 17/12/97 (S Schneider, JM Kueffer, D Roessli, L Excoffier)	Windows 3.1 or later	RFLPs, microsatellites, allozymes, RAPDs, AFLPs, allele frequencies, DNA sequences	Calculates gene and nucleotide diversity, mismatch distribution, haplotype frequencies, linkage disequilibrium, tests of Hardy-Weinberg equilibrium, neutrality tests, pairwise genetic distances, analyses of molecular variance (AMOVA).	Freeware from http://anthropologie.unige.ch/arlequin Schneider et al. (1997)
DNASP v. 2.52, 9/97 (J Rozas, R Rozas); v. 2.9 is available as a beta version	Windows 3.1 or later	DNA sequences	Estimates several measures of DNA sequence variation within and between populations (in noncoding, synonymous or nonsynonymous sites), and also linkage disequilibrium, recombination, gene flow, and gene conversion parameters. Also can conduct several tests of neutrality.	Freeware from http://www.bio.ub.es/~julio/DnaSP.html Rozas & Rozas (1995, 1997)
FSTAT v. 1.2, 12/95; Fstat for windows v. 2.3, is available as beta upon request (J Goudet)	DOS; new version will be Windows compatible	Allozymes, microsatellites, mtDNA RFLPs	Calculates gene diversity statistics of Weir and Cockerham (Weir, 1996). Computes jackknife and bootstrap confidence intervals of the statistics or can test gene diversity statistics using a permutation algorithm.	Freeware by writing to J. Goudet at jerome.goudet@izea.unil.ch Goudet (1995)

Appendix 2: Continued

Package name, latest update (author)	Operating system	Types of data handled	Analyses supported	Availability, literature citation
GDA, 11/7/97 (PO Lewis, D Zaykin)	Windows 3.1 or later	Allozymes, microsatellites	Calculates standard gene diversity measures, Wright's F-statistics using the method of Weir and Cockerham (Weir, 1996), genetic distance matrices, UPGMA and neighbour-joining dendrograms, exact tests for disequilibrium	Freeware; http://chee.unm.edu/gda Designed to accompany *Genetic Data Analysis* (Weir, 1996)
GENEPOP v. 3.1b, 12/97 (M. Raymond, F. Rousset)	DOS	Allozyme, microsatellites	Calculates exact tests for Hardy-Weinberg equilibrium, population differentiation, and genotypic disequilibrium among pairs of loci. Computes estimates of classical population parameters, such as allele frequencies, F_{ST}, and other correlations. Includes LINKDOS (Garnier-Gere & Dillmann, 1992), which is a program for testing pairwise linkage disequilibrium.	Freeware from 3 ftp sites: ftp://ftp.cefe.cnrs-mop.fr/genepop/ ftp://ftp2.cefe.cnrs-mop.fr/pub/pc/msdos/genepop/ ftp://isem.isem.univ-montp2.fr/pub/pc/genepop/ Raymond & Rousset (1995a, b)
GENETIX v. 3.3, 14/05/98 (K Belkhir, P Borsa, L Chikhi, J Goudet, F Bonhomme)	Windows95/NT	Allozymes, microsatellites	Calculates estimates of classical parameters (e.g., genetic distances, variability parameters, Wright's fixation indices, linkage disequilibrium) and tests their departure from null expectations through permutation techniques. The interface is not user-friendly for everyone, because it is currently only available in French.	Freeware from http://www.univ-montp2.fr/~genetix/genetix.htm Belkhir *et al.* (1998)
IMMANC, 17/10/97 (JL Mountain)	Windows 3.1 or later, MacOS (PowerPC), NeXT HP-RISC, Sun UltraSPARC	Allozymes, microsatellites, RFLPs	Tests whether or not an individual is an immigrant or is of recent immigrant ancestry. The program uses Monte Carlo simulations to determine the power and significance of the test.	Freeware from http://mw511.biol.berkeley.edu/software.html Rannala & Mountain (1997)

Appendix 2: Continued

Package name, latest update (author)	Operating system	Types of data handled	Analyses supported	Availability, literature citations
MIGRLIB v. 1.0 (J Tufto)	Unix (available as a collection of S-Plus functions and some C code)	Allele frequencies	Estimates the pattern of migration in a subdivided population from genetic differences generated by local genetic drift. Functions are also provided for carrying out likelihood ratio tests between alternative models such as the island model and the stepping stone model.	Freeware from http://www.math .ntnu.no/~jarlet/ migration Tufto *et al.* (1996)
PMLE12 v. 1.2, 4/3/96 (B Rannala)	Windows 3.1 or later, MacOS (PowerPC or 68K), NeXTStep	Allozymes, mtDNA RFLPs	Estimates the gene flow parameter theta for a collection of two or more semi-isolated populations by (pseudo) maximum likelihood. For discrete-generation island model, theta=2Nm. For a continuous-generation island model, theta is the ratio of the immigration rate phi to the individual birth rate lambda.	Freeware from http://mw511.biol .berkeley.edu/ bruce/exec.html Rannala & Hartigan (1996)
POPGENE v. 1.21, 22/12/97 (F Yeh, RC Yang, T Boyle)	Windows 3.1 or later	Co-dominant or dominant markers using haploid or diploid data	Calculates standard genetic diversity measures, tests of Hardy-Weinberg Equilibrium, Wright's F-statistics, genetic distances, UPGMA dendrogram, neutrality tests, linkage disequilibrium	Freeware from http://www.ualberta. ca/~fyeh/ index.htm Yeh & Boyle (1997); Yeh *et al.* (1997)
RSTCALC v. 2.2, 6/10/97 (SJ Goodman)	DOS, Windows 3.1 or later	Microsatellites	Performs analyses of population structure, genetic differentiation, and gene flow. Calculates estimates of Rst, tests for significance and calculates 95% CI.	Freeware from http://helios.bto.ed .ac.uk/evolgen Goodman (1997)
TFPGA (Tools for Population Genetic Analyses), 12/5/98 (MP Miller)	Windows 3.1or later	Codominant (allozyme) and dominant (RAPD, AFLP) genotypes	Calculates descriptive statistics, genetic distances, and F-statistics. Performs tests for Hardy-Weinberg equilibrium, exact tests for genetic differentiation, Mantel tests, and UPGMA cluster analyses.	Freeware from http://herb.bio.nau .edu/~miller No citation available

Appendix 3: List of software packages that will analyse geographically structured populations using estimators based on coalescence.

Package name, latest update (author)	Operating system	Types of data handled	Analyses supported	Availability, literature citation
BOTTLENECK v. 1.1.03, 27/11/97 (JM Cornuet, G Luikart, S Piry)	Windows95	Allele frequencies	Detects recent reductions in effective population size from allele frequency data. Tests whether a set of loci shows a significant excess of heterozygosity (*i.e.*, the observed heterozygosity is larger than the heterozygosity expected at mutation-drift equilibrium and assuming a given mutation model).	Freeware from http://www.ensam. inra.fr/~piry Cornuet & Luikart (1997)
FLUCTUATE v. 1.50B, 6/2/98 (M Kuhner, J Yamato)	Windows 95/NT, MacOS (PowerMac); UNIX; available also as C source code	DNA sequences	Estimates the effective population size and an exponential growth rate of a single population using maximum likelihood and Metropolis-Hastings importance sampling of coalescent genealogies.	Freeware from http://evolution. genetics.washington .edu/lamarc.html Kuhner *et al.* (1995, 1998)
GENETREE, 9/6/98 (M Bahlo, RC Griffiths)	Windows 95/NT, Dec Alpha; available also as C source code	DNA sequences	Finds maximum likelihood estimates of population sizes, exponential growth rates, migration matrices, and time to the most recent common ancestor.	Freeware from http://www.maths. monash.edu.au/ ~mbahlo/mpg/ gtree.html Griffiths & Tavaré (1996) Bahlo & Griffiths (1998)
MIGRATE-0.4 v. 0.4.3, 25/5/98 (P Beerli)	Windows 95/98/NT, MacOS (PowerMac), Dec Alpha, LINUX/Intel, NeXTStep; available also as C source code	Allozymes, microsatellites, DNA sequences	Menu driven, character-based program that finds 4+1 maximum-likelihood estimates of population parameters for a two-population model: effective population sizes, migration rates between the two populations, and for multilocus data, a shape parameter for the distribution of the mutation rate.	Freeware from http://evolution. genetics.washington .edu/lamarc.html Beerli, this volume

Appendix 3: Continued

Package name, latest update (author)	Operating system	Types of data handled	Analyses supported	Availability, literature citation
MIGRATE-n v. Alpha-3, 25/5/98 (P Beerli)	Windows 95/98/NT, MacOS (PowerMac), Dec Alpha, LINUX/Intel, NeXTStep; available also as C source code	Allozymes, microsatellites, DNA sequences	Menu driven, character-based program that finds maximum-likelihood estimates of population parameters for a multi-population model: effective population sizes for each population, migration rates between populations, and for multilocus data, a shape parameter for the distribution of the mutation rate.	Freeware from http://evolution. genetics.washington .edu/lamarc.html Beerli, this volume
RECOMBINE v. 1.0, 17/6/98 (MK Kuhner, J Yamato, J Felsenstein)	MacOS (PowerMac), Windows95/NT available as C source code that will compile on DEC ULTRIX, DEC alpha, INTEL machines, NeXT, SGI, but needs gcc to compile on Suns	DNA or RNA sequences, single nucleotide polymorphisms	Fits a model which has a single population of constant size with a single recombination rate across all sites. It estimates $4N_e\mu$ and r, where N_e is the effective population size, μ is the neutral mutation rate per site, and r is the ratio of the per-site recombination rate to the per-site mutation rate.	Freeware from http://evolution. genetics.washington .edu/lamarc.html No citation available
SITES v. 1.1, 21/4/98 (J Hey)	DOS, MacOS; also available as ANSI C source code	DNA sequences	Generates tables of polymorphic sites, indels, codon usage. Computes numbers of synonymous and replacement base positions, pairwise sequence differences, and GC content. Performs group comparisons and polymorphism analyses and estimates historical population parameters. Primarily intended for data sets with multiple closely related sequences.	Freeware from http://heylab.rutgers .edu/index.html #software Hey & Wakeley (1997) Wakeley & Hey (1997)

Glossary of Terms

Alignment The juxtaposition of amino acids or nucleotides in homologous molecules to maximise similarity or minimise the number of inferred changes among the sequences. Alignment is used to infer positional homology prior to or in parallel with phylogenetic analysis.

Allele One or more alternative forms of a gene, each possessing a unique **nucleotide** sequence. In diploid cells, a maximum of two alleles will be present, each in the same relative position or **locus** on homologous chromosomes of the chromosome set.

Allozymes Enzymes differing in electrophoretic mobility as a result of allelic differences at a single gene (*cf.* **Isozyme).**

Amplify (in the molecular sense) To increase the number of copies of a nucleotide sequence using the **polymerase chain reaction.**

Ancient DNA (aDNA) DNA found in palaeontological, archaeological, museum, forensic, and clinical specimens. The unifying component is that preserved DNA is damaged over time by processes such as oxidation and hydrolysis, leaving only trace amounts of DNA containing cross-links and modified bases.

Anneal (in the molecular sense) To bring together individual strands of DNA that pair due to the sharing of some complementary base pairs.

Apomorphy A derived character state.

Autapomorphy A derived character state unique to a particular taxon.

Autoradiograph Image on an X-ray film created by radioactive or chemiluminescent labelled DNA fragments.

Bacteriophage (= phage) A virus that infects bacteria.

Band-sharing coefficient A pairwise measure of similarity which is often used to estimate relatedness using multibanded **DNA fingerprints**. It is calculated simply as twice the number of bands in common divided by the total number of bands scored.

Base composition The relative proportions of the four respective nucleotides in a given sequence of DNA or RNA.

Base pairs (bp) The bases adenine (A) and thymine (T), or cytosine (C) and guanine (G), linked by hydrogen bonds (A = T; C = G) binding complementary strands of DNA.

Bifurcation A node in a tree that connects exactly three branches. If the tree is directed (rooted), then one of the branches represents an ancestral lineage and the other two branches represent descendant lineages.

Biparental inheritance Genes and genetic elements in sexual organisms which are inherited from both parents.

Cloning of gene sequence Involves the replication of an isolated gene sequence by incorporating it into a bacterial or viral host (or more rarely into a eukaryotic cell) and growing up that host. Most frequently, such cloning involves the insertion of the sequence into a plasmid **vector.**

Coalescence The evolutionary process viewed backward through time, so that allelic diversity is traced back through mutations to ancestral alleles. Coalescent theory can be used to make predictions about effective population sizes, ages and frequencies of alleles, selection, rates of mutation, or time to common ancestry of a set of alleles.

Codon A sequence of three nucleotide bases along a DNA or RNA chain which represents the code of a single amino acid.

cDNA (= **complementary DNA**) DNA reverse transcribed from an RNA template.

Complementary sequence A sequence of nucleotides related by the base-pairing rules. For example in DNA, a sequence A-G-T in one strand is complementary to T-C-A in the other. A given sequence defines the complementary sequence.

Concerted evolution The generation and maintenance of homogeneity among members of a family of DNA repeats within a species or population.

Congruence Agreement among data or data sets.

CpDNA Chloroplast DNA.

Denature To break the hydrogen bonds between two **complementary** strands of DNA, separating them into two single-stranded molecules.

Directional selection Selection which acts on individuals showing a phenotypic distribution in such a way that those individuals towards, or at the end of, the distribution are favoured.

Disruptive (= diversifying) selection Where individuals with an intermediate phenotype are as a selective disadvantage and extreme phenotypes are favoured.

D-loop A non-coding region of (vertebrate) **mitochondrial DNA** (mtDNA) that serves as the initiator of mtDNA replication and is often more variable than the coding regions of mtDNA.

DNA fingerprinting In original usage, the use of multilocus probes to reveal hypervariability (see **Hypervariable sequence**) at many loci in the human genome. More generally used to refer to the characterisation of an individual's genome by developing a DNA fragment band (allele) pattern. If a sufficient number of different-sized fragments are revealed, these banding patterns, which resemble a bar-code profile, will usually be unique for each individual except identical twins.

DNA ligases One of the enzymes involved in DNA replication in prokaryotes by catalysing nucleotide phosphodiester bond formation.

Effective population size (N,) The effective size of a population is defined as the size of an idealised population (a random mating population of self-compatible hermaphrodites, with no selection, mutation or genetic migration occurring) which behaves in *the same way* as the real population under consideration. It is important to understand that effective population size does not mean something as simple as that fraction of the population able to reproduce (*e.g.* it does not mean total population minus juveniles and senescent adults), but incorporates information on mating patterns and the extent of population subdivision.

Electrophoresis The separation of macromolecules (*e.g.* enzymes or DNA) in the presence of an electric current. In molecular genetics, differences in charge, size or shape (i.e. differences in electrophoretic mobility) of the macromolecules are used to estimate genetic differentiation.

Electromorph Protein or **microsatellite** variant detected by its distinct electrophoretic mobility.

Endonuclease See **Restriction enzyme**

Exon That portion of a DNA strand within a gene that codes for a protein. Coding regions that are broken up into one or more segments within a gene, are separated by regions of non-coding DNA called **introns.**

Fishery stock A group of individuals exploited in a particular area or by a specific method. The definition takes no account of the biological basis of stock identity or extent of stock integrity (*cf.* **Genetic stock** and **Harvest stock**). See also **Stock.**

Fixed In population genetics, a gene is said to be fixed when it has a frequency of 100%.

F_{ST} This was defined by Wright as the correlation between random gametes, drawn from the same subpopulation, relative to the total. For a two-allele locus, $F_{ST} = V_P/pq$, where V_P is the variance of one allele over subpopulations, and p is the average frequency of that allele in the total population. This was generalised by Nei for any number of alleles to $G_{ST} = 1 - (H_S/H_T)$, where H_S is the average Hardy-Weinberg expected heterozygosity per subpopulation, and H_T is the Hardy-Weinberg heterozygosity of the total population. Effectively, G_{ST} *and* F_{ST} measure the same quantity. See G_{ST}.

Gel A supporting matrix used for sample application during electrophoresis. Gels are most commonly composed of starch, cellulose acetate, polyacrylamide or agarose.

Gene A hereditary unit consisting of a **nucleotide** sequence and occupying a specific position or **locus** within the **genome.**

Gene flow (= **migration** in population genetic terms) The movement of genes into or out of a population by interbreeding, or by migration (of individuals or their propagules) and interbreeding. It is important to distinguish migration in the genetic sense from animal movement, because the latter may not necessarily lead to gene flow due to death or failure of migrants to reproduce.

Gene pool All the alleles (pool of eggs and sperm) in a population at a particular time. The extent to which individuals in a population share a common gene pool will determine the extent of genetic differentiation among taxa.

Gene tree A branching diagram that depicts the known or (usually) inferred relationships among historically related groups of genes or other nucleotide or amino acid sequences.

Genetic distance The quantitatively measured differences between taxa (between genes, individuals, populations, or species) in terms of their allele frequencies.

Genetic drift Variation in allele frequency from one generation to another due to chance fluctuations. It is generally greater in populations with small **effective population size** and high inbreeding.

Genetic fingerprinting See **DNA fingerprinting.**

Genetic management The incorporation of information on the levels and distribution of genetic variability into management programmes, with the overall aim of conserving genetic resources (levels of allelic diversity and associated genotypic variance in ecologically significant traits).

Genetic marker (= **molecular marker**) A genetically inherited variant from which the genotype can be inferred from the phenotype as identified during genetic screening.

Genetic stock A reproductively isolated unit* that is genetically different from other stocks. The degree of integrity here is high, since very few migrants are sufficient to prevent the development of genetic differentiation between monospecific stocks. *The reproductive isolation referred to above is not usually absolute and operative over evolutionary time, as in the case of interspecific stocks. *Cf.* **Stock, Harvest stock** and **Fishery stock.**

Genome All the genetic material contained in an individual.

G_{ST} The proportion of total genetic diversity attributable to subpopulation differentiation. See F_{ST}.

Gynogenesis Unisexual reproduction in which the egg is stimulated to commence cleavage by the sperm but without fertilisation, and therefore no genetic contribution from the male. Gynogenetic offspring therefore are genetically identical to the mother.

Haplotype Nucleotide sequence of an individual's mtDNA genes characterised by **restriction fragment length polymorphisms (RFLPS)** or direct sequencing. It is the multilocus analogue of an **allele.**

Hardy-Weinberg equilibrium Ratio of genotype frequencies expected in a population when mating is random and neither selection nor drift is operating. For two alleles (A and a) with frequencies p and q there are three genotypes $AA, Aa, and aa;$ and the expected Hardy-Weinberg ratio for the three is $p^2 AA, 2pq Aa, q^2 aa$. Genotypic frequencies obtained from molecular genetic analysis of natural populations can be compared with predicted frequencies calculated from allele frequencies to determine whether samples are drawn from large, randomly mating populations.

Harvest stock Locally accessible fish resources in which fishing pressure on one resource has no effect on the abundance of fish in another contiguous resource. This definition does not imply any genetic, nor any phenotypic, differences between stocks, but describes a group of individuals whose abundance depends to a very much larger degree on recruitment and mortality, especially that caused by fishing, than on immigration and emigration. *Cf.* **Stock, Genetic stock** and **Fishery stock.**

Heritability In the 'narrow sense', the ratio of the additive genetic variance (differences that will be inherited consistently by the offspring) to the total phenotypic variance.

Heterologous Homologous molecule from a species other than that which is being examined.

Heteroplasmy The containment by one cell or individual of more than one type of a particular organellar DNA (*e.g.* cpDNA, mtDNA).

Heterozygosity Proportion of individuals in a population that are heterozygous (see **Heterozygote**) at a given locus. Can be calculated: $HL = 1 -$ sum. xi^2, where x_i is the frequency of the ith allele at a locus. The mean heterozygosity per locus, H_L is the sum of H_L over all loci (including loci with two identical alleles where $H_L = 0$), divided by the total number of loci examined. An observed heterozygosity (H_o) can be determined from a direct count of the frequency of heterozygous genotypes in a sample. H_L and H_o can be compared statistically to determine whether genotypic ratios are in accordance with Hardy-Weinberg expectations (see **Hardy-Weinberg equilibrium**).

Heterozygote The presence of two dissimilar alleles at a given genetic locus.

Homology Common ancestry of two or more genes or gene products (or portions thereof).

Homoplasy Similarities in character states due to reasons other than inheritance from a common ancestor. These include convergence, parallelism or reversion. At the gene level, two alleles are homoplasic when they are identical in state, though not identical by descent.

Homozygote Two identical alleles at a genetic locus.

Hotspot Position on a gene where nucleotide substitutions are particularly common.

Hybridization (in the breeding sense) Crossing of inbred lines or individual organisms of differing genetic constitution or species.

Hybridisation (in the molecular sense) To induce, experimentally, the pairing of complementary nucleic acid strands, often from different individuals or species, to form a DNA-DNA or RNA-DNA hybrid molecule.

Hybridogenesis A form of unisexual reproduction where an ancestral genome from the maternal line is transmitted to the egg without recombination, whereas paternally-derived chromosomes are discarded premeiotically, only to be replaced each generation through fertilisation by sperm from a related sexual species.

Hypervariable sequence A segment of a chromosome characterised by considerable variation in the number of tandem repeats at one or more loci. See **Tandem array.**

Iceman Name given by the mass-media to the Neolithic (5100-5300 BP) human body found on 19 September 1991 in an Alpine glacier.

Imperfect microsatellite Microsatellite for which one of the motif(s) has mutated (*e.g.* AGAGACAGAGAG).

Indel Insertion/deletion event.

Infinite allele model (IAM) Mutation model which assumes an infinite number of possible alleles at a given locus, so that any new allele arising by mutation is different from those previously present in the species.

Insertion Mutation in which one or more nucleotides are inserted into DNA sequence.

Interrupted microsatellite Microsatellite with an inserted base(s) separating motifs (*e.g.* AGAGAGTAGAGAG).

Introgression The sexual transfer of genes between genetically differentiated populations.

Intron The non-coding sequence in a gene between the **exons.** Because introns never code for a protein, they are expected to have few functional constraints, and tend therefore to evolve more rapidly (and are correspondingly more variable) than coding regions.

Isoloci Two or more loci of a multilocus enzyme system that produce products of the same electrophoretic mobility.

Isozymes Enzymes differing in electrophoretic mobility but which share the same substrate. Isozymes may arise from genetic (multiple loci or alleles) or epigenetic (post-translational) sources. It is therefore essential to exclude epigenetic variability if isozymes are to be used as **genetic markers.**

K-allele model (KAM) Mutation model which assumes that there are exactly K possible allelic states and that any allele has a constant probability $[\mu/(K-1)]$ of mutating towards any of the other K-1 allelic states.

Linkage A measure of the degree to which alleles of two genes do not assort independently at meiosis or in genetic crosses. Those loci on different chromosomes are non-linked, whereas those close together on the same chromosome are closely linked and are usually inherited together.

Linkage disequilibrium Departure from the predicted frequencies of multiple locus gamete types assuming alleles are randomly associated. When there is no deviation, the population is said to be in linkage equilibrium.

Linkage map A chromosome map showing the linear order of the genes associated with the chromosome.

Local adaptation A process that increases the frequency of traits which enhance the survival or reproductive success of individuals in a particular environment.

Locus A physical position of a gene on a chromosome.

Mapping Determination of the position of genes (genetic map), or of physical features such as restriction endonuclease sites (restriction map, physical map).

Marker Any diagnostic feature (*e.g.* allozyme, mtDNA haplotype, meristic, morpho-metric) of an individual, population or species. See **genetic marker.**

Maximum likelihood A criterion to find parameter values by maximising the probability of observed data under an explicit model.

Metapopulation A group of populations in a local geographic area.

Microsatellite (= simple sequences) Tandem array of short (1-6 base pairs) repeated sequences, with a total degree of repetition of five to about one hundred at each locus, and usually scattered randomly throughout the genome. For example, the repeat unit can be simply CA, and might exist in a tandem array of, for instance, 50 repeats, denoted by $(CACACACACA \dots)_{50}$. The number of repeats in an array can be highly variable, giving rise to extensive **polymorphism.**

Migration rate The rate at which subpopulations exchange migrants per generation. For genetic studies this is often synonymous with the rate of gene flow.

Minisatellite Tandem array of from two to several hundred copies of a short (9- 100 base pairs) sequence of DNA, usually interspersed but often clustered in telomeric regions of the chromosome. Arrays generally have different numbers of copies on different chromosomes, which when cut by restriction enzymes produce DNA fragments of differing lengths, thereby potentially giving rise to a **DNA fingerprint.**

Mitochondrial DNA (mtDNA) DNA located in the mitochondrion. In animals it is generally a small circular molecule, 16 000 to 18 000 base pairs long, and is, with rare exceptions, solely maternally inherited.

Mixed stock analysis (MSA) The use of markers to determine the relative proportions of identifiable stocks in a mixed-stock fishery. MSA is widely employed in the management of Pacific salmon.

Molecular drive (= meiotic drive) Any one of a number of mechanisms that produce unequal numbers of the two gametic types formed by a heterozygote.

Multilocus probe Used typically to refer to probes used in **DNA fingerprinting** (*e.g.* minisatellites) where many loci are visualised simultaneously, producing a banding pattern comprising many DNA fragments. In such cases it is usually not possible to identify loci or assess levels of heterozygosity.

Mutation rate Number of mutations (alteration of a DNA sequence) arising in an individual per **gene** or per **nucleotide** site per unit time (for example per generation).

ND genes Sequences of DNA in the mitochondrial genome that code for enzymes in the NADH dehydrogenase complex.

nDNA Nuclear DNA, the DNA contained in the chromosomes within the nucleus of eukaryotic cells, and inherited from both maternal and paternal parents.

Neutrality The state of being free from the effects of selection.

Non-synonymous substitution A nucleotide substitution that results in an amino acid replacement.

Normalizing (= balancing) selection The situation in which individuals with an intermediate phenotype are at a selective advantage.

Nucleotide One of the monomeric units from which DNA molecules are constructed, consisting of a purine (adenine and guanine) or pyrimidine (thymine and cytosine) base, a pentose sugar, and a phosphoric acid group.

Null alleles at microsatellite loci Alleles that give no **PCR** product due to mutations (base **substitution** or **deletion**) occurring at one or both **primer** site(s).

Oligonucleotide Short DNA fragment typically of 10-20 nucleotides. Generally refers to single-stranded, synthetic DNA molecules used as a **probe** or **primer.**

Parallel substitution(s) Independent occurrence of the same mutation in two or more evolutionary lineages.

Perfect microsatellite Microsatellite with a stretch of **tandem** repeats having no interruption in the run of repeats (*e.g.* AGAGAGAGAGAGAG).

Phylogeny The historical relationships among lineages of organisms or their parts (*e.g.* genes).

Phylogeography The principles and processes governing geographical distributions of genealogical lineages, especially at the intraspecific level.

Plasmid A self-replicating extrachromosomal circular DNA.

Plesimorphy An ancestral character state.

Polymerase An enzyme that assembles the subunits of macromolecules. DNA polymerases have the ability to synthesise the **complementary** strand of single-stranded DNA template. Synthesis only extends from existing double-stranded sequences across a single-stranded template.

Polymerase chain reaction (PCR) The amplification of particular regions of DNA using **primers** (which flank the region of DNA to be amplified) and the DNA **polymerase** of the thermophilic bacterium *Thermus aquaticus.* PCR involves a cycle of denaturation to single strands (around 94°C, primer annealing (37-60 °C), and primer extension (around 72°C). Thirty or more cycles are typically carried out to create a large number of copies of the target DNA sequence.

Polymorphism Existence at the same time of two or more different classes of a morph within a population, that is, individuals with discrete phenotype differences. In the molecular sense, polymorphism may be detected as alternative forms of a gene (*e.g.* allozymes or nucleotide sequence), and is sometimes defined as variants with a frequency of > 1% or 5% in the population. The latter criterion is employed more often to exclude the incidence of rare mutations.

Population size Number of individuals in a population (census population size).

Primer A short single-stranded sequence of DNA which binds to a complementary sequence and initiates the extension of adjacent DNA regions (DNA strand synthesis, *e.g.* in **PCR**) using DNA polymerase. Primers can be designed so that they will bind to a very specific region of the DNA, and will thus initiate synthesis of a targeted sequence (as in **PCR** or DNA sequencing).

Probe A length of RNA or single-stranded DNA radioactively (or otherwise) labelled and used to locate complementary sequences by base-pairing in a heterogeneous collection of sequences. The probe therefore **hybridises** with the target sequence (one or many repeat copies) making it visible to the naked eye (*e.g.* through **autoradiography**), so allowing the degree of variability to be assayed.

Random amplified polymorphic DNA (RAPD) A technique allowing detection of DNA polymorphisms by randomly amplifying multiple regions of the genome by PCR using single arbitrary primers. The primers are generally between 10 and 20 base pairs long, of an arbitrary but known sequence.

rDNA Ribosomal DNA.

Repetitive DNA Nucleotide sequences occurring repeatedly in chromosomal DNA. Repetitive DNA can belong to the highly repetitive (sequences of several nucleotides repeated millions of times) or middle repetitive (sequences of 1-500 base pairs in length, repeated 100 to 10000 times each) categories.

Restriction enzyme (= endonuclease) An enzyme that cleaves double-stranded DNA. Type I are not sequence specific; type II (the type used routinely in molecular genetic analyses) cleave DNA at a specific sequence of nucleotides known as **restriction** or **recognition sites.** The enzymes are named by an acronym that indicates the bacterial species from which they were isolated, followed by a roman numeral that gives the chronological order of discovery when more than one enzyme came from the same source. Most restriction enzymes currently employed in molecular ecology recognize sequences of either four, five or six bases.

Restriction fragment length polymorphism (RFLP) Variations occurring within a species in the length of DNA fragments generated by a specific **restriction enzyme.** Such variation is generated either by base substitutions that cause a gain or loss of sites, or by insertion/deletion mutations that change the length of fragments independent of **restriction site** changes.

Restriction site (= recognition site) A specific sequence of nucleotide bases which is recognised by a **restriction enzyme.** The enzyme will cleave both DNA strands at a specific location within that sequence. Variation in the presence and absence of restriction sites among individuals generates **restriction fragment length polymorphisms (RFLPs).**

Reticulate evolution The fusing of previously separated branches on an evolutionary tree.

Reversion Mutation resulting in a come back to the ancestral state.

rRNA Ribosomal RNA.

Satellite DNA DNA from a eukaryote that separates on gradient centrifugation as a distinct fraction. The separation results from differences in the base composition of the distinct fraction and main band of genomic DNA (i.e. the A + T or G + C content is higher in the satellite than in the main band). Many satellites consist of **highly repetitive** DNA, usually millions of tandem repeats of a relatively short sequence (**tandem array**).

scnDNA (single copy nuclear DNA) Sequences that occur once, or very few times, in a genome.

Silent mutation A change in the DNA structure that has no effect on the phenotype of the cell.

Single-locus probe (SLP) A **probe** consisting of short repeat sequences (*e.g.* **minisatellites**) that identify allelic products at a single locus, thus producing banding patterns typically consisting of either one (homozygote) or two (heterozygote) DNA fragments. (*cf.* **Multilocus probe**).

Size homoplasy Identity of microsatellite alleles by state not by descent. Microsatellite variation is essentially revealed through **electrophoresis** of **PCR** products and allelic classes differ by the length (in bp) of the amplified fragments. Two PCR products of the same length may not be a copy of the same ancestral sequence without mutation, introducing the possibility of size homoplasy.

Southern blot A membrane (*e.g.* nitrocellulose or nylon) onto which DNA has been transferred directly from an electrophoretic gel. The transfer is facilitated by simple diffusion of salts across the membrane, or by using automated vacuum blotters. The membrane can then be exposed to a labelled **probe** that will bind to the specific fragments of interest, allowing their visualisation independent of thousands of other fragments from the gel.

Stepwise mutation model (SMM) Mutation model which assumes that alleles are represented by integer values and that a mutation either increases or decreases the allele value by one. For **variable number tandem repeats** loci (**VNTR**), the **allele** value is generally taken as the number of tandem repeats in the DNA sequence.

Stock Unit of an exploited species that is employed in **stock assessment**. Definition depends on management aims and time scale of interest (see **Fishery stock, Genetic stock** and **Harvest stock**).

Stock assessment The use of various statistical and mathematical calculations to make quantitative predictions about the reactions of exploited populations to alternative management options.

Substitution Mutation in which one nucleotide is substituted for another.

Symplesimorphy A shared ancestral character state.

Synapomorphy A shared derived character state that is indicative of a phylogenetic relationship among two or more operational taxonomic units (OTU).

Synonymous substitution Nucleotide substitution which does not alter the amino acid composition of a gene because of the redundancy of the genetic code.

Tandem array Multiple copies of a sequence of DNA that are arranged one after another in series. Repeat units can be short nucleotide sequences or entire sets of genes.

Taphonomy Grecian neologism created in the 1940s by the Russian palaeontologist, Efremov, meaning literally "the law of the tomb". Taphonomy is usually described as a subdiscipline of palaeontology, but its methods and data are often applied to more recent, that is, archaeological, contexts.

Template The use of a nucleic acid strand to carry the information required for the synthesis of a new (**complementary**) strand.

Transposon A segment of DNA flanked by transposable elements that is capable of moving its location in the genome.

Transition A nucleotide substitution from one purine to another purine (*e.g.* adenine (A) to guanine (G)), or from one pyrimidine to another pyrimidine (*e.g.* thymine (T) to cytosine (C)).

Transversion A nucleotide substitution from a purine to pyrimidine (*e.g.* adenine (A) to cytosine (C)), or vice versa.

Two-phase model (TPM) Mutation model in which mutations introduce a gain/loss of X repeats. With probability p, X is equal to one (this corresponds to the **SMM**) and with probability, $1\text{-}p$, X follows a geometric distribution defined as Proba(X=k) = $Z\alpha^k$, in which a specified variance $V(X)=\alpha/(1-\alpha)^2$ or expectation $E(X)=1/(1-\alpha)$ determines the value of α and of the normalisation constant $Z=(1-\alpha)/\alpha$.

Vector A self-replicating DNA molecule capable of transferring foreign DNA into a cell. For example, the human insulin gene can be cloned into the plasmid vector pBR 322 which in turn will replicate in *Escherichia coli* cultures.

Vicariance The fragmentation or fusion of a species range as a consequence of processes such as plate tectonic or glacial movements.

VNTR loci (variable number of tandem repeats) The variable number of repeat core base pair sequences at specific loci in the genome. Variation in the length of the alleles formed from the repeats provides the basis for the detected **polymorphism**.

Wright-Fisher population model An idealised population with a fixed number, N, of individuals living only one generation without migration and selection. Each individual produces a large number gametes, and all reproduce at the same time. In the gamete pool of a diploid species, : $2N$ gametes are drawn randomly, and random pairs form N diploid individuals in the next generation. In the gamete pool of haploid species, N gametes are drawn randomly and form N individuals in the next generation. There are many extensions of this basic model to include additional population parameters.

UNIVERSITY COLLEGE

SCARBOROUGH